Health, Wellness
&
Longevity

Handboook

By

Steve Dimon

ISBN-10: 1-939534-37-2

ISBN-13: 978-1-939534-37-8

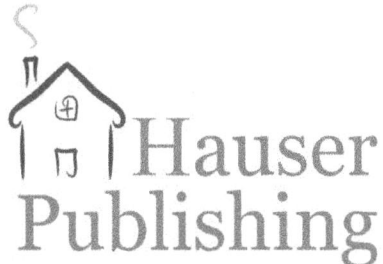

Hauser
Publishing

Disclaimer

The author and the publisher make no representation or warranties with respect to the accuracy or completeness of the content in this book and specifically disclaim all warranties and liabilities, including loss and risk, resulting directly or indirectly from the use or application of any of the strategies and information discussed. We further disclaim all warranties, including without limitation warranties of fitness for a particular purpose and accept no responsibility or liability of any kind.

No statement in this book should be construed as a claim for cure, treatment, or prevention of any disease. The information in this book is for informational and educational purposes only and is not intended to diagnose, treat, cure, or prevent any diseases. This book solely expresses the opinion and the experiences of the author. The author is not a doctor of medicine and the information contained herein is not a substitute for medical advice from a licensed physician, healthcare professional, or healthcare provider and provides general health information only.

Under no circumstance is the information intended to be used instead of a medical consultation. The reader should always consult a doctor, physician, or healthcare provider before starting a diet, nutrition, vitamins, supplements, or exercise program or before adapting any of the suggestions in this handbook. The author and the publisher disclaims all responsibility for any liability, loss, or risk, which is experienced as a consequence, directly or indirectly, from the use, misuse, or application of any of the contents in this handbook, as every individual is different, every application is different, and outcomes may vary.

Especially if you are pregnant, if you are nursing, or if you are taking medication, it's absolutely crucial that you consult your healthcare professional before using any products based on this content. The same applies if you have a medical condition, anticipate surgery, or are under any type of medical supervision.

While we do our best to ensure that the information is up-to-date at the time of publishing, we make no representations or warranties with respect to the accuracy of the content; all the information is subject to change without notice. Further, readers should be aware that internet websites listed in this work may have changed or disappeared between when this work was written and when it's read.

We would further like to point out that listing of a company or website in this book is solely for the purpose of information; we do not endorse them or the information they provide.

Table of Contents

Acknowledgements

I'd like to thank my many friends and professionals who helped me in my time of need and who gave me the support I needed to get to this point, to not only save my life and give me new purpose, but also the empowerment to give back and to help save others' lives. My intent is to make a difference!

Devin Haman and Dan Holtz, BHRC, Alex Nicol, Paul Knapp, Cheryl Dimon George (sister), Jeff Dimon (brother), Morry Karp, Berry Bly, Jeff Bozz, Brett Clark, Dave Meyering, Marjan Consari, Denise Haman, Scott Schilling, Mike Ortiz, Chi Wai Eng, Dr. Garth Fisher, Mary Chu, Ron Smith, Chris Whalley, Chris Tesara, Scott Bader, Chris Brake, Jim Atchison, Travis Corby, Shernoff Law Firm, my team of doctors: Dr. Nerses Sanossian, (Neurologist), Dr. Shervin Eshaghian, (Cardiologist), Dr. P.K. Shah, (Cardiologist), Dr. Reza Nazemi, (Endocrinologist), Dr. Christopher Ng (Urologist), Dr. Ashkan Naraghi, (Internal Medicine), Dr. Bita Shokouh O.D., Dr. Ellis Wong, (DDS), Dr. Rita Metrikin, (DDS), Dr. Aarmir Wahab (DDS), Dr. Philip Goglia, PhD (Nutritional Science), Dr. Tom Marinaro, (Chiropractor), Dr. Dan Tehari (Dermatologist), Deborah McMahon, (Homeopath & Feldenkrais Practitioner), Maureen Harrington, (Author), Cedars Sinai Hospital, Rancho Los Amigos National Rehabilitation Center, Covey Lazouras, (Physical Therapist), Suzanne Lai, (Occupational Therapist), Amanda Dufresne, (Occupational Therapist), Adnan Haidar, (Head Nurse) and the entire staff at Rancho, my editor, Greg Gubi, Enrique Almeida and Nicole Spohn-Almeida, Hauser Publishing. Thank you. Thank you. Thank you, to all.

About the Author

I suffered a stroke on April 22, 2012. Paralyzed from head to toe on my left side, I spent nearly a month in two different hospitals in Los Angeles, California, followed by three months in outpatient therapy.

I was 63 years old, 100 pounds overweight, and suffered from of metabolic syndrome, high blood pressure, high cholesterol, type 2 diabetes, morbid obesity, and diet-induced inflammation.

In 1986 I moved to Los Angeles from Des Moines, Iowa, to be an actor and a model. Over the years I transitioned into producing live shows, special events, concerts, festivals, films, and TV shows. Eventually, though, all that success, stress, and Hollywood glamour caught up with me and I paid the price with an ischemic stroke on that spring afternoon in 2012.

Being paralyzed on my left side, including a facial disfigurement and slurred speech, I had to relearn how to walk, talk, eat, swallow, cut my food, dress myself, tie my shoes, and go to the bathroom. I even had to relearn to wipe my butt.

Now, 68 years old and 100 pounds lighter, I have a 32-inch waistline, 6.5% body fat, and at six feet in height, I weigh 175 pounds. I have essentially turned back the clock and reversed all of the metabolic syndrome symptoms that caused my stroke through lifestyle change diet, nutrition, exercise, and supplementation.

My doctors use two words to describe my recovery: miraculous and amazing, but I don't believe in miracles. I believe in hard work. Amazing things can happen as a result of commitment to hard work.

As a former college football and baseball player with strong Midwestern values and a solid work ethic, I have recovered nearly 100% of my physical capacity. I attribute this not only to hard work, mental toughness, and discipline, but to the power of the human spirit and the will to live; perhaps, even, a higher power.

To look at me now, you wouldn't know I had a life-threatening stroke just a few years ago. I truly believe I lived through my stroke and got my health back in order to motivate and inspire others.

The handbook takes readers through the occurrence and the causes of heart attacks, strokes, cancers, diabetes and obesity, then describes the hospitalization and rehab process, and finally explains the vital importance of lifestyle changes in diet and nutrition, vitamins, supplements, and exercise. Also discussed are tests to save lives, tools for disease prevention and reversal, stress reduction, weight loss and weight management, brain health, and finally, the psychology of lifestyle change.

The book will inform readers which valuable tests I believe they must have their doctors perform, because they save lives. I will discuss many new and cutting-edge tests, how to read those tests, and what best results are. I will also show you how to maintain new-found health and how to live a longer, more productive life.

My stroke didn't happen TO me – it happened FOR me. My stroke does not define who I am. It did, however, make me want to work harder to thrive and overcome life's challenges. It inspired me to live a normal, productive, healthy, long life. It challenged me to discover the "whys" of stroke and its prevention.

Don't wait for a near-death experience or a life-threatening or life-changing event to trigger your lifestyle change. The first symptom of a heart attack or stroke can literally be death. Eighty percent of all heart attacks and strokes are preventable. Life is worth living. Take command and control of your own health.

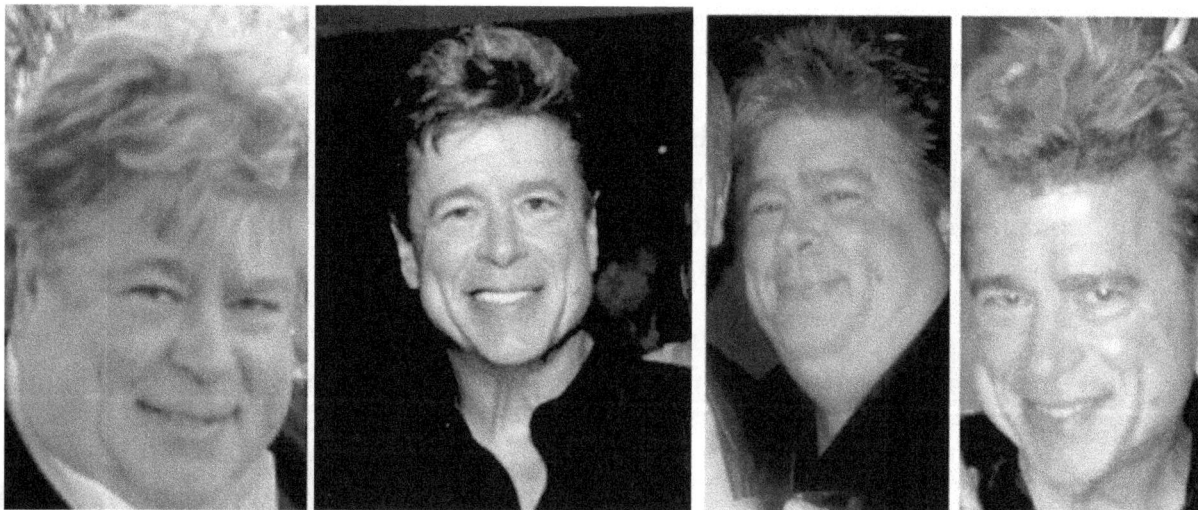

"Today I will do what others won't, so tomorrow I can accomplish what others can't." - Eleanor Roosevelt

Forward

FAST:

In the event of a stroke it is very important to act fast. Receiving treatment quickly can limit the effect a stroke has on a person's speech, movement, memory and permanent damage or disability, paralysis and loss of independence. FAST is a helpful acronym to recognize symptoms of a stroke.

F=FACE

Numbness in the face, especially one side

Sudden trouble seeing in one or both eyes or the onset of a severe headache with no known cause.

Look at the person's face. Ask them to smile. Is one side of their mouth drooping?

A=ARM

Ask the person to raise both arms. Does one arm drift downward or not respond?

Numbness or weakness of face, arm, or leg, especially on one side of the body.

Trouble walking, dizziness and loss of balance or coordination.

S=SPEECH

Speech difficulties, trouble speaking or understanding. Sudden confusion.

Ask the person to talk or repeat a simple phrase; slurred speech.

T=TIME

Stick out tongue. Does it go to one side or the other of the mouth?

If you observe any of these signs, time to call 9-1-1 immediately!

Note the time when symptoms were first observed. Knowing when a stroke first occurred can affect treatment decisions, such as life saving and damage reduced clot busters, known as tpa (tissue plasminogen activator). Time is brain. Time is life.

ANOTHER STROKE SYMPTOM ACRONYM:
STR:

S: smile

T: talk

R: raise arm

Stick out tongue

Call 9-1-1

STROKE TEST:

Talk

Wave

Smile

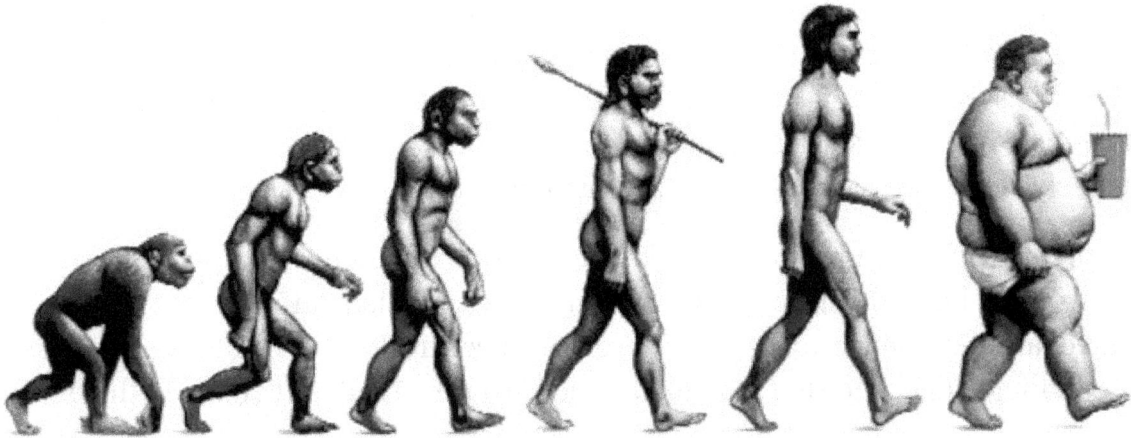

Photocredit: Penguin-Random House Publishers, Barry Popkin 2009

Introduction

"Let food be thy medicine and medicine be thy food."

Hippocrates

All truth goes through three stages: First, it is ridiculed. Second, it is violently opposed. Finally, it is accepted as self-evident. This is not only true for health but all areas of life.

"All great truths begin as blasphemies." - George Bernard Shaw

There is so much information on health and nutrition today, but who and what do you believe? What I strive for in this handbook is science fact and common sense, not science fiction. However, science does not supersede nature, so I will give you my latest scientific research and nature's remedies and a "how's" and "why's" to guide you.

"All of science is nothing more than refinement of everyday thinking." – Albert Einstein

There is much to learn about the details of diet and health.

This book is a little bit about a lot of things. But it's not about credentials, diplomas or initials after my name. It's about my personal experience with the fundamentals of health that I had to learn to take command and empower myself to what I call optimal health, wellness and longevity. Join me and personalize your pursuit of the same. This is evidence-based, non-biased, scientific information, as well as anecdotal experience I have exhaustively researched and lived for the past few years.

Improving my health has been my job since my stroke. I became my own experiment in regaining my health. I have been my own guinea pig, lab rat, and crash test dummy. My near-death experience was a catalyst to seize control of my health and find my new purpose in life, which is to share my experience, awareness, and insights with you.

My mission with this handbook is to educate, inform, and teach you not only how to lose and maintain weight, but to prevent and reverse disease and rid the body of diet-induced inflammation. Inflammation is the root cause of most modern diseases. The one thing you have the most control of in your environment today is the food you choose to eat.

"Tell me what you eat and I'll tell you who you are." – Jean n Anthelm Brillat-Savarin

I also cover cardiovascular disease, heart attack, stroke, cancer, obesity, type 2 diabetes, and Alzheimer's disease, environmental toxins, heavy metals, and funguses. This information will help you take control of your health now and not wait for a life-threatening, near-death experience or catastrophic life-changing event to trigger you into action. It could be too late by then. The first symptom of a heart attack or stroke is often death.

This handbook is a mosaic of contemporary research from my study of hundreds of books and articles since 2012, as science is continually changing and updating with new discoveries and information, much of it contradictory and confusing.

This is not just a "how to" book, but a "why" book. What if the things you thought were good for you actually harm your health?

Let's never be afraid to look at evidence that threatens our beliefs. That's how we grow and expand. The same factors that lead to good health are the ones that are needed to recover lost health.

"It's not what we know that hurts us; it's what we don't know." – Anonymous

I was a nutritional perfect storm, a ticking time bomb. Many of you are the same; you just don't know it – yet. When was the last time you had your blood tested? In this handbook you will learn the tests that will save your life, and how to decipher them; how to recognize proper levels, not just clinical ranges based on average Americans. You do not want to be an average American when it comes to health, as the average American is sick, fat, tired, and dying.

Don't wait. Don't gamble with your life. Even if you think you're bulletproof. Father Time is undefeated.

It's not so much what you know that can hurt you; it's what you don't know that can have the most severe consequences. Just like it's not so much what you eat, as what you don't eat. So connecting the dots between education and nutrition will provide you with the best results.

Knowledge isn't power unless it is put into action.

Why should you care? "I'm too young to worry. All I want to do is party and have a good time. Drugs, alcohol, rock & roll." But time marches on. These are progressive diseases.

Many of you are ticking time bombs like I was, waiting for a health event to happen, and then BOOM! It happens and you are flat on your back in a hospital bed or diagnosed with cancer or worse, dead from a heart attack or stroke.

Let me tell you, when you are paralyzed and hooked up to oxygen, monitors, IV's, bells and whistles, you have lots of time to think. How'd I get myself into this mess and how do I get myself out?

"An ounce of prevention is worth a pound of cure." – Benjamin Franklin

In America, we don't have healthcare, we have sick care and disease management. Western doctors are trained to treat symptoms, not causes. That's why there is such a movement in this country to move from "traditional" medicine controlled by Big Pharma to functional medicine; to treat the cause, not the symptom, and move into preventative medicine, which will also save our bankrupt Medicare/Medicaid system, not to mention millions of lives.

Illnesses happen because of us, and not to us – a big difference, which comes down to lifestyle factors, diet, nutrition, exercise, and supplementation.

Everyone knows that you need more prevention than treatment, but few reward acts of prevention, especially in the medical, pharmaceutical and healthcare business where they are reactive, not proactive or preventative. This seems to be very evident, as 80% of heart attacks, strokes and cancer, the leading causes of death in the U.S., are preventable.

What we do with our feet, forks, fingers, sleep, stress, and love will determine 80% of our mortality. An 80% reduction in all chronic diseases would count as one of the most stunning advances in the history of public health. Better than any pharmaceutical drug.

"Prevention is better than cure." – Desiderius Erasmus

You can't change your genes, but you can change how they perform by creating a gene-supportive environment through your diet, the fuel your cells and DNA thrive on to create either health or illness. You're not stuck with the way your genes perform. You control their environment through the fuel that you feed them in your diet. It's called "epigenetics."

Exercise is a wellness tool, not a weight loss tool. Weight loss is 80% diet, 20% exercise. You cannot exercise away a bad diet. Requiring overweight people to exercise is punitive. Empowering overweight people to focus on losing weight first then becoming fit afterward is a smart strategy. Most people feel better and function better when they get a modest amount of exercise. In general, thin people get more exercise than heavy people. People who exercise regularly throughout a lifetime live longer than those who don't.

Combining a well-formulated low-carb, high-healthy-fat, and moderate-healthy-protein diet, with high-interval, high-intensity exercise of cardio and resistance training, is a roadmap to optimal health, wellness and longevity.

The information in this book is empirical and designed through science-based research and my real-life experience, to help guide you to be the CEO of your own health. The bottom line is, you have to be your own advocate and your own master when it comes to your health. No one else can do it for you.

With information and your God-given right you can become a PhD in Self, as I did in my stroke recovery journey. Trust me, you do not want to go through what I did. I believe it's very different when you get advice from someone who has researched it, studied it, lived it and breathed it, as opposed to a doctor, nurse, therapist, nutritionist or hospital administrator, who has been trained, but has not lived through a life-threatening illness and come out of it stronger and healthier than before.

"There is one consolation in being sick and that is the possibility you may recover to a better state than you were in before." – Henry David Thoreau

The food you eat today will become the cellular chemistry of your body tomorrow. The food you put into body becomes your body. You are not only what you eat, but how your body metabolizes what you eat – how your body burns it, stores it and excretes it, how it affects your genes and your gene's expression, and ultimately, whether you are sick or healthy.

Just because you do not currently exhibit any signs of disease, does not mean you will not develop disease. Degenerative, deadly diseases are the result of imbalances in the body that are present and building up for 30 or more years before they become noticed. Some can even begin before birth and may have developed in a toxic womb environment. You may be struck down in your 20s or 30s, when, if you had known beforehand through blood tests, you could have reversed or prevented the disease. This imbalance is generally caused by chronic long-term inflammation, which in turn, is diet-induced.

"Knowledge is power." – Sir Francis Bacon

Most of us have a profound lack of knowledge about what our bodies need to function healthfully. We find ourselves out of balance and susceptible to all kinds of illnesses. Each of us must take an active role in the maintenance of our own health and prevention of disease. The more we know about nutrition, the better prepared we are to take an active role. If you use nutrition as medicine, there is no prescription required.

PREPARATION + OPPORTUNITY = SUCCESS

Lifestyle, desire, and belief must come together. But we must also take action. Armed with the right knowledge we can confidently take steps, see results, and reap rewards.

Eighty percent of the costs of an average HMO go to pay for the disease conditions associated with diet-induced inflammation. Type 2 diabetes is an epidemic, followed by obesity, cardiovascular disease, heart attack, stroke, and cancer. Health insurance costs are rapidly rising and we are increasingly unable to pay for them. We live in the richest country in the world, yet 40 million people are uninsured. Our healthcare system is collapsing.

One-third of the children born after 2000 will develop type 2 diabetes at some point in their lives. They will suffer obesity, cardiovascular disease, heart attack, strokes, and cancer at earlier ages and become the first American generation in history to live a shorter lifespan than their parents.

The primary cause of our crisis in America's healthcare system is the continued disconnect with our genes and our diets. Aging Americans, baby boomers, and retirees on Medicare, are far less healthy than their predecessors, even though living longer, due to medical advances. Older people are full of diet-induced inflammation, the leading cause of all major diseases – obesity, type 2 diabetes, cardiovascular disease, heart attack, stroke, cancer, and Alzheimer's disease – from decades of eating poorly. However, this is all reversible or preventable through proper nutrition and lifestyle changes.

The proper diet or well-managed eating strategy outlined in this book can be the "miracle" drug you are waiting or searching for, to reduce diet-induced inflammation and turn on genes that promote cellular rejuvenation and cellular repair. Understand the value of nutrition and supplementation for healthcare intervention and therapy. The food we eat causes genetic expression of inflammation and we can turn off or turn on those expressions, simply by eating the right foods – eating smart.

In many ways, our current healthcare problems can be attributed to a mismatch between our genes and a pro-inflammatory diet to which these genes are exposed, resulting in diet-induced inflammation and toxic fat in the organs and brain, thereby giving rise to all these modern chronic diseases and faster aging as a result. The good news is: it's never too late to change.

We must un-brainwash ourselves from decades of nutritional propaganda and misinformation, some of it well-intended but deadly wrong.

Low-fat diets are the equivalent of the flat-earth theory of nutrition. The body has a remarkable ability to respond to healthy habits, so it's never too late to develop them. The body will heal itself with proper nutrition. As always, prevention is the best cure.

The psychology of lifestyle change can be broken down into several stages; however, if you are reading this handbook or are at a seminar you have already started to prepare yourself for lifestyle change, because you have the desire and commitment to move forward and you are starting to educate yourself to take action. Just keep on moving on, until it becomes habit and transformative for a lifetime, when it's a true lifestyle change.

Don't wait for a life-threatening, life-changing event or a near-death experience to trigger or to motivate you to make a lifestyle change, as the first symptoms of heart attack or stroke is often death. The symptoms build up over years of damage and neglect, so it will take time to reverse them as well. The sooner you start, the sooner you will be on your pathway to enjoying life as it was meant to be.

Delaying or slowing the aging process and disease prevention would more than pay for itself in reduced healthcare costs, rescuing America's healthcare system from the brink of disaster. Disabled life expectancy is now rising faster than total life expectancy, decreasing the number of years you can expect to live in good health. Studies show that if we can slow the aging process, we can delay the onset and progression of many fatal and disabling diseases simultaneously. Treat the cause, not the symptom. The underlying cause of fatal and disabling diseases is aging itself.

Diet-induced inflammation is not only the primary cause of disease and 80% preventable as a human health disaster – it is also a preventable economic disaster for the country. The increase in healthy years of life from an investment of slowing aging and preventing diseases would generate an economic benefit of as much as $7.1 trillion over the next 50 years – enough to rescue our collapsing healthcare system.

There are no shortcuts to good health. The sooner you test and measure your body's numbers and symptoms, the sooner you will be able to prevent and reverse disease. Do this instead of waking up one day when a condition you have been carrying around unknowingly for decades rears its ugly head. By then it's too late. Many times the first symptom of a heart attack or stroke is death.

You say good health is expensive. Have you checked into hospitalization or funerals lately? Pay me now or pay me later.

You say you're too busy to eat right and exercise; you'd rather take a pill, potion, tonic, or cream, the easy way out. Prescription drugs can do long-term damage as well. All you have to do is eat the right nutrition, supplement with vitamins, and exercise a little, and you'll build a foundation for a lifetime of wellness instead a lifetime of illness.

Good nutrition has a powerful effect on your health and is the number one integrative medicinal tool. Learn to build your health foundation with brick and mortar, not sand – one day and one brick at a time.

Further proof that one diet does not fit all is the Mediterranean Diet which is generally promoted by many doctors as healthy. The Mediterranean region includes 16 countries, all of whom have different eating habits, but are lumped together as part of the "Mediterranean Diet." Granted, it is far superior to the colossal failure that is America's low-fat, high-carb diet, but you can improve and fine-tune it with the information in this book.

We are only alive in the now. Be aware. Be present. Live in the moment. Learn from the past and plan for the future. Test, measure, and use all available tools. Be mindful that your future is in your own hands. Be your own advocate for your health.

I plan to live to be 100, so join me in a health revolution, one person at a time, for one great cause, to overcome America's and the world's diet-induced health epidemics. I received a wake-up call, a second chance at life. You may not be so lucky. You don't want to spend endless hours in rehabilitation therapy testing your resolve. Write your own powerful story of transformation, a renewal of lifestyle evolution and a lifestyle overhaul. Don't just survive – thrive!

I am not a stroke survivor, nor a stroke victim. I am a stroke victor. You too, can become a health victor.

"The greatest wealth is health." – Virgil

"Unless you change how you are, you will always have what you've got." – Jim Rohn

The true definition of anti-aging and wellness is simultaneously decreasing the body's pro-inflammation responses while increasing its internal anti-inflammatory responses. This leads to continual cellular rejuvenation and cellular repair for a longer lifespan, the benefit of an anti-inflammatory diet.

Think of your food as medicine to take in the right quantity and the right dosage, at the right time. Your choice of food is either a poison pill or a healing pill – pro-life or pro-death. Once you establish your new lifestyle and eating strategy, your body will automatically choose and crave healthy choices.

The more we understand the molecular biology of our genes and the bioavailability of nutrients and supplements, the more power we have with our food choices to direct the expression of our genes through what we eat.

The food list and eating strategies in this book are great for most people trying to lose weight or maintain proper weight and improve their diet and health, while creating nutritional sufficiency. Everyone has different biochemistry and metabolism. Each person's eating strategy may vary and require modifications or adjustments to individualize and personalize. The low-carb, higher healthy fats and moderate to higher healthy proteins will definitely serve as a template for the majority of people.

Fine-tuning your diet and supplementation program from time to time is essential as your body chemistry changes. Your metabolism is subject to occasional shifts. Listen to your body. It will give you signals. It will crave healthy choices.

Many people tend to be out of touch with their bodies and are not conscious what genuinely good health feels like. Our diets have been nutritionally substandard and deficient for so long that many people have either forgotten or never experienced what robust health really feels like. Most people have failed to live up to their genetically endowed and genetically engineered potential because they lack the proper fuel for a healthy life.

Simple lifestyle changes by one person at a time, one day at a time, can start a healthcare revolution, save lives, and save America's healthcare system. You must take control of your health: no one else can do it for you. Good nutrition has a powerful effect.

Eat to live. Don't live to eat. Enjoy natural, permanent weight loss, weight control, and maintenance. Prevent chronic diseases and reverse chronic and degenerative health disorders. Enhance your immunity and resistance to colds, flu, and infections.

You want your biological age to be younger than your chronological age and to slow the aging process down. You can do this by eating smart – allow your genes to work for you rather than against you.

The human body is the greatest machine on earth. It is a complex organism that has the ability to heal itself. Nerve signals travel through muscles and tissues at 200 miles per hour, while the brain produces enough electric power to light a 20-watt light bulb. Healthy bone is stronger than most building materials, including concrete. The body is composed of millions of tiny little engines and for those engines to work properly, they require specific fuels. If the fuel is given in the wrong combination, the engine will not perform at full capacity and efficiency. With the help of proper nutrition, a well-formulated eating strategy, exercise, and smart supplementation, you can slow the aging process, reverse and prevent diseases and live a happy, healthier, longer life.

The quality of the food we eat (the micronutrients we absorb from macronutrients) is the most important factor in our health.

Sugar, grains, starchy carbohydrates, vegetable oils, trans fats, processed foods and fast foods, are all poisonous to our system. They cause most modern diseases, obesity, type 2 diabetes, heart attacks, strokes and cancers.

I have studied most popular diets, bearing in mind that no one diet fits all: Atkins for Life, Beat Life, DASH, Paleo, Primal, South Beach and Mediterranean. These popular weight loss and lifestyle diets are on average 50% micronutrient deficient, meaning they do not provide half the nutrients required to prevent or reverse disease. You can become nutrient sufficient with a well-formulated eating strategy.

If everyone would take control of their personal health, the world will be a much healthier and wealthier place.

Some studies have shown that animals in zoos live a much shorter lifespan than the same animals in the wild. Why? Because of their diet and lifestyle. The analogy is that we humans, with our industrialized diet and environment, are similarly enclosed in a zoo. We eat the Standard American Diet ("SAD") full of diet-induced-inflammation, we are bombarded by environmental chemicals, toxins, pollution and stress, we are sedentary at both work and play, and we don't exercise, so, it's no wonder we are fat, sick, tired, and dying.

There is a sea of misinformation about diet, nutrition, vitamins, supplements and exercise, leaving people confused and frustrated. I hope this book and my seminars will help clarify it for you.

Make up your mind to put your health first. Be selfish. Demand optimal health.

One sure way to know you are making progress and positive lifestyle changes is when relatives, friends, coworkers, and even strangers start commenting and complimenting you on the difference they notice in your appearance. Take note and use this as positive reinforcement, inspiration, and motivation to continue. A great human quest is the journey to becoming the best possible you.

When it comes to health, wellness, nutrition, diet, vitamins, supplementation, exercise and longevity, challenge your boundaries and expand your horizons. Reeducate yourself. You won't be sorry.

Have faith that your health will truly improve. You will feel it and see it – your life re-imagined. You will now have the nutritional knowledge to attain the health you have dreamed of and to reverse and heal damage, and reclaim control of your health.

Do you want to lead a reactive lifestyle or a well-designed healthy lifestyle? It all adds up in the end. Each step and lifestyle change you make will bring you one step closer to your goal.

Your food affects every aspect of your life. It is the single most powerful influence on the future of your health. Decades of poor eating habits and lifestyle choices accumulate and lead to all major modern diseases and early death from causes like obesity, type 2 diabetes, heart attack, stroke, and cancer. Most of these diseases are preventable.

In the US alone, more than 1 million people will suffer heart attacks, with one-third of them resulting in death, and 800,000 strokes with 130,000 resulting in death. Stroke is the most debilitating disease in the world, with over 50 million people disabled or impaired. By age 20, most people begin developing atherosclerosis, with a 15–25% narrowing of the arteries due to plaque formation and buildup. By age 40, this increases to 30–50% clogging of the arteries.

When you are eating and living a healthy lifestyle, weight loss becomes a beneficial side effect. It's far more important to be consistent and emphasize what makes you healthy and well in the long term. Weight loss will quickly follow as a result, almost effortlessly. You cannot out-exercise a bad diet or deficient nutrition. Don't use exercise as a weight loss tool. Weight loss is 80% diet, 20% exercise.

Empower yourself. 80% of heart attacks, strokes and cancers are preventable. Get your immune system, inflammation, insulin, and leptin under control. Cut the sugar, cut the stress. Heal from within. Education, not medication.: take control of your health!

Make well-informed dietary choices: Nurture nature. Eat fresh, whole, real foods. Love the foods that love you back.

Lifestyle is the medicine; culture the spoon, anti-aging the prize. No Nobel required.

A note to baby boomers: Life begins at 65. You have Medicare and Social Security. You're retired if you want to be, on a pension if you have one, kids gone if you have any – your job now is your health, because if you don't have your health, you have nothing. The greatest gift you can give to yourself and your family is optimal health, wellness, and longevity.

"A wise man should consider that health is the greatest of human blessings."
– Hippocrates

"Giving is the greatest gift: When you learn, teach. When you get, give."
- Maya Angelou

CHAPTER 1
Foods Journey

Our diet starts in the field, garden, farm, or ocean. From there, the food moves to the plate, fork and mouth, sip or drink, before it ends up in our stomach, gut and digestive system, eventually hitting the bloodstream, cells and tissues. Here good nutrition works its magic before being excreted through sweat, urine and feces.

Not only do you need to know what you're eating, but what was eaten by what you're eating, ate.

It's a long journey, but you have control of the journey. You are the captain of your own ship, your own advocate, your own master. Along the journey, there are toxins, pesticides, herbicides, chemicals, hormones, bacteria, and GMOs to name a few. However, by eating wild fish, grass-fed beef, organic chicken, pasture-raised eggs, organic vegetables and fruits – in other words, whole, real, nutrition-rich foods and meats – you can win the war. I promise.

Food is information and the primary delivery system of vitamins, minerals, nutrients, antioxidants, and anti-inflammatories, which are vital to your health.

The process of change from what you are to what you would like to become can be either arduous and frustrating or easy and rewarding. The effort required for both paths is the same. Choose the first and you will probably have an endless cycle of yo-yo dieting and yo-yo weight loss and gain, with no stability. Eat from a nutrient-rich list of foods, cut the sugar and wheat, eat a low-carb, moderate-protein, higher-healthy-fats, higher-fiber diet, and what was once arduous and frustrating will become easy and rewarding as new lifestyle habits emerge and you crave healthy choices instead of unhealthy choices. You are not only receiving the rewards of good health:

you are reducing your risk of heart attack, stroke and cancer, so change, once thought as only a distant possibility, now becomes an absolute certainty. The choice is yours. When you start introducing proper nutrition into your body and it starts to burn fat instead of sugar, it's your body's version of spring cleaning. Diet also has a huge impact on dental health, which will be covered in detail in the chapter about dental health and hygiene segment.

The knife and fork are powerful tools for improving well-being. Use them wisely.

Timing and frequency of eating throughout the day is important, by creating thermogenesis and calorie burning to keep your furnace revved up and your energy abundant, while keeping blood sugar and insulin low, on a slow steady burn, with a faster, hotter metabolism that will work for many people. Intermittent Fasting (I.F.) is described in later chapters and may help your individual metabolism and weight-loss goal even more.

CHAPTER 2
Knowing What You Are Eating Ate

"It's not what you know that kills you; it's what you don't know."

- Anonymous

Food can be a medicinal nutrient or a toxic irritant. Simply replace bad foods with good foods – a food swap. You now have the knowledge and power to do so.

Consider the journey from the farm or ocean to your plate, your fork, your mouth, your gut, and your cells. Learn to become healthy for life: it took years to tear your body down with the accumulation of toxins, inflammation, and weight gain, so it will take time to build it back up to prime health, but believe me, it can be accomplished.

The quality of the food we eat comes from the quality of the food that our food eats.

"If you are what you eat and you don't know what you are eating, do you know who you are?" – Claude Flischler

Calorie-counting is not the key to healthy weight; the source of those calories is the most important factor. All calories are not the same. It's no longer simply a "calories in/calories out" mentality. Not only do you need to know what you are eating, but what you are eating ate.

In America we think it's cool to outsource everything, including our food. Over 50% of our meals are eaten away from our homes, where we've been brainwashed by the food industry into believing that healthy food is just a drive-thru or microwave away. We think that our harried schedules don't allow us the time to cook; that it is all too easy to pick up conveniently pre-made, packaged, processed "diet" foods, shakes, snack bars, or restaurant foods, all prepared by someone else with a list of ingredients we have no clue of or control over. The end result is "Franken Foods."

Outsourcing our food means outsourcing our health and it's making us sick. The healthiest people are those who cook at home using fresh, whole food ingredients, thereby avoiding thousands of unwanted and unhealthy food additives, many of which are known obesogens, carcinogens, and toxins. They not only make us fat, but sick and tired and dying. Some of these chemicals increase the number of fat cells, others expand the size of fat cells, while even others influence appetite, cravings, fullness, and how well our bodies burn and store fat and calories. Preparing your own meals promotes a good relationship with your food.

Just as what you eat affects your health, what animals eat also affects their health. In turn this impacts the health of their meat, eggs, and milk, which we then consume.

What about plants? What are they eating and absorbing from pesticides, herbicides and fungicides and the chemicals in the water they are showered with? Is it any wonder we are sick, tired, fat, and dying?

There are diets with variations based on your blood type, metabolic type, or genetic type, but the only one that seems to be backed by scientific evidence and much research is gene expression – epigenetics. Epigenetics has to do with what you eat and how your genes decide how you metabolize your food intake. You can measure your genetic type through a simple blood test called APOE.

I strongly believe in controlling insulin. By controlling insulin, you will control diet-induced inflammation, which is the main cause of most modern diseases.

Pasture-raised, free-range, cage-free, organic chicken eggs contain 2 times more omega-3s, 4-6 times more vitamin D, 2/3 more vitamin A, 3 times more vitamin E, 7 times more beta-carotene, 170% more vitamin B12, and 150% more vitamin B9 (Folate) than eggs from confined, commercially-raised chickens. It also goes to reason that the chickens that produce the healthiest eggs would also be the healthiest chickens to eat.

Ninety percent of salmon eaten in the US is from factory aqua farms, many of which are in China or elsewhere outside the US. Atlantic salmon are being fed food pellets full of GMO corn and soy and artificial color dyes. Because these fish are so sick and nutrient-depleted, they can't even produce their natural red color. They are full of omega-6s from their food supply, as opposed to the healthier omega-3s. The next time you go to the store, compare the color of a wild-caught Sockeye salmon with an aqua farm-raised Atlantic salmon. The Atlantic salmon will look sick in comparison. Wild-caught fish have up to

380% more omega-3s than farm-raised fish. Aqua farmed fish are raised in pens, do not get exercise, are fed grain and given antibiotics.

Not only do you need to know where your food comes from and who made it, but, you need to know what you are eating and what you are eating ate.

There are differences between products derived from grain-fed animals versus grass-fed animals. Avoid meat and organs coming from animals that are grain-fed or grain-finished. Many grain-fed livers are "condemned," whereas this does not happen with grass-fed livers. Meats can be grass-fed, but then grain-finished, so you have to ask your meat provider or butcher. If they don't know, pass and go on to someone who does. Your good health is at stake, so it's vital to know what your meat animals ate. Restrict all of your meats to pastured, or at the very least, grass-finished animals. In the wake of mad cow disease, it is particularly important to consume animals raised on pasture and fed a biologically appropriate diet, which virtually eliminates their risk of mad cow disease, as well as many other dangerous contaminants.

Learn the difference between grass-fed/grass-finished vs. grass-fed/grain-finished but advertised as "grass-fed!" Sometimes grass-fed doesn't mean grass-fed right up until slaughter. Grain-finished cattle are grass-fed most of their lives, but grain-finished to fatten them up for slaughter to increase the beef company's bottom-line profits – their meat is sold by the pound, after all. However, when this occurs it robs the meat of the omega-3s and healthy nutritional values that 100% grass-fed meats have. Grain-fed/grain-finished feedlots introduce unhealthy omega-6s and potentially GMOs, plus all the other nasty components contained in GMOs, as well as hormones and antibiotics added to grain feed. So, it's important to ask the butcher or meat counter clerk when meat is advertised or marked "grass-fed," if it also "grass-finished."

Ask the same question when buying buffalo or bison, as they are not always grass-fed and grass-finished, but sometimes grass-fed and grain-finished. You'll be surprised by the answers. New Zealand lamb is generally 100% grass-fed. Again, you want grass-fed and grass-finished. It makes a big difference in your health and in the quality of the nutrition in the meat.

Grass-fed and grass-finished means the animal stays on a pasture eating a grass and foraging diet for its entire life and is not moved to a grain feedlot before market. It is never fed grains. It takes 24-36 months for 100% grass-fed beef to reach the market, but only 18-20 months for grain-fed. This is one of the primary reasons grass-fed/grass-finished products are more expensive.

Know what you're eating ate!

CHAPTER 3
Eating Organic

"There is only one good, knowledge; and one evil, ignorance." – Socrates

Eat organic. Give your body the best. It deserves it. You live inside it. We can pay our doctor to make us better or we can pay the farmer to keep us healthy. Pay me now or pay me later.

Eat as if your life depends on it, because it does. We are not only what we eat, but we are what we don't eat. A bonus of eating organic is that the food is also more nutritious and tasty. By eating organic, you will become literally hungry for change and crave nutritious foods.

Eating organic protects you from toxic pesticide residue, herbicides, chemical fertilizers, chemical food additives, industrial solvents, sewage sludge, hormones, and the antibiotics used in conventional agriculture. It guarantees that your food is not GMO and has not lost its nutrient value content due to irradiation. Factory farmed and processed foods are far more likely to cause illness, both acute and chronic, than organically grown foods.

Pay the farmer now or pay big pharma later.

Be a food creator not a food consumer. Buying food products with your wallet is a vote for organic and sustainable food products, forcing Big Food Manufacturers and Big Agra to change their ways and create healthy food products instead of poison that causes illnesses, diseases and premature death. With every bite we are either eating life or death. Vote for life!

Scientists have proposed that one of the most widely used herbicides in the world, glyphosate (the active ingredient in Monsanto's Roundup), may be dramatically contributing to the rise of chronic disease.

Glyphosate was also recently reclassified as a Class 2A "probable human carcinogen." The International Federation of Gynecology & Obstetrics and a US Endocrine Society task force warn that pesticides pose a major threat to human health and should be avoided by everyone.

Glyphosate is in 80% of the food supply in the US, and some scientists believe it may well be the most toxic chemical ever approved for commercial use. Glyphosate causes both toxins and nutritional deficiencies in our bodies and is now linked to kidney disease, antibiotic resistant bacteria, inflammatory bowel disease, obesity, depression, ADHD, autism, Alzheimer's disease, Parkinson's disease, ALS, multiple sclerosis, cancer, cachexia, infertility, and developmental malformations. It destroys the microbiome of humans and plants, which is the root cause of many modern diseases.

Recent studies confirm that eating an organic diet can significantly reduce your toxic load by as much as 65%. The goal is to rid your body of toxins and inflammation, as they are the root of most modern diseases and deaths from heart attack, stroke, and cancer.

In addition to its toxic effects, glyphosate also denatures the food by blocking nutrient uptake and killing the microorganisms in the soil responsible for the plant's natural defense systems against pests of all kinds.

A Stanford University meta-analysis published in 2012 found that people who eat an organic diet tend to have far lower levels of toxic pesticides in their systems. Other studies have found that organic grass-fed meats are far less likely to contain multi-drug resistant bacteria. Hundreds of studies have shown that organic produce contains greater amounts of nutrients than conventional produce. The widely adopted factory farm in the "bigger is better" food system has reached a point where the fundamental weaknesses are becoming more and more visible, as we become a nation of food-induced illness.

Do not buy pre-sliced produce, fruits and vegetables. They will have lost some of their micronutrient value and will have started to oxidize (think apples turning brown.). Do not buy frozen or canned foods that contain added sugar, citric acid, maltodextrin, dextrose, or refined salt. Make sure all canned goods are BPA-free.

CHAPTER 4
Organic Versus Conventional Farming

The use of pesticides and herbicides in conventional farming reduces the levels of polyphenols in plants, vegetables, and fruits, and the soil is depleted of vital minerals and nutrients. The less a plant has to fight off microbes, diseases, and pests, the fewer polyphenols there are.

This is why conventionally raised vegetables and fruits look picture-perfect and larger, with no defects, while organic produce often looks imperfect in shape and smaller in size and have a lack of uniformity in color and shape, with scars on the surface. It is the collateral damage of polyphenols organically fighting off pests and microbes in the environment in the absence of herbicides and pesticides, thereby producing higher levels of polyphenols in organic vegetables and fruits. The end product is a healthier, more nutritional product.

Eating organic is not a health fad. It's a scientifically healthier choice. Eating organic can reduce chemicals and toxins in your body in just two weeks.

Just because it's organic, however, doesn't mean it is gluten-free.

Many processed food products are made with water that is not filtered. Not only do you get all the chemicals inherited in the processed foods themselves, you also get all the chemicals in that polluted water supply.

When you analyze production of a can of soda, it's not only the sugar and water in the contents, but also the water and chemicals to grow the sugar, sugar beets, corn, and corn syrup (HFCS), most of which are GMOs. That pathway is not listed on the labels of the products you are eating or drinking. This causes a cascade of unhealthy ingredients into our food supply. No wonder we are getting fatter and sicker. Not only do we have hidden sugar in our labels, we also have hidden ingredients and chemicals in processed foods.

There is a solution. Eat whole, real foods. If Mother Nature made it, eat it organically. If man made it, pass on it, and educate our kids not to eat it.

Organic bone broth (chicken or turkey) should be on your shopping list, as its benefits are innumerable, including:

- Helps heal and seal your gut.

- Promotes healthy digestion.

- Attracts and holds liquids, including digestive juices, thereby supporting proper digestion.

- Inhibits infection caused by cold and flu viruses.

A study published over a decade ago found that chicken soup does indeed have medicinal qualities, significantly mitigating infection and reducing joint pain and inflammation, courtesy of chondroitin sulphates, glucosamine, and other compounds extracted from the boiled-down cartilage. It fights inflammation. Amino acids lycine, proline, and arginine all have anti-inflammatory effects. Arginine has been found to be particularly beneficial for the treatment of sepsis (whole-body inflammation).

Glycine also has calming effects, which may help you sleep better. It promotes strong, healthy bones. Bone broth contains high amounts of calcium, magnesium, and other nutrients that play an important role in healthy bone formation, and the gelatin in the broth promotes healthy hair and nail growth. It also contains healthy doses of sodium, which are important when your body transforms into burning fat as opposed to sugar. I buy organic bone broth at Whole Foods, but you can also make batches from recipes at home.

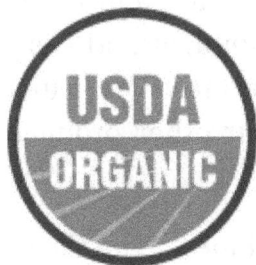

USDA Organic certification addresses a growing worldwide demand for organic food. It is intended to assure quality, prevent fraud, and promote commerce. While such certification was not necessary in the early days of the organic movement, when small farmers would sell their produce directly at farmers' markets, as organics have grown in popularity, more and more consumers are purchasing organic food through traditional channels, such as supermarkets. As such, consumers must rely on third-party regulatory certification.

For organic producers, certification identifies suppliers of products approved for use in certified operations. For consumers, "Certified Organic" serves as a product assurance. Certification is essentially aimed at regulating and facilitating the sale of organic products to consumers.

National organic labels also exist in Australia, Canada, France, Germany, and Japan. It's clearly a world-wide movement, not just a fad, but a fact.

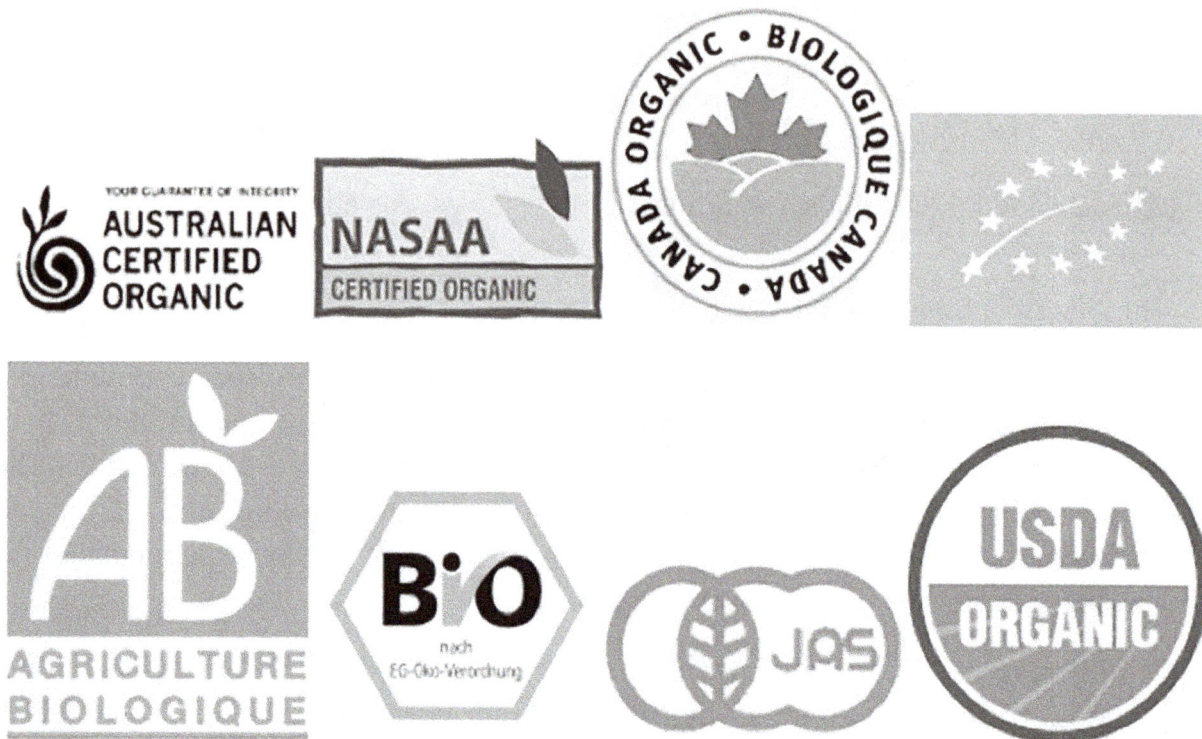

Organic is not only about having lower levels of pesticides, herbicides, and GMOs in our bodies. It's not just about the soil, vitamins, minerals, phytonutrients, phytochemicals, and antioxidants. It's also about the taste. You can taste the difference. Organic tastes healthy, tastes better – and that's a mouthful!

Buying organic costs more but is better for you nutritionally, tastes better, and keeps pesticides and herbicides out of your system. However, if you need to budget and can't always eat 100% organic, you might opt to limit your organic purchases to those fruits and vegetables that have the most pesticide residues and purchase your other produce conventionally grown.

"The Filthy Fourteen" is a list of produce with the most pesticide residues. "The Clean Fifteen" is a list of produce with the lowest residues. Always buy the organic version of The Filthy Fourteen.

Filthy Fourteen:

- Apples
- Celery
- Tomatoes
- Cucumbers
- Grapes
- Nectarines
- Peaches
- Potatoes
- Spinach
- Strawberries
- Blueberries
- Sweet Bell Peppers
- Green beans
- Kale

The Clean 15 are fruits and veggies you can eat conventionally (if you must, for budget or availability reasons), because they are not sprayed as heavily with pesticides.

Clean 15:

- Onions
- Avocado
- Sweet Corn (if GMO, don't eat.)
- Pineapple
- Mango
- Sweet Peas
- Eggplant
- Cauliflower

- Asparagus

- Kiwi

- Cabbage

- Watermelon

- Grapefruit

- Sweet Potatoes

- Honeydew Melon

Corn is a grain, not a vegetable. There are no healthy grains.

The only milk products you should be consuming are raw and unprocessed, if you consume them at all. Pasteurization kills beneficial enzymes and nutrients that help boost your immune system. Homogenization renders the butterfat in milk toxic and pro-inflammatory due to changes in its molecular structure.

"Never doubt that a small group of thoughtful, committed citizens can change the world, indeed, it's the one thing that ever has." - Margaret Mead

CHAPTER 5
GMO

The most common GMO ingredients found in food include: Corn, including corn flour, corn starch, corn oil, and corn syrup (as well as high-fructose corn syrup). Corn derivatives that may be of GMO origin include vitamin C supplements, citric acid, dextrose, and xylitol. Soybeans, including soy flour, soy lecithin, and soy protein isolates and concentrates. Soy derivatives that may be of GMO origin include vitamin E supplements, textured vegetable protein, monosodium glutamate (MSG), and Cottonseed oil.

Read the labels. Make sure your vitamins and supplements are soy free.

It's important to realize that genetically engineered (GMO) foods have never been proven safe for human consumption over a lifetime, let alone over generations. Monsanto and its advocates claim genetically engineered crops are "the most-tested food product that the world has ever seen." What they don't tell you is:

Industry-funded research predictably affects the outcome of the trial. This has been verified by dozens of scientific reviews comparing funding with the findings of the study. When industry funds the research, it's virtually guaranteed to be positive. Therefore, independent studies must be done to replicate, and thus verify, results.

The longest industry-funded animal feeding study was 90 days, which recent research has confirmed is FAR too short. In the world's first independently funded lifetime feeding study, massive health problems set in during and after the 13th month, including organ damage and cancer.

Companies like Monsanto and Syngenta rarely, if ever, allow independent researchers access to their patented seeds, citing the legal protection these seeds have under patent laws. Hence, independent research is extremely difficult or nearly impossible to conduct. If these scientists get seeds from a farmer, they sue them into oblivion, as one of their favorite tactics is to use the legal system to their advantage. Additionally, virtually all academic agricultural research is controlled by Monsanto, because they are the primary supporters of these departments and none will risk losing their funding from them.

There is no safety monitoring of GMOs. This means that once the item in question has been approved, not a single country on earth is actively monitoring and tracking reports of potential health effects.

Feedlot-farmed meat and milk contains growth hormones, steroids, and antibiotics fed from grains full of GMOs, herbicides and pesticides.

Wheat, corn, and soy are not only GMO, they are also sprayed with pesticides and herbicides – a toxic dump, to say the least.

The Non-GMO Project lists the following foods as the most common GMO foods to avoid in the American food supply:

- Soy
- Corn
- Canola
- Sugar beets
- Hawaiian papaya
- Alfalfa (as fed to conventional livestock)
- Yellow squash
- Zucchini

You also need to watch out for hidden additives in processed food made from GMOs, which include:

- Citric acid (GMO corn)
- Vegetable oil (GMO soy, corn, and canola)
- Caramel color (GMO corn)
- Dextrose (GMO corn)

- Isoflavones (GMO soy)

A good rule of thumb: if you can't pronounce an ingredient and if the product isn't labeled as certified organic or non-GMO, it probably contains cancer-causing GMOs and should be avoided.

Choosing organic fruits and vegetables to consume assures that you will avoid two potentially cancer-causing problems: high pesticide residues and the potential hazards of genetically modified foods.

CHAPTER 6
Pantry Purge, Cleanse, and Swap

G et rid of bad foods that create toxicity and inflammation. Replace them with good foods that are detoxifying and anti-inflammatory. It's a simple formula and you won't be tempted to cheat.

Quality food equals quality health. Swap bad, unhealthy foods for good, healthy foods. Love the food that loves you back. Rehab your taste buds, they will adapt. Food swap. Trade up. Pantry cleanse and purge. To eat right, you need to shop right. Get optimal nutrition from the grocery shelf to your dining table.

CHAPTER 7
Weight Loss/Weight Gain/Body Fat Loss

Dieting usually does not work, and most people gain back the weight they lose and more. Many fad diets work short-term, but for long-term weight loss and weight management, it takes habit changes or lifestyle changes and eating from a list of nutritious, whole, live foods and preparing them right. No processed foods, no fast foods, no sugar, no wheat or grains, no dairy, no soy, no trans fats, no vegetable oil and no fried foods.

Most overweight people and nearly all obese people are not leptin deficient, but produce too much leptin and become leptin resistant. When a person becomes leptin resistant, it takes more and more leptin to tell the brain it is satisfied and full and that you don't need more food, so you don't overeat on your way to obesity. Leptin is made from fat cells, so your body has to make more and more fat to get the message to the brain to stop being hungry and stop storing fat and that you are full and to stop eating. It's a vicious cycle leading to eating more, getting fatter and becoming more insulin and leptin resistant. Carbohydrates are the worst offenders. Carbohydrates that aren't burned are treated by the body the same way as sugar and the excess, unburned sugar is turned into saturated fat, which is resistant to burning, producing even more leptin and leptin resistance.

Beef and chicken (protein) from grain-fed animals that are not grass-fed and pasture raised are much higher in saturated fat. The fat in grain-fed animals is second-generation starch from the starchy carbohydrates that the animals are fed to fatten them up and then, stored as fat, which is ultimately stored as fat in our bodies. Thus, the old nutritional advice of a high-carbohydrate, low saturated fat diet was a double whammy, causing much harm from heart attacks, strokes, cancers, obesity and type 2 diabetes. Know what you are eating ate!

If your metabolism is functioning at full capacity, weight loss becomes relatively easy. If it's not, however, which is the case for most people, losing even a single pound can become seemingly impossible.

We each have a unique metabolism. If you chose foods from a nutrition-rich list, you will be healthier over the long-term, and once you establish your ideal weight and are in the maintenance stage, then you can customize and personalize and design a diet just for you. It may include carbs such as rice, but if you gain 4-5 pounds, you must get back on a restricted carb diet before the momentum starts to swing towards weight gain. Weight loss has many overlapping dimensions and benefits: social, job productivity, interpersonal, metabolic, hormonal, good health. You gain a lot in the process of losing.

It's not a diet but a "live it" – a way to live your life forever. Insulin sensitivity always improves when you lose weight. When you control insulin, you hugely increase the odds that you will control your weight. To lose weight you must control insulin and leptin, turning off the hunger switch. A diet containing adequate amounts of good fat and low in starchy carbs and sugar, will accomplish weight loss goals long-term for most people.

Low-carb, higher healthy fat and moderate healthy protein is what we are trying to attain. Low-fat diets generally accomplish weight gain, not weight loss, because the low fat is replaced by carbs, sugars, and grains, causing insulin resistance and weight gain.

The problem with obesity is carbohydrates, not fat, which is the exact opposite of its intention. Low fat, fat-free, cholesterol-free, and sugar-free foods are driving the obesity and type 2 diabetes epidemic in the world. The Standard American Diet (SAD) is the cause.

"Diabesity" is a combination term used for the epidemic in America of obesity and type 2 diabetes.

A low-carb diet is a permanent lifestyle, not just a temporary weight loss tool. You'll likely lose a lot more weight for the same caloric price. Once you reach your goal weight you may be able to add back some carbs, but if you are carbohydrate intolerant and not good at processing or metabolizing carbs, you will add weight, so you must not let carbs and weight creep back into your diet. If you've accomplished converting your body into a fat-burning machine as opposed to a sugar-burning machine and you lost weight in the process, why revert to old eating habits?

Lower fat in the diet is not the answer to obesity. A number of recent studies have shown that weight loss is actually greater on a low-carb diet than on a conventional low-fat diet with the same number of calories, with the added benefit of better blood chemistry. A lower-carb diet is much more satiating and easier to maintain over the long term as a lifestyle eating strategy than a diet that simply reduces fat. Long-term maintenance is the ultimate goal.

There is no RDA for carbohydrates. They are not necessary to sustain life; this is especially true for sugars and starches. However, protein and fat are necessary to sustain life. Getting your carbs from healthy fruits and vegetables, seeds, and nuts will be all you need to sustain your life and maintain your ideal weight. Add healthy fats and protein from olive oil, coconut oil, avocados, wild-caught fish such as Sockeye Salmon, grass-fed beef, pasture-raised, organic chicken and eggs, and you will have the perfect foundation of a permanent lifestyle diet for weight loss and weight maintenance. Toss in some exercise, vitamins, minerals and supplements and the new you will arrive.

Sixty-five percent of the US population is considered overweight. Our fat cell numbers generally don't increase after puberty. They just grow bigger and fatter. (There is new research indicating adults may grow new fat cells as well. Oh no.)

"Overweight" is considered a BMI of 25-29.9 (Body Mass Index). "Obese" is a BMI of 30 and above.

One key is to consume fewer calories while experiencing less hunger, and at the same time gaining more energy and enjoying your food. The moral of the story is that insulin levels must be controlled to create an environment of fat mobilization, resulting in natural loss of body fat.

Even if nothing else has worked before, or you lost weight but gained it back plus more, or have been on a yo-yo up and down cycle for years, the Food List, Food Choices and Swaps in this handbook, will put the majority of people on a pathway to weight loss and weight maintenance for a lifetime.

A diet based on low-carb, low-glycemic load, moderate healthy protein and higher healthy fats is the complete opposite of a low-fat, high-carbohydrate diet that has been promoted for nearly 50 years and is killing people one bite, one fork, one sip at a time. Most diets succeed because you are eating fewer calories and fewer carbohydrates and more greens and more vegetables.

The eating strategy I promote does not starve you or make you crave your old eating habits, but individualizes a well-formulated, balanced eating strategy that puts the right fuel into your body. You will lose weight if that's your goal, or maintain your ideal weight. You will feel energized. Your skin, hair and nails will look vital. You will be proud and happy about your lifestyle change because that's the only way you will maintain it for a lifetime.

Most dairy products (milk and cheese) will slow or stall weight and fat loss. Eliminating sugar (starches), wheat, dairy, and alcohol are your fastest track to weight loss.

"A calorie is a calorie" is simply not true, so it stands to reason that all carbohydrates, all fats and all proteins are not the same. Weight gain and weight loss are dependent on the knowledge of dietary strategy and practice.

Volume measuring is a technique to track your progress. It's not so much your weight as what your weight is made of: fat, water and lean muscle.

Your weight can fluctuate 4-5 pounds based on water weight alone. However, if you gain more than that, restrict your carbs and get back on a low-carb diet.

High-intensity interval training and weight resistance exercise are superior because they not only build muscle – they burn fat. (See HIIT and resistance/strength training under exercise segment.)

Exercise will recompose and re-sculpt your body mass. You don't merely want to lose weight – you want to lose fat and become lean and healthy with tight skin.

Whether you're a man or a woman, adding muscle will aid you in losing body fat.

Even though scale weight is important psychologically for us to measure progress and results, volume is important too. Six pounds of fat takes up about a gallon of space in volume. So, take a pair of pants that you can no longer fit into and try them on from time to time to measure your volume. Another way is to take a small rope or cord and wrap it around your waist and cut it where it meets, so you have a volume measurement with the length of the rope to compare from time to time to track your results. It will amaze you, just like on "The Biggest Loser."

Recent research confirms that the best diet to eat to lose weight, restricting fattening carbohydrates, is also the one that best prevents CVD (cardiovascular disease.).

Most diets don't work. The ones that do, do not have beneficial results for cardiovascular disease and diabetes risk factors because they are geared to rapid weight loss as opposed to health and wellness.

Men tend to gain weight above their waist as a beer belly and love handles. Women tend to gain weight below the waist in their hips, butt and thighs, until after menopause, when they gain it in the stomach, too.

The very worst foods for us are sugars, wheat, high-fructose corn syrup in sodas, and even artificial sweeteners. The worst combination of all may be fries, a soda and a Big Mac – an order of dietary and nutritional suicide. It's a heart attack just waiting to happen – truly a Big Mac Attack.

While our bodies are accumulating fat, our fuel requirements are increasing. When we get fatter we add muscle to support the additional fat. So as we fatten, our energy demand increases, therefore our appetite increases, especially for carbohydrates, because this is the only fuel our body will burn when our insulin is elevated. It's a vicious circle and it's precisely what we want to avoid. Otherwise we'll be driven to crave exactly those carb-rich foods that make us fat. Food manufacturers know this and advertise accordingly. They say, "Bet you can't eat just one," and they're right.

Keep your body cool – keep your thermostat down. This creates internal heat loss which in turn causes your body to burn calories to create heat to keep your core temperature warm to 98.6 degrees. I keep my doors and windows open year-round to breathe fresh air. Even when I lived in Iowa and Minnesota, I always cracked a window open near my bed, even in winter, for continued cold, fresh air. I rarely ever caught colds or flu. If your house breathes, you breathe. The coolness also helped me with better quality sleep.

Sleep, particularly that obtained before midnight, stimulates release of growth hormone, production of testosterone, and repair of cells, all of which is conducive to fat loss. Sleeping with the thermostat at 68 degrees promotes deeper sleep and an accelerated rate of calorie burn. Couple that with strength training and lean muscle gain, and you will burn calories and lose fat in your sleep.

Adequate sleep and the absence of stress send a physiological message of "all is well" to your body, which in turn allows your body to release stress-stored fat more easily.

There are a number of reasons to stay hydrated every day. Weight loss is one of them. As the thermal cost of heating water to the body temperature of 98.6 degrees, the body burns calories in the process. As the water cools the core body temperature, it requires calories to be expended to heat the body back up to normal. Hence, calories are burned. That's why drinking plenty of water daily helps you to lose weight. Drink at least eight 8-ounce glasses per day or up to 100 ounces per day if you're able. Another rule of thumb that can be used is to drink 0.5 ounces of water per pound of bodyweight. If you weigh 150 pounds, drink 75 ounces of water per day.

A further benefit of adequate hydration is an expansion of circulating blood volume. Blood plasma is 92% water. Expanded blood volume allows hormonal efficiency and for hormones to come into play that promote fat loss by interacting with various tissues, including your fat cells. Dehydration compromises circulating blood volume, compromising this process. Maintaining fully expanded blood volume and increased circulation of fat loss hormones aids the fat loss process. Dehydrated hormones don't circulate as well. Keeping well-hydrated also aids the liver in processing mobilized body fat so that it can be burned as fuel.

Another reason to eat a diet rich in fruits and vegetables is their naturally high water content, helping you to stay hydrated.

And finally, staying hydrated sends a biological message to the body that there is no threat of famine and no need to store fat. Drought precedes famine. If the body thinks famine is coming it will automatically slow its metabolism and you will start to store fat. This is the wrong message to send, so stay hydrated and it will help you lose weight. Staying well-hydrated sends the body physiology a message that all is well and there is no need to slow metabolism or raise appetite, because famine is not forthcoming.

Weight loss is not the same as fat loss. No diet in history has worked long-term for more than 2% of the population.

Once you lower leptin levels and regain leptin sensitivity, leptin can then begin doing its vital job of turning off the hunger switch and turning on the fat-burning switch.

Better health and well-being should be your goal. If your 3 best friends are overweight, there's a 50% chance you'll be overweight. Surround yourself with positive-thinking people with good habits – or enlist your friends to join you in your new lifestyle.

Add more years to your life and more life to your years. Health is a life-long investment.

With a lower carb, moderate protein, higher fat and higher fiber diet, your body won't have enough sugar coming in to burn as fuel. Your body will have to make its own, mostly from fat and some amino acids. This will make it easier for your body to switch from burning sugar to burning fat so you will lose weight. That's what you want: your body to switch from burning sugar to burning fat as fuel. You will also improve your lipid profile, with lower triglycerides, higher HDL and insulin sensitivity. You will lose fat and your risk for cardiovascular disease and hypertension will decrease.

The only side- effects of a lower-carb, moderate-healthy protein, higher-healthy fat, higher fiber diet are weight loss, better health, wellness and longevity. Talk about a winning strategy!

"Tell me what you eat and I shall tell you what you are." – Jean Anthelme Brillat-Savarin, 1825.

Two urges must be balanced to maintain ideal weight in the long term: hunger and satiety. When these two urges are balanced, permanent weight control becomes a habit or lifestyle. If you can lose weight without hunger, aren't you more likely to maintain that eating pattern, than one of indefinite starvation and deprivation?

It's not willpower or exercise, but control of your hormones, particularly insulin, through your diet that accelerates hunger (overeating) or reducing hunger (satiety). Excess or "bad" carbohydrates are the primary culprit for generating hunger, while protein and fat are the primary agent in generating satiety.

Fat does not impact insulin secretion or affect blood sugar levels. Many people lose inches before they lose weight. If energy intake is greater than energy expenditure, fat gain occurs.

Lose the wheat, lose the weight.

Seventy-five percent of your ability to gain weight or become obese is a result of your genetics. You can't change your genes, but you can change their expression by your diet, which determines whether they are turned on or turned off, and by reducing insulin levels in your bloodstream, thereby, not storing more fat. Reduced insulin levels allow the fat to be released from your cells to be burned as energy.

Insulin is known as the fat storage hormone. Excess insulin and insulin resistance traps fat in the cells, not allowing it to be burned as energy (ATP) in your cells and muscles, so you just keep accumulating fat until you reach obesity. This is especially true if you are pre-programmed with obesity genes. Treating obesity is not solved by "eating less and exercising more," but by reducing insulin levels generated by the diet, so fat stores can be released and used for ATP production.

Obese people tend to overeat carbohydrates and are obsessed with food. Their overeating is not the primary cause of their obesity, but rather is a secondary consequence of their genetics interacting adversely with excess insulin being produced by their diet from consuming too many of the wrong carbohydrates. This increases insulin levels, which increases fat storage. So those who were genetically programmed to be obese are adding fuel to the fire and getting sicker and fatter.

ATP: Adenosine Triphosphate is a source of energy for physiological reactions in every cell and muscle. It stores and supplies the cell with energy needed for sustaining life. Energy is the currency of life.

Excess insulin causes diet-induced inflammation, which is a primary risk factor for high blood pressure, cardiovascular disease, heart attack, stroke, obesity, elevated cholesterol level, elevated triglycerides, and diabetes. Weight gain is a gradual process. Many illnesses are progressive over a lifetime.

You cannot exercise your way out of a bad diet. SOFI is an acronym for Skinny on the Outside, Fat on the Inside. You may look skinny on the outside of your body, but you are fat on the inside where it matters most, with visceral fat in and around your major organs. This means you are actually not well and will probably eventually become sick with a major disease.

Low-fat diets generally accomplish weight gain, not weight loss, because the low fat is replaced by carbs, sugars and grains, causing insulin resistance and weight gain. The problem with obesity is carbohydrates, not fat, the exact opposite of its intention. Low fat, fat-free, cholesterol-free, and sugar-free foods and diets are driving the obesity and type 2 diabetes epidemic in the world.

You don't want your body to go into starvation mode, because then weight loss is difficult. Protein and fat are key ingredients. You can live without carbs but you can't live without fat and protein.

Alcohol has 7 calories per gram, approximately 200 calories per ounce. The liver will process alcohol before anything else, so if you want to lose weight you must cut your alcohol consumption. You can resume once you have reached your ideal weight and are in maintenance mode.

One pound of fat contains about 3,500 calories of energy. Two pounds equals 7,000 calories. So if you are lean at 25, but overweight at 50, here's the math:

20 calories per day times 365 days per year is a little more than 7000 calories stored as fat every year or 2-lbs of excess fat gained, times 25 years, equals 50 lbs. This is why a simple calories in/calories out equation does not work.

No matter how hard you work, you cannot exercise away a bad diet. All calories are not created equal and all carbohydrates are not created equal. If you burn calories, they are not stored as fat. If you have a calorie deficit diet, you will lose weight. If you balance your calories you maintain weight. A well-formulated low-carb, healthy higher-fat, healthy moderate-protein diet turns your body into a fat burner as opposed to a sugar burner, since you have eliminated most of the foods that are turned into sugar, thereby controlling your blood sugar and insulin, hence diminishing your fat stores.

Losing body fat efficiently requires heeding the laws of thermodynamics, which means calories must be restricted. In energy, you can't get something for nothing, and that's what calories are, energy and fuel. If you consume 2,000 calories of refined carbohydrates, the metabolic cost of converting carbs into stored energy (body fat) is close to zero. However, if you consume lean meats, vegetables and fruits, the metabolic cost converting these foods into energy is high, from the thermic cost of digestion. Consuming a diet composed of real, whole foods and unrefined foods increases the thermic cost of digestion, stabilizing blood sugar along the way, as this is a more metabolically expensive process compared to the near zero cost of metabolizing carbs. As a result, there is simply a greater caloric cost of maintaining stable blood glucose with these real foods than there is with consuming refined sugars and carbohydrates to accomplish the same process. In addition, consuming real foods as opposed to processed foods ensures blood glucose levels within the bloodstream rise and fall more gradually, maintaining serum insulin levels at a much lower level. Part of the reason is the fiber in vegetables and fruits, as fiber does not affect glucose levels.

This formula will allow you to lose weight simply by the laws of dynamics – how calories are digested and converted into energy, by consuming real foods and restricting carbohydrates. A real-foods diet provides a double metabolic advantage by promoting a higher thermic cost of digestion while keeping insulin levels low, enabling fat loss to occur naturally in the process of a calorie deficit. Simply put, if your calories are in excess of your energy expenditure, it's going to be a colossal task to lose body fat.

Insulin trumps several other metabolic hormones necessary for fat mobilization, including glucagon, epinephrine, norepinephrine, growth hormone and testosterone. All are shut down by elevated insulin levels.

Some people may be able to lose weight on a diet of calorie restriction, but are still consuming too many carbohydrates, resulting in elevated insulin levels, making mobilization or losing body fat more difficult. That's why many diets work at first through decreased calorie consumption, calorie restriction, and calorie deficit. But if you don't restrict carbs or if you resume eating carbs, the weight will always come back over the long term. Ninety-five percent of all dieters gain the weight back and more. It's from the refined carbs and sugar in processed foods. Simply keep it real and your body will thank you with sustained weight management.

CHAPTER 8
Balance/Optimize Hormones

If you are overweight or obese, how many times have you been told that it was your fault because you lacked will power and motivation or were just too lazy and didn't care? The psychology of change was just too difficult to overcome. Or worse yet, every diet you tried failed and you gained more weight afterward than before, and you just accepted your plight of being fat. Or maybe you thought your weight problem was genetic and you were stuck with your DNA, so you were unhappy, depressed, and lacking in self-confidence.

What if I told you it wasn't your fault? It wasn't your lack of willpower or that you were stuck with your genes. You were addicted and it was your hormones making you fat.

What if I told you that it's reversible and preventable? No more cravings or binges. Insulin is known as the fat and fat storage hormone. Controlling your insulin controls your diet and controls your weight. We truly are what we eat, but even more so, we are what we don"t eat.

It has nothing to do with willpower. Sugar and wheat are addictive. They increase your hunger and drive you to overeat and gain weight. Eliminate the sugar, wheat, processed foods, fast foods, fried foods, starchy carbohydrates, and HFCS sodas and you will control your insulin, thereby controlling your weight.

Hormones ultimately control activation of inflammatory genes in your body. Diet controls these key hormones. Homeostasis and diet can unbalance them as well. The gut is your second brain, so if your stomach is distressed, your body is not getting the right signals from your food. Remember, food is information for your cells. If your thyroid is not activating properly and your hormones are imbalanced you've got chaos and a body out of control – all because of a distressed stomach!

Insulin, the "fat storage" hormone, is the main hormone to control through diet, but leptin and gherelin need to be controlled as well. Leptin is the satiety hormone that curbs appetite. Leptin is produced by fat cells and exerts its appetite-satiating effects by acting on the brain. Leptin resistance means you are starving your brain. If you're eating or drinking a lot of HFCS, your brain doesn't recognize it and even though your fats cells are full, your brain doesn't send the satiety signal and you keep eating and craving more in a vicious cycle leading to obesity. Obese people have more fat cells but experience leptin resistance, so they don't receive its appetite-suppressing effects. So, when you eat that whole bag of chips or that second serving of pie and ice cream, it's your brain telling you that you are addicted and craving more, hence a cycle of overeating and weight gain.

The lack of satiety comes from disruption in the gut-brain communication involving hormones such as insulin, leptin and ghrelin, and is accompanied by cellular inflammation. This leads to obesity, diabetes, and chronic diseases such as heart attack, stroke, cancer. It also sets the stage for Alzheimer's disease. When this lack of communication occurs, you gain weight, you accelerate the development of chronic diseases, and you age faster.

Leptin, discovered in 1994, is a hormone that plays a crucial role in appetite and weight control and is produced by the body's fat cells. It crosses the blood-brain barrier and binds to receptors in the appetite center in the brain, regulating brain cells that tell you how much to eat. It's called the obesity hormone or fat hormone.

Cortisol is like cyanide to your body. Stress will kill you. High levels of cortisol shrink your brain, increase insulin resistance, promote metabolic syndrome and heart disease, and lower your immune system – all known longevity robbers.

Hypothyroidism: 27 million Americans are estimated to have thyroid disease, 60% undiagnosed. Hypothyroidism affects 50% of the American population. Why? Diet and environment. Our bodies must deal with hormone and antibiotic residues in meat, dairy, and soy; food-borne bacteria; chemicals in cleaning products, food additives, and cosmetics; metabolic byproducts of unfriendly gut bacteria; and fluoride and chlorine in drinking water. In addition, there are some 80,000 registered chemicals in use in the US, including pesticides, herbicides and the like, most of which are toxic.

Your thyroid is one of the endocrine glands, a small, butterfly-shaped gland situated at the base of the front of your neck, just below your Adam's apple. The thyroid controls how your body's cells use energy from food, a process called metabolism. Hormones produced by the thyroid gland - triiodothyronine (T3) and thyroxine (T4) - have an enormous impact on your health, affecting all aspects of your metabolism. They maintain the rate at which your body uses fats and carbohydrates, help control your body temperature, influence your heart rate, and help regulate the production of proteins.

Hypothyroidism results when the thyroid gland fails to produce enough hormones

(TSH, T3 and T4.) Hypothyroidism may be due to a number of factors, including auto-immune disorders, viral infection, radiation therapy, certain medications to treat heart problems, psychiatric conditions, cancer, iodine deficiency, pituitary gland disorder, hypothalamus disorder, and simply aging.

TSH: Thyroid stimulating hormone is a pituitary hormone that stimulates the thyroid gland to produce thyroxine (T4), and then triiodothyronine (T3) which stimulates the metabolism of almost every tissue in the body.

Hypothyroidism may also be associated with an increased risk of heart disease; primarily because it increases levels of low-density lipoprotein (LDL) cholesterol - the "bad" cholesterol - can occur in people with an underactive thyroid. Too much bad cholesterol can lead to atherosclerosis (hardening of the arteries), which increases your risk of heart attacks and strokes. Even subclinical hypothyroidism, a mild or early form of hypothyroidism in which symptoms have not yet developed, can affect the health of your heart, with the buildup of fluid around the heart (a pericardial effusion), which may make it harder for the heart to pump blood. Hypothyroidism can also lead to an enlarged heart, heart failure, and increased rates of cardiovascular disease; arrhythmia in particular.

Depression may occur early in hypothyroidism and may become more severe over time. Hypothyroidism can also cause slowed mental functioning. The symptoms of hypothyroidism can take a mental toll if left untreated. Without treatment, the symptoms of hypothyroidism will increase. This can directly affect your mental state and your depression may intensify as a result.

Hypothyroidism signs and symptom may include:

- Fatigue

- Increased sensitivity to cold

- Constipation

- Dry skin

- Weight gain

- Puffy face

- Hoarseness

- Muscle weakness

- Elevated blood cholesterol level

- Muscle aches, tenderness and stiffness

- Pain, stiffness or swelling in your joints

- Heavier than normal or irregular menstrual periods

- Thinning hair

- Slowed heart rate

- Depression

- Impaired memory

Millions of Americans suffer from fatigue, weight gain, depression, and cognitive impairment. Many believe that they have no choice but to accept these seemingly "age-related" declines in quality of life.

Underactive thyroid (hypothyroidism) is often overlooked or misdiagnosed and can be the underlying cause of these symptoms. Patients and their doctors often disregard these common signs of thyroid hormone deficiency, mistaking them for normal aging.

Fortunately, a simple blood test for TSH, T3, and T4 can reveal an underlying thyroid condition and help direct treatment to improve the symptoms.

NASA has mission control; the thyroid is yours – your master switch. Diagnosed or undiagnosed thyroid disease can lead to heart disease, heart attack, and stroke if not treated. Environmental toxins are a leading cause. Multiple dental X-rays have been linked to thyroid disease. Ask for a thyroid or neck cover shield for your next dental X-ray, just like the chest protector.

The thyroid, adrenal, and pituitary glands affect your hormonal balance and must be tested for health. Balancing your hormones, for both men and women, is essential for weight loss, weight control, and weight maintenance. As your master switch, the thyroid may be the trickiest to balance. You must have an endocrinologist on your team of physicians. The thyroid is a specialized gland that only an endocrinologist or functional M.D. should be entrusted to balance and treat.

Insulin resistance is actually a hormone imbalance. Until you balance your hormones, especially insulin, which is secreted at the highest levels with carbohydrate consumption, you will not be able to lose weight. In fact, you will just keep getting fatter.

A sudden increase in blood-sugar level from a high glycemic load of carbohydrate, sugar, wheat, or starch causes your pancreas to produce more insulin. Eventually you develop insulin resistance. If your diet continues on this destructive path over a long period of time, type 2 diabetes results. If the pancreas is pushed even further, pancreatic cancer can develop. Insulin is probably the easiest hormone to balance through your diet.

I had borderline type 2 diabetes, which was one of the metabolic syndrome factors that contributed to my stroke. My insulin was elevated and I probably suffered from insulin resistance as well. Immediately after getting them under control, I lost nearly 100 pounds in four months. It was almost effortless with proper diet and nutrition.

Since elevated insulin levels shut down testosterone production, my first blood test for testosterone post stroke was 97, far below suboptimal levels for T. Studies show that when men maintain testosterone levels in the 550-750 range, they stopped having cardiovascular events, heart attacks, and strokes. I'm not sure of the cause and effect science here, but needless to say I now maintain my testosterone above 750 and have never felt healthier.

It's estimated that 13.9 million American men, one in four over age 30, have low testosterone levels, yet only 9% of men are being treated with testosterone replacement therapy. Low testosterone has been associated with serious medical conditions including diabetes, cardiovascular disease, and metabolic syndrome, which leads to stroke. By 2025 as many as 6.5 million American men between the ages of 30-79 will be testosterone hormone deficient, an increase of 38% from 2000.

One reason men get a beer belly and love handles is because they secrete less testosterone as they age. Less testosterone equates to more fat. High free testosterone does not promote prostate cancer. Low free testosterone and high estrogen promote prostate cancer. Low thyroid causes hardening of the arteries (atherosclerosis), leading to heart attacks and stroke.

The most accurate way to balance your hormones is through a blood test. If you don't test, you're left to guess. If you can't measure it, you can't improve it.

CHAPTER 9
Alkaline Water/Hydration

Considering that water makes up more than 75% of our muscular system and upwards of 93% of our bloodstream, water is an essential component of a healthy, cancer-free lifestyle.

Benefits of alkaline water:

- An alkaline environment is important for tissue health, repair, and growth, but not the blood. Blood pH stays constant at 7.4

- Alkaline water is a foundation of good health

Alkaline vs. acidic: Much of the SAD (Standard American Diet) is acidic, so an alkaline environment is important to maintain and reverse the overly acidic environment that most American's maintain

- Antioxidant

- Anti-inflammatory

- Detoxifier

- Weight management tool

- Lemon water (add some lemon to your water for taste as well as a detox agent)

- Apple cider vinegar (in concert with alkaline water as another detox agent)

Water improves energy, increases mental and physical performance, removes toxins and waste from your body, keeps skin healthy and glowing, and can help with weight loss. Most people are under-hydrated so their blood is thicker and as a result their body has to work harder to circulate the thicker blood. As a result, your brain becomes less active, concentration is more difficult, and you feel fatigued. Water lubricates and cushions joints and muscles and reduces cramping and fatigue during and after exercise. A good rule of thumb is to divide your bodyweight by 2 and drink that number of ounces per day of water. If you eat 10-13 servings of fresh vegetables and fruits a day you will add to your water consumption and good health.

Whether your water is alkaline or filtered, add a pinch of Himalayan pink rock salt or sea salt to your water. It helps efficiently transport water into your cells, improving their ability to flush the toxins out. A pinch of sodium is also a good compliment to a low-carb diet and exercise regimen, so the kidneys will not hold onto sodium and water weight. It adds a little sodium and trace minerals to your body that it may crave, especially if you work out and sweat a lot. You may think you are having a sugar or carbohydrate craving, when in fact it is sodium.

The foods that we eat can have either an alkalizing or acidic effect on our bodies. Alkalizing foods are primarily leafy greens, vegetables, grasses, sprouts, herbs, and most seeds, nuts, and fruits. Acidic foods are primarily meat, dairy, sugar, wheat, alcohol, and processed foods.

Tap water causes harm. It's not the water itself that causes the damage, but what's in it.

Tap water: (municipal water) from all over the world (including the US) is contaminated with heavy metals and toxins that can cause cancer and other serious illnesses. Every informed person knows you should NEVER drink the tap water. Nearly all bottled water is just filtered tap water!

Fluoride is an industrial waste product. Chlorine is a toxin. Chlorine in municipal water supplies kills the good gut bacteria of the microbiome.

Chlorine and fluoride are in our water supply, so if you don't drink filtered (not just bottled water, as some bottled water is not pure or filtered), you are drinking a toxin that kills your good microbiome (chlorine), a toxin that is considered industrial waste (fluoride), as well as runoff from pesticides and herbicides that are deposited into our water supply. Know your water.

Why you should never trust tap water:

The recent Flint, Michigan scandal revealed that many water plants in the US contain alarmingly high levels of toxic metals such as lead.

Many municipal water systems add toxic fluoride to the water supply.

Fluoride is a known neurotoxin that's been linked to lower IQ scores in children.

Fluoride promotes corrosion of water pipes, releasing even more lead or other toxic elements into your tap.

More than 60% of Americans are exposed to lead and fluoride-contaminated water. Are you one of them?

Tap water is filled with chloride and chlorine. It's added by water quality operations to kill bacteria, but it can also affect our own health.

The EPA in 2016 just announced its plan to allow gigantic increases in the allowable radioactivity in drinking water ... increasing it by over 3,000 times in the case of radioactive Iodine-131 ... while calling it "safe" to drink even though it's almost certain to give you cancer.

Far too little credit is given to the awesome nature that alkaline ionized water has on our bodies:

- Your body is 83% water

- Muscles are 75% water

- Brain is 74% water

- Bones are 22% water

- Water is needed for every metabolic process in the body

- Water is necessary to digest and absorb nutrients and vitamins

- Water carries away metabolic waste

Water flushes fat and toxins through the liver and kidneys and out of the body. An interesting theory, observation, and conclusion about your body and water: Doesn't it make sense to constantly replenish and feed your body the equivalent of a clean, fresh mountain stream, rather than to let 83% of your body sit and recycle like a stagnant pond?

Hydrate your body on a cellular basis to keep it fresh, not stagnant and aging. It's not just what we are eating, but also what we are drinking that is killing us – not just one fork and one bite at a time, but one sip and one drink at a time, from both water and sodas.

Chromium VI: In a recent study, the Environmental Working Group (EWG) found measurable levels of chromium VI in the tap water of 31 out of 34 cities sampled. In addition to being a carcinogen, chromium VI is a skin irritant and can cause contact dermatitis and allergic reactions.

Heavy metals: Tap water contains heavy metals like iron, copper, magnesium, and zinc. Though they are present at very small levels, they can interact with free radicals and damage collagen fibers in the skin. They can also cause a reaction with the skin's natural oils, clogging pores.

Minerals: Most American homes have hard water, which is full of minerals. If you don't have a water softener in your home, you've likely seen the hard water stains on your shower door or curtain – those white, chalky marks. That same water can leave a soapy layer on the skin that clogs pores, increasing acne breakouts, while leaving skin itchy and dry. With repeated use, hard water can also increase risk of redness and eczema. A 2014 study, for example, found that infants living in areas with high calcium content in the water supply (hard water) were at an increased risk for eczema. Researchers also found that those living in hard-water areas were at a greater risk for damage to the skin barrier, resulting in dryness.

Chlorine: According to the Environmental Protection Agency (EPA), to protect water from disease-causing organisms, water suppliers often add a disinfectant, like chlorine. Unfortunately, chlorine is bad for your skin (and your hair). It's an irritant, and because of its abrasiveness, can cause itchiness and even rashes. It strips the skin of its natural oils and damages the outer layer, leading to increased dryness and flakiness. Over time, it can exacerbate the appearance of fine lines and wrinkles, accelerating the aging process.

Fluoride: Fluoride is also added to drinking water to "protect public health" as the EPA says – mainly to promote dental health. Like chlorine, it's irritating to skin, but it can also disrupt the production of collagen, which can have aging effects.

We want to rid our bodies of all diet-induced inflammation and all environmental toxins, including in our municipal water supply or tap water. Drink filtered, alkaline, spring, or glacier water. Bottled water is not always pure or filtered. Read the labels and know your sources. Do your research and drink whichever one makes you feel the healthiest.

Drink a minimum eight 8-oz glasses per day (64 oz) and shoot for 100 oz per day. A rule of thumb that can be used is 0.5-oz per pound of bodyweight. If you weigh 140 pounds, drink 70 ounces of water per day. Water is very important for weight loss and anti-aging. Stay hydrated or you will wrinkle and shrink. If you are wrinkling on the outside, you are wrinkling on the inside, so hydration not only helps your external skin health, but your internal system of veins, arteries, tissues muscles, organs, and bones.

Research from Mayo Clinic suggests:

- 2 glasses of water after waking up helps activate internal organs

- 1 glass of water 30 minutes before a meal helps digestion

- 1 glass of water before taking a bath helps lower blood pressure

- 1 glass of water before going to bed helps prevent stroke or heart attack

- water at bed time helps prevent night time leg cramps. Leg muscles are seeking hydration when they cramp and wake you up with a Charlie Horse.

Most heart attacks occur generally between 6 A.M. and noon. Having one during the night, when the heart should be most at rest, means that something unusual went wrong. Sleep apnea may be to blame for nighttime heart attacks and strokes.

Why do people need to urinate so much at night time? Gravity holds water in the lower part of your body when you are upright. When you lie down and the lower body is level with the kidneys; it is then that the kidneys remove the water because it's an easier function for the kidneys to perform. I still like drinking water at night before and during bedtime, even though there are those who advocate no water before or during bedtime because it interrupts sleep. I believe the health benefits of being hydrated outweigh those negatives of peeing like a racehorse.

Don't drink tap water. I personally prefer alkaline water and find it the foundation to my good health for all the reasons discussed above. Most people and pets love the taste of alkaline water.

CHAPTER 10
Reading Labels & How to Interpret Them

If cane sugar, corn syrup or any other type of sugary sweetener, including fruit juice, is listed in the first 3 ingredients, avoid the product.

When one lives in a society where people can no longer depend on institutions to tell them the truth, then the truth must come from the culture.

Fewer than 50% of Americans read food labels when making a food product purchase and even fewer know how to accurately read and interpret them.

Reading labels is a tricky business. Consumers are more health-conscious than ever, so food manufacturers use misleading tricks to convince people to buy their products. They often do this even when the food is highly processed and unhealthy. The regulations behind food labeling are complex, so it's not surprising that the average consumer has a hard time understanding them.

Don't be duped by the marketing claims on the front of the package. Front labels try to lure you into purchasing products by making health claims. Manufacturers want to make you believe that their product is healthier than other, similar options. This has actually been studied. Research shows that adding health claims to front labels affects people's choices. It makes them believe a product is healthier than the same product that doesn't list health claims.

Manufacturers are often dishonest on their labels. They tend to make health claims that are misleading, and in some cases downright false. Avoid foods that have sugars or starches listed in the first 5 ingredients.

Ninety-five percent of Americans eat processed foods. There are 10,000 chemical ingredients listed by the US government as GRAS (Generally Regarded as Safe) that are allowed in processed foods and don't have to be listed on the label. However, many of these chemicals have never been tested through proper scientific clinical trials as to their safety and efficacy for human consumption. So, on top of GMOs and trans-fats, we have 10,000 GRAS chemicals that don't even have to be listed on the labels. No wonder America is sick, tired, fat, and dying.

Europe tends to take a much more precautionary approach with food additives, approving only those shown to be safe. The U.S. takes a more reactionary approach. Unless you can prove a chemical is unsafe, then it's fair game.

The simple message is: eat real, whole, unprocessed foods. Prepare your food at home with real, fresh, whole food ingredients. The healthiest people are those who eat and prepare their own food, in their own kitchens, in their own homes. If it comes in a bag, box, can, carton or container and has a bar code or label, it is most likely processed food and is full of harmful, unhealthy chemicals that are making you sick.

More than 3,000 food additives, preservatives, flavorings, colors, and other ingredients are added to US foods. This is another reason to avoid most of the processed foods that contain them. While many well-meaning nutritionists will teach you the importance of reading food labels, the easiest way to eat healthy is to stick with foods that need no food label at all.

There are 10,000 registered chemicals that do not have to be listed on labels. Real, whole foods do not have labels. The food is the label.

Modern food manufacturers have hijacked our food supply. Most food labels list so many chemicals and ingredients that you'd need a PhD in chemistry to understand exactly what you're eating. US processed foods in the US may be even worse than those in other countries. Manufacturers don't care about your diet or your health. All they want is your money and astronomical profits.

Ninety percent of fresh produce at the grocery store has been processed just like a packaged food, unless it is specifically labeled "organic" or "non-GMO." Commercial agriculture is a multi-billion-dollar industry. Seeds modified in a lab are planted in soil that has been chemically treated and as the plants develop and grow, they absorb all these artificial nutrients and are constantly showered with pesticides, fungicides and herbicides. The food is then rinsed in water with bleach and bathed in wax to try to kill some bacteria and to make it look pretty and edible for consumers. By the time these foods reach the grocery store, they have spent days or weeks in trucks, trains, or boats in transit, longer than you'd be comfortable knowing about, either ripening or being tricked into not ripening by artificial means and exposed to heat and light, which further damage the quality of the food before it even reaches your plate.

Commercially raised meats, unless labeled "organic" and "grass-fed and grass-finished," are generally fed GMO grain enhanced with growth hormones and grown in chemically treated and pesticide-filled soil, then injected with antibiotics, growth hormones, and other dangerous compounds that infuse the meat you ultimately consume. Some foods and meats are then irradiated (exposed to ionized radiation), before hitting the store shelves. Irradiated-exposed foods are dangerous and originate from nuclear waste products. By eating organic food choices, you eliminate all this, helping build your immune system to fight off bacteria and bio-accumulative toxins at the cellular level, resulting in a healthier you. Ideally, the only hands to touch your foods should be the farmer's and yours.

Freshness dating:

- "Sell by" date means nothing more than telling the store how long to display the product for sale. Never buy the product after this date.

- "Best if used by" date means the flavor, taste, and quality of the product will be at its optimum before this date. It has nothing to do with freshness or safety.

- "Use by" date means just that — don't consumer the product after this date.

If you eat processed foods, the knowledge of reading labels is invaluable.

The worst:

- Artificial sweeteners

- Synthetic Trans fats

- Artificial flavors

- Monosodium glutamate (MSG)

- Artificial colors

- High-fructose corn syrup (HFCS)

- Preservatives

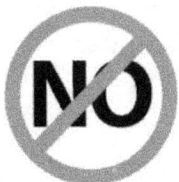

If it's labeled "No Fat" or "Low-Fat," it's probably bad for you.

"All Natural" is marketing hype word. So are the rest of these:

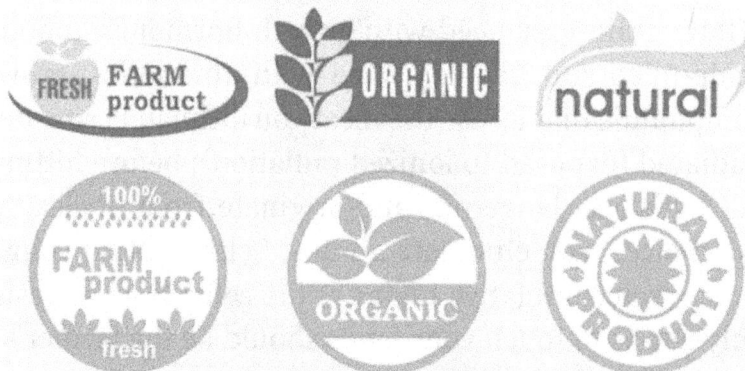

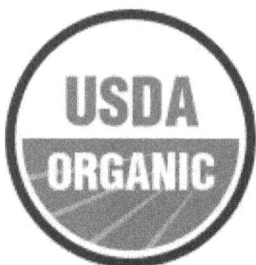

To be "Certified Organic," the little tag on organic produce must start with the number 9. The number 8 means GMO and should be avoided at all costs. All the other starting numbers are conventionally grown and are not organic.

Ingredients for a healthier you are simply healthy food choices, swaps of good foods for bad. It's that easy.

If food were just calories it wouldn't make any difference where they came from; as long as they provided enough energy to sustain us and it tasted good, it would be fine. Good health results from the quality of information we have about our fuel – food –that we put into our bodies, and not disease-causing misinformation from hidden ingredients in modified, processed and chemically derived foods.

Examples include labels on many high-sugar breakfast cereals, like "whole grain." Despite the label, these products are not healthy. Not falling for this kind of deception requires a working knowledge of and a thorough inspection of the ingredients list.

Product ingredients are listed by quantity, from highest to lowest amount. This means that the first listed ingredient is what the manufacturer used the most of. A good rule of thumb is to scan the first three ingredients, because they are the largest part of what you're eating. If the first ingredients include refined grains, some sort of sugar or hydrogenated oils, you can be pretty sure that the product is unhealthy. Instead, try to choose items that have whole foods listed as the first three ingredients. Another good rule of thumb is if the ingredients list is longer than 2–3 lines, you can assume that the product is highly processed.

There is considerable evidence that artificial sweeteners contribute to weight gain. Studies have shown that the brain does not recognize artificial sweeteners as food, since they are man-made and non-caloric. So the body over-compensates to fill the void by eating more food and becoming obese. Artificial sweeteners also fake the pancreas into believing the body is receiving sugar, so it cranks up insulin production, and obese people are already insulin resistant and insulin stores as fat. Artificial sweeteners are non-caloric and are not burned as sugar, so they are stored in cells as a man-made, foreign toxin that the body does not recognize, maybe for years. So, the next time you want to drink a "sugar-free" or "diet" soda, think again.

Watch out for serving sizes. The backs of nutrition labels state how many calories and nutrients are in a single serving of the product. However, these serving sizes are often much smaller portions than people generally eat in one sitting. In this way, manufacturers try to deceive consumers into thinking that the food has fewer calories and less sugar than it actually does. Many people are completely unaware of this serving size scheme. They often assume that the entire container is a single serving, while it may actually consist of two, three, or more servings. To calculate the nutritional value of what you're eating, you have to multiply the serving size given on the back by the number of servings you consume.

Net carb count of vegetables should be 5 grams or less per serving. Net carb count of meats or condiments should be 1 gram or less per serving. Avoid foods that have any form of sugar or starch listed in first 5 ingredients. Health claims on packaged food are designed to catch your attention and convince you that the product is healthy. Some of the most common claims to watch for include:

Light: Light products are processed to reduce either calories or fat, and some products are simply watered down. Check carefully to see if anything has been added instead; most notably, sugar.

Multigrain: This sounds very healthy, but basically just means that there is more than one type of grain in the product. These are most likely refined grains, unless the product is marked as whole grain.

Natural: This does not necessarily mean that the product resembles anything natural. It simply means that at some point the manufacturer had natural sources to work with.

Organic: This label says very little about whether the product is healthy or not. For example, organic sugar is still sugar. Only certified organically grown products can be guaranteed to be organic.

No added sugar: Some products are naturally high in sugar. The fact that they don't have added sugar doesn't mean they're healthy. Unhealthy sugar substitutes may also have been added.

Low-calorie: Low-calorie products have to contain 1/3 fewer calories than the same brand's original product. However, one brand's low-calorie version may contain similar calories as the original of another product.

Low-fat: This label almost always means that the fat has been reduced at the cost of adding more sugar. Read the ingredients listed on the back.

Low-carb: Recently, low-carb diets have been linked with improved health. However, processed foods that are labeled low-carb are usually just processed junk foods, similar to processed low-fat junk foods. Junk is still junk.

Made with whole grain: There is probably very little whole grain in the product. Check the ingredients list and see where the whole grain is placed. If it is not in the first 3 ingredients, then the amount is negligible.

Fortified or enriched: This basically means that some nutrients have been added to the product. Vitamin D is often added to milk.

Gluten-free: Just because it says "Gluten Free" on the label does not mean it's healthy. It simply means that the product doesn't contain wheat, spelt, rye or barley. Many foods are gluten-free, but can be highly processed and loaded with unhealthy fats and sugar. Gluten is a poison/toxin and should not be consumed. It could have other ingredients that raise your blood sugar just like wheat, so read the ingredients label and not just the package marketing label on the front.

Fruit-flavored: Many processed foods have a name that refers to a natural flavor, such as strawberry yogurt. However, there may not be any fruit in the product; only chemicals designed to taste like fruit.

Zero trans fat: "Zero trans fat" actually means "less than 0.5 grams of trans fat per serving." So if serving sizes are misleadingly small, the product can actually contain a lot of trans fats.

So, just having labels printed on the package does not guarantee that a product is healthy. Most are simply marketing tools for processed junk foods that make you fat and unhealthy.

Sugar is disguised by many names:

Types of sugar: beet sugar, brown sugar, buttered sugar, cane sugar, caster sugar, coconut sugar, date sugar, golden sugar, invert sugar, muscovado sugar, organic raw sugar, rapadura sugar, evaporated cane juice and confectioner's sugar.

Types of syrup: carob syrup, golden syrup, high fructose corn syrup, honey, agave nectar, malt syrup, maple syrup, oat syrup, rice bran syrup and rice syrup.

Other added sugars: barley malt, molasses, cane juice crystals, lactose, corn sweetener, crystalline fructose, dextran, malt powder, ethyl maltol, fructose, fruit juice concentrate, galactose, glucose, disaccharides, maltodextrin and maltose. If it ends in an 'ose' it usually sugar-derived.

If you see any of these in the top spots on the ingredients lists, or several kinds of sugar throughout the list, then you can be sure that the product is high in added sugars. Always choose whole foods whenever possible.

Obviously, the best way to avoid being misled by these labels is to avoid processed foods altogether. If you decide to buy packaged foods, it is necessary to sort out the junk from the higher quality products and probably the most unrecognized and under-calculated label factor is the hidden sugars on food labels.

"Whenever you see the words 'Fat-Free' or 'Low-Fat,' think "chemical shit storms." – Rory Freedman

In the grocery store, try to avoid the boxed, bagged and packaged food in the center aisles. Instead, shop the periphery of the grocery store aisles where the fresh, real, whole foods are located. The middle of the store is where the mass manufactured, chemically engineered, processed foods are located. The worst choices are generally eye-level and the healthier choices are usually obscured or hidden on the top or bottom shelves. Take time to read the labels, as these middle-aisle choices are generally science fair projects. They're Frankenfoods, not real foods.

Avoid nitrates, sulfites, bromates and MSG. No Olestra.

Be an avid and informed food label reader. Your health depends on it. Whole food doesn't need an ingredients list, because the whole food "is" the ingredient. Eat real foods.

"If you can't explain it simply, you don't understand it well enough." – Einstein

CHAPTER 11
Hidden Sugar Calculator

New nutrition labels by mid-2018 will be amended to show added sugars, but what about hidden sugars?

The hidden sugar calculator is: Total Carbohydrates minus Dietary Fiber equals Net Carbs minus Label Sugar equals Hidden Sugar.

(TC – DF = NC – LS = HS).

Total sugar needs to be accounted for in reading and interpreting labels.

Total sugar and net carbs are the same for purposes of hidden sugar calculations. Sugar grams listed on product labels rarely, if ever, are the same as the net carbs/total sugars. The difference between the two numbers is the hidden sugar.

For example, if the label reads:

Total carbohydrates   35g

Dietary fiber   7g

Sugars   20g

The hidden sugar is 5g. (35g – 7g = 28g - 20g = 8g of hidden sugar)

An alternative method to determine the hidden sugar calculation is:

#1: Add Dietary Fiber and Sugars together.

#2: Subtract that number from total carbs.

#3: That number is the hidden sugar.

Added sugars hide in 74% of processed foods, under 60 different names. Average

Americans consume 37 teaspoons of sugar daily and if eating a fast food diet, as many as 86 teaspoons daily. Both categories are far too high. Ouch.

HFCS is classified by the government as GRAS and it's in nearly everything. HFCS is not "safe" because it kills mitochondria, your cells energy production plant.

Know your sugars: brown sugar, corn syrup, dextrin, dextrose, fructose, fruit juice concentrate, high-fructose corn syrup, galactose, glucose, invert sugar maltose, lactose, sucrose (basically, anything that ends in "ose"), honey, hydrogenated starch, manitol, maple syrup, molasses, polyols, raw sugar, sorghum, sorbitol and turbinado.

Forms of sugars to avoid are sucrose, dextrose, fructose, maltose, lactose, glucose, honey, agave syrup, high fructose corn syrup, maple syrup, brown-rice syrup, molasses, evaporated cane juice, cane juice, fruit-juice concentrate, corn sweetener, and all artificial sweeteners, including succralose.

Sugars are hidden in cough syrups, cold aids, chewing gum, tomato sauce, baked beans, soups, salad dressings, condiments, ketchup, mustard, relishes, protein bars, many protein powders and lunch meats.

Avoid the following:

- Whole or skimmed milk
- Canned soups
- Dairy substitutes
- Ketchup, sweet condiments or relishes
- Coleslaw
- Foods labeled fat-free, lite, natural, sugar-free, or Great for Low-Carb Diets

These products contain hidden sugars and starches, as do some cough drops, syrups and over-the-counter medications.

Wheaties

Nutrition Facts

Serving Size	¾ cup (27g)	
Servings Per Container	about 16	

Amount Per Serving	Wheaties	with ½ cup skim milk
Calories	100	140
Calories from Fat	5	5
% Daily Value		
Total Fat 0.5g*	1%	1%
Saturated Fat 0g	0%	
Trans Fat 0g	0%	
Polyunsaturated Fat 0g		
Monounsaturated Fat 0g		
Cholesterol 0mg	0%	1%
Sodium 190mg	8%	11%
Potassium 90mg	3%	8%
Total Carbohydrates 22g	8%	10%
Dietary Fiber 3g	12%	12%
Sugars 4g		
Other Carbohydrates 16g		
Protein 2g		
Vitamin A	10%	
Vitamin C	10%	
Calcium	2%	
Iron	45%	
Vitamin D	10%	
Thiamin	50%	
Riboflavin	50%	
Niacin	50%	
Vitamin B 6	50%	
Folic Acid	50%	
Vitamin B12	50%	
Phosphorus	8%	
Magnesium	6%	
Zinc	50%	

*Amount in cereal. A serving of cereal plus skim milk provides 0.5g total fat, less than 5mg cholesterol, 250mg sodium, 290mg potassium, 28g total carbohydrates, (10g sugars), and 6g protein.

**Percent Daily Values are based on 2,000 calorie diet. Your daily values may be higher or lower depending on your calorie needs:

	Calories	2000	2500
Total Fat		Less than	65g
Sat fat	Less than	20g	25g
Cholesterol	Less than	300mg	300mg
Sodium	Less than	2,400mg	2,400mg
Potassium		3.500mg	3,500mg
Total Carbohydrates		300g	375g
Dietary Fiber		25g	30g

Ingredients: Whole Grain Wheat, Sugar, Salt, Corn Syrup, Trisodium Phosphate. BHT Added to Preserve Freshness.

Vitamins and Minerals: Calcium Carbonate, Zinc and Iron (mineral nutrients), B Vitamin (niacinamide), Vitamin C (sodium ascorbate), Vitamin B6 (pyridoxine hydrochloride), Vitamin B2 ((riboflavin), Vitamin B1 (thiamin mononitrate), Vitamin A (palmate), B Vitamin (folic acid), Vitamin B12, Vitamin D3.

CONTAINS WHEAT. MAY CONTAIN ALMOND INGREDIENTS.

DISTRIBUTED BY GENERAL MILLS SALES, INC.

Cheerios

Nutrition Facts

Serving Size	1 cup (28g)		
Children Under 4	¾ cup (21g)		
Servings Per Container	about 14		
Children Under 4	about 19		

Amount Per Serving	Cheerios	with ½ cup skim milk	Cereal for Children under 4
Calories	100	140	80
Calories from Fat	15	20	10
	% Daily Value **		
Total Fat 2g*	3%	3%	1.5g
Saturated Fat 0g	0%	3%	0g
Trans Fat 0g			0g
Polyunsaturated Fat 0.5 g			0g
Monounsaturated Fat 0.5 g			0g
Cholesterol 0mg	0%	1%	0mg
Sodium 190mg	8%	10%	140mg
Potassium 170mg	5%	11%	130mg
Total			
Carbohydrates 20g	7%	9%	15g
Dietary Fiber 3g	11%	11%	2g
Soluable Fiber 1g			0g
Sugars 1g			0g
Other Carbohydrates 16g			12g
Protein 3g			2g

			% Daily Value**
Protein			9%
Vitamin A	10%	15%	10%
Vitamin C	10%	10%	10%
Calcium	10%	25%	8%
Iron	45%	45%	50%
Vitamin D	10%	25%	8%
Riboflavin	25%	35%	35%
Niacin	25%	25%	35%
Vitamin B6	25%	25%	45%
Folic Acid	50%	50%	60%
Vitamin B12	25%	35%	30%
Phosphorus	10%	25%	8%
Magnesium	10%	10%	10%
Zinc	25%	30%	30%
Copper	2%	2%	2%

*Amount in cereal. A serving of cereal plus skim milk provides2g total fat 90.5g saturated fat, 1g monounsaturated fat), 0mg cholesterol, 250mg sodium, 370mg potassium, 26g total carbohydrate (7g sugars) and 7g protein.

** Percent Daily Values are based on a 2,000 diet. Your daily values may be higher or lower depending on your calorie needs.

	Calories	2,000	2,500
Total Fat	Less than	60g	80g
Sat Fat	Less than	20g	25g
Cholesterol	Less than	300mg	300mg
Sodium	Less than	2400mg	2400mg
Potassium		3500mg	3500mg
Total Carbohydrates		300g	375g
Dietary Fiber		25g	30g

INGREDIENTS: WHOLE GRAIN OATS. MODIFIED CORN STARCH, SUGAR, OAT BRAN, SALT, CALCIUM CARBONATE, OAT FIBER, TRIPOTASSIUM PHOSPHATE, CORN STARCH, WHEAT STARCH, VITAMIN E (MIXED TOCOPHEROLS) ADDED TO PRESERVE FRESHNESS.

VITAMINS AND MINERALS: IRON AND ZINC (MINERAL NUTRIENTS), VITAMIN C (SODIUM ASCORBATE), B VITAMIN (NIACINAMIDE), VITAMIN B6 (PYRIDOXINE HYDROXCHICLORINE), VITAMIN B2 (RIBOFLAVIN), VITAMIN b1 (THIAMIN MONONITRATE), VITAMIN A (PALMATE), B VITAMIN (FOLIC ACID), VITAMIN B12, VITAMIN D.

DIST. BY GENERAL MILLS CEREALS, LLC

Grape Nuts

Nutrition Facts

Serving Size	1/2 cup (58 g)	
Amount Per Serving	GrapeNuts	Cereal with ½ cup Fat Free Milk
Calories	210	250
Calories from Fat	10	10
	% Daily Value**	
Total Fat 1g*	2%	2%
Saturated Fat	0%	0%
Polyunsaturated Fat 0.5g		
Monounsaturated Fat		
Cholesterol 0mg	0%	0%
Sodium 270mg	11%	14%
Potassium 90mg	3%	8%
Total Carbohydrates 47g	16%	18%
Dietary Fiber 7g	28%	28%
Soluable Fiber 1g		
Insoluable Fiber 6g		
Sugars 5g		
Other carbohydrates 35g		

Post Foods, LLC

Raisin Bran

Nutrition Facts

Serving Size	1 cup (59 g)	
Amount Per Serving	Raisin Bran	Cereal with ½ cup Fat Free Milk
Calories	190	230
Calories from Fat	10	10
Total Fat 1g*	2%	2%
Saturated Fat 0g	0%	0%
Trans Fat 0g		
Polyunsaturated Fat 0g		
Monounsaturated Fat 0g		
Cholesterol 0mg	0%	0%
Sodium 230mg	10%	13%
Potassium 310mg	9%	15%
Total carbohydrates 47g	16%	185%
Dietary Fiber 8g	32%	32%
Soluable Fiber <1g		
Sugars 19g		
Other Carbohydrates 20g		

Ingredients : Wheat Bran, Raisins, Sugar, High Fructose Corn Syrup, Salt, Malt Flavoring

Buttermilk Pancakes

Nutrition Facts

Serving size	3 Pancakes (116g)
Amount Per Serving	
Calories	280
Calories from Fat	80
	% Daily Value*
Total Fat 9g	14%
Saturated Fat 1.5g8%	8%
Trans Fat 0g	
Cholesterol 15mg	5%
Sodium 590mg	25%
Potassium 65mg	2%
Total Carbohydrate 45g	15%
Dietary Fiber 1g	4%
Sugars 12g	
Protein 6g	
Vitamin A	20%
Vitamin C	0%
Calcium	8%
Iron	25%
Thiamin	20%
Riboflavin	20%
Niacin	20%
Vitamin B6	20%

*Percent Daily Values are based on a 2,000 calorie diet. Your daily values may be higher or lower depending on your calorie needs:

	Calories	2,000	2,500
Total Fat	Less than	65g	80g
Sat fat	Less than	20g	25g

Cholesterol	Less than	300mg	300mg
Sodium	Less than	2,400mg	2,400mg
Potassium		3,500mg	3,500mg
Total Carbohydreates		300mg	300mg
Dietary Fiber		25g	30g

Ingredients: Enriched flour (wheat flour, malted barley, niacin, reduced iron, vitamin b1 (thiamin mononitrate), vitamin B2 (riboflavin), folic acid, water, high fructose corn syrup, soybean and/or canola oil, buttermilk, eggs, contains 2% or less of leavening (baking soda, sodium aluminum phosphate), salt, soy lecithin.

Vitamins and Minerals: Vitamin A palmitate, reduced iron, niacinamide, vitamin B12, vitamin B6 (pyridoxine hydrochlorine), vitamin B1 (thiamin hydocloride), Vitamin B2 (riboflavin).

CONTAINS WHEAT, MILK, EGG AND SOY INGREDIENTS.

Turkey Breast

Nutrition Facts

Serving size:	1 slice (28g)

Servings Per Container: Varied

Calories 30

   Fat Cal 0.5

*Percent Daily Values are based on 2,000calorie diet.

Amount/serving	%DV*
Total Fat 0.5g	
Total Carb 2g	1%
Fiber og	0%
Sugars 1g	
Protein 5g	
Sat Fat og	
Trans Fat 0g	
Cholesterol 10mg	3%
Sodium 220g	9%
Vitamin A	0%
Vitamin C	0%
Iron	2%

INGRDIENTS: TURKEY BREAST, WATER, MODIFIED FOOD STARCH, CONTAINS 2% OR LESS OF THE FOLLOWING: DEXTROSE, SALT, POTASSIUM LACTATE, SODIUM PHOSPHATE, SODIUM DIACETATE, SODIUM ERYTHORBATE, SODIUM NITRATE, FLAVORING.

Bagels

Nutrition Facts

	1 Deli Baked
Serving Size	(128g)
Servings Per Container	1
Amount Per Serving	
Calories	370
Calories from Fat	100
	% Daily Value*
Total Fat 18g	20%
Saturated Fat 7g	
Trans Fat 0.5g	
Cholesterol 40mg	13%
Sodium 680mg	28%
Total Carbohydrates 38g	13%
Dietary Fiber 3g	12%
Sugars 6g	
Protein 15g	
Calcium	0%
Iron	4%

*Percent Daily Values are based on 2,000 calorie diet. Your daily values may be higher or lower depending on your calorie needs:

	Calories	2000	2500
Total Fat	Less than	40g	40g
Saturated Fat	Less than	20g	25g
Cholesterol	Less than	300mg	300mg
Sodium	Less than	2,400mg	2,400mg
Total carbohydrates		300g	375g
Dietary Fiber		24g	30g

Sara Lee Whole Wheat Bread

Nutrition Facts

Serving Size	1 Slice (26g)
Servings Per Container	22
Amount Per Serving	1 Slice
Calories	60
Calories from fat	10
	100% Daily Value

Total Fat 1g	
Saturated Fat 0g	
Trans Fat 0g	
Polyunsaturated Fat 0g	
Monounsaturated Fat 0g	
Cholesterol 0mg	0%
Sodium 170mg	7%
Total Carbohydrates 22g	7%
Dietary Fiber 5g	
Sugars 2g	
Protein 5g	
Vitamin A	0%
Vitamin C	0%
Calcium	4%
Iron	6%
Thiamin	6%
Riboflavin	4%
Niacin	8%
Folic Acid	4%

*Percent Daily Values are based on 2,000 calorie diet. Your daily values may be higher or lower depending on your calorie needs:

	Calories	2,000	2,500
Total Fat	Less than	65g	80g
Saturated Fat	Less than	20g	25g
Cholesterol	Less than	20g	25g

Sodium	Less than 2,400mg	2,400mg
Total Carbohydrates	300g	375g
Dietary Fiber	25g	30g

Ingredients: Whole wheat flour, water, **High Fructose Corn Syrup**, sugar, wheat gluten, yeast, salt, soybean oil, wheat bran, datem, calcium propionate (preservative), monoglycerides, calcium sulfate, soy lecithin, critic acid, grain vinegar, potassium iodate, soy flour.

Gluten Free Bread

Nutrition Facts

Serving Size	1-2/5 oz or 40g	
Servings Per Container	22	
Amount Per serving		
Calories	140	
Calories from Fat	5	
		% Daily Value*
Saturated Fat	0.5g	1%
Trans Fat	0g	0%
Cholesterol	0mg	0%
Sodium	0mg	0%
Total Cabohydrate	32g	11%
Dietary Fiber	2g	10%
Sugars	5g	
Protein	2g	
Vitamin A		0%
Vitamin C		0%
Calcium		0%
Iron		4%

*Percent Daily Values are based on 2,000 calorie diet. Your daily values may be higher or lower depending on your calorie needs:

	Calories	2,000	2,500
Total Fat	Less than	65	80g
Sat Fat	Less than	20g	25g

Cholesterol	Less than	300mg	300mg
Sodium	Less than	2400mg	2,400mg
Total Carbohydrates		300g	375g
Dietary Fiber		25g	30g

Calories per gram:	
Fat	9
Carbohydrate	4
Protein	4

Ingredients: Sorghum Flour, Tapioca Flour, Sucanat, Rice Flour, White Rice Flour, Millet Flour, Guar Gum, Brown Rice Flour, Yeast, Sea Salt.

Subway Tuna Sandwich (6 inch)

Nutrition Facts

Serving Size	252g	
Amount Per Serving		
Calories	530	
Calories from Fat	270	
		% Daily Value
Total Fat	30g	46%
Saturated Fat	6g	30%
Trans Fat	0.5g	0%
Cholesterol	45mg	15%
Sodium	930mg	40%
Total Carbohydrates	46g	15%
Dietary Fiber	5g	20%
Sugars	5g	
Protein	21g	
Vitamin A	10%	
Vitamin C	20%	
Calcium	10%	
Iron	20%	

*Percent Daily Values are recommendations based on a 2,000 calorie diet.

Ingredients: Contains soy and wheat. ITALIAN (WHITE) BREAD Enriched flour (wheat flour, niacin, iron, thiamin mononitrate, riboflavin, folic acid), water, yeast, sugar, contains 2% or less of: soybean oil, calcium carbonate, wheat gluten, salt, sunflower lecithin, ascorbic acid, yeast extract, Vitamin D2, enzymes. Contains wheat.

Subway Turkey Sandwich (6 inch)

Nutrition Facts

Serving Size	226g	
Amount Per Serving		
Calories	280g	
Calories from Fat	30g	
		% Daily Value
Total Fat	3.5g	5%
Saturated Fat	1g	5%
Trans Fat	0g	0%
Cholesterol	20mg	7%
Sodium	920mg	40%
Total Carbohydrates	47g	16%
Dietary Fiber	5g	20%
Sugars	6g	
Protein	18g	
Vitamin A	8%	
Vitamin C	20%	
Calcium	6%	
Iron	15%	

*Percent Daily Values are recommendations based on a 2,000 calorie diet.

Ingredients: Contains soy and wheat. ITALIAN (WHITE) BREAD Enriched flour (wheat flour, niacin, iron, thiamin mononitrate, riboflavin, folic acid), water, yeast, sugar, contains 2% or less of: soybean oil, calcium carbonate, wheat gluten, salt, sunflower lecithin, ascorbic acid, yeast extract, Vitamin D2, enzymes. Contains wheat.

Nacho & Cheese Doritos

Nutrition Facts

Serving Size	1 oz (28g) or about 12 chips	
Servings Per Container		
Amount Per Serving		
Calories	150	
Calories from Fat	70	
		% Daily Value*
Total Fat	8g	12%
Saturated Fat	1.5g	7%
Trans fat	0g	0%
Cholesterol	omg	0%
Sodium	180mg	7%
Total Carbohydrate	17g	6%
Dietary Fiber	1g	6%
Sugars	1g	
Protein	2g	
Vitamin A	0%	
Vitamin C	0%	
Calcium	2%	
Iron	0%	
Thiamin	4%	
Vitamin B6	2%	
Phosphorous	6%	

*Percent Daily Values are based on 2,000 calorie diet. Your daily values may be higher or lower depending on your calorie needs.

	Calories	2000	2500
Total Fat	Less than	65g	80g
Sat Fat	Less than	20g	25g
Cholesterol	Less than	300mg	300mg
Sodium	Less than	2400mg	2400mg
Total Carbohydrates		300g	375g
Dietary Fiber	25g		30g

Calories per gram:	
Fat	9
Carbohydrate	4
Protein	4

Ingredients: Whole corn, vegetable oil (corn, soybean, and/or sunflower oil), salt, cheddar cheese (milk, cheese cultures, salt, enzymes), maltodextrin, wheat flour, whey protein isolates, monosodium glutamate, buttermilk solids, romano cheese (part skim cow's milk, cheese cultures, salt, enzymes), whey protein concentrate, onion powder, partially hydrogenated soybean and cottonseed oil, lactose, dextrose, sugar, non-fat milk solids, corn syrup solids, citric acid, sodium casemate, yellow 5, Red 40%, natural and artificial flavors.

Contains Milk and Wheat ingredients.

Sour Cream & Onion Lays

Nutrition Facts

Serving Size	1oz	
Amount Per Serving		
Calories	160	
Calories from Fat	90	
		% Daily Value*
Total Fat	10g	15%
Saturated Fat	1g	5%
Polyunsatyrated Fat	4.5g	
Monounsaturated Fat	4.5g	
Trans Fat	0g	
Cholesterol	0mg	0%
Sodium	210mg	12%
Potassium	410mg	12%
Total Carbohydrates	15g	5%
Dietary Fiber	1g	4%
Sugars	1g	
Protein	2g	
Vitamin A	0%	
Vitamin C	10%	
Calcium	0%	
Iron	0%	
Vitamin E	6%	
Thiamin	4%	
Niacin	6%	
Vitamin B6	4%	
Phosphorus	4%	
Zinc	2%	

*Percent Daily Values are based on 2,000 calorie diet. Your daily values may be higher or lower depending on your calorie needs:

	Calories:	2,000	2,500
Total Fat	Less than	65g	80g

Sat Fat	Less than	20g	25g
Cholesterol	Less than	300mg	300mg
Sodium	Less than	2,400mg	2,400mg
Potassium		3,500mg	3,500mg
Total Carbohydrates		300mg	375mg
Dietary Fiber		25mg	30mg

Ingredients: Potatoes, Vegetable Oil (Sunflower, Corn, And/Or Canola Oil), Sour Cream & Onion Seasoning (Skim Milk, Salt, Maltodextrin [Made from Corn], Onion Powder, Whey, Sour Cream [Cultured Cream, Skim Milk], Canola Oil, Parsley, Natural Flavor, Lactose, Sunflower Oil, Citric Acid, Whey Protein Concentrate, Monosodium Glutamate, Palm Oil, Citric Acid, Partially Hydrogenated Soybean or Cottonseed Oil, Lactose, Lactic Acid, Buttermilk, Natural and Artificial Flavors, Salt.

Contains Milk Ingredients.

Salt & Vinegar Pringles

Nutrition Facts

	1oz
Serving Size	(15 chips)
Servings Per Container	16
Amount Per Serving	
Calories	150

	% Daily Value*
Total Fat	9g
Saturated Fat	3g
Polyunsaturated Fat	0g
Monounsaturated Fat	0g
Trans Fat	0g
Cholesterol	0mg
Sodium	180mg
Potassium	0mg
Total carbohydrates	15g
Dietary Fiber	1g
Sugars	1g
Protein	1g
Vitamin A	0%
Vitamin C	6%
Calcium	2%
Iron	0%

*Percent Daily Values are based on a 2000 calorie diet. Your daily values may be higher or lower depending on your calorie needs.

Ingredients: Dried Potatoes, Vegetable Oil (Contains One Or More of The Following: Corn Oil, Cottonseed Oil, Soybean Oil, And/Or Sunflower Oil), Corn Flour, Wheat Starch And Maltodextrin. Contains 2% Or Less of: Rice Flour, Salt, Dextrose, Lactose, Malic Acid, Vinegar, Sodium Diacetate And Turmeric (Color).

Sara Lee Chocolate Brownies

Nutrition Facts

Serving Size	1 Cake (85g)	
Serving Per Container	1	
Amount Per Serving		
Calories	300	
Calories from Fat	100	
		% Daily Value**
Total Fat	11g	16%
Saturated fat	2.5g	13%
Trans Fat	0g	0%
Cholesterol	35mg	12%
Sodium	340mg	14%
Total Carbohydrates	46g	15%
Dietary Fiber	1g	5%
Sugars	30g	
Protein	4g	
Vitamin A		0%
Vitamin C		0%
Calcium		4%
Iron		8%
Thamin		6%
Riboflavin		8%
Niacin		4%
Folic acid		8%

*Percent Daily Values are based on 2,000 calorie diet. Your daily values may be higher or lower depending on your calorie needs.

	Calories	2,000	2,500
Total Fat	Less than	65g	80g
Sat Fat	Less than	20g	25g
Cholesterol	Less than	300mg	300mg
Sodium	Less than	2,400mg	2,400mg
Total Carbohydrate		300g	375g

Dietary Fiber	25g	30g

Calories per gram:	
Fat	9
Carboydrate	4
Protein	4

Ingredients: Sugar, Bleached Wheat Flour, (Wheat Flour malted Barley Flour, Niacin, Iron, Thamin Mononitrate, Riboflavin, Folic Acid, Eggs, High Fructose Corn Syrup, Soybean Oil, Water, Chocolate Chips [Sugar, Chocolate Liquor, Cocoa Butter, Dextrose, Chocolate Liquor (Processed With Alkali), Soy Lecithin, Vanillin], Corn Syrup, Chocolate Liquor (Processed With Alkali), Palm Oil, Fructose, Whey (Milk), Modified Cornstarch, Dextrose, Natural and Artificial Flavors, Natural Cocoa Extract, Carmel Color, Modified Corn Starch, Leanening (Sodium Aluminum Phosphate, Baking Soda, Monocalcium Phosphate, Corn Starch, Potassium Sorbate (Preservative), Gums (Xanthin, Gellan), Wheat Starch. Soy Lecithin, Soy Flour.

Allergen Statement: Contains Wheat, Eggs. Milk and Soy

CHAPTER 12
Foods with More Sugar than a Doughnut

Doughnuts are one of the worst foods you can eat, and they're also one of the most sugar-laden, so they serve as a good baseline for sugar content. If the food you're eating contains more sugar than a doughnut, it's probably not good for your health. There's more to a food's nutritional value than its sugar content, as eating a piece of whole fruit with 10 grams of fructose is going to offer you far more nutritional value than a doughnut with 10 grams of pure sugar. However, even some "healthy-sounding" foods are even too high in sugar for your good health.

Sugar is our enemy.

Krispy Kreme's original glazed doughnut contains 10 grams of sugar. Here are 31 foods, that you may be eating, that have more.

- Chili's Caribbean Chicken Salad with Grilled Chicken = almost 7 doughnuts (67 grams of sugar)

- Starbucks Caramel Frappuccino = 6 doughnuts (64 grams of sugar)

- Jamba Juice Banana Berry Smoothie, small = 6 doughnuts (60 grams of sugar)

- Odwalla Superfood Smoothie, 15.2 ounces = 5 doughnuts (50 grams of sugar)

- Sprinkles Red Velvet Cupcake = 4.5 doughnuts (45 grams of sugar)

- California Pizza Kitchen Thai Chicken Salad = 4.5 doughnuts (45 grams of sugar)

- Kraft French Style Fat Free Dressing = 4 doughnuts (42 grams of sugar)

- Dunkin' Donuts Reduced-Fat Blueberry Muffin = 4 doughnuts (40 grams of sugar

- Snapple Peach Tea = 4 doughnuts (39 grams of sugar)

- Burger King Chicken, Apple, and Cranberry Garden Fresh Salad with Chicken = 4 doughnuts (38 grams of sugar)

- Craisins Dried Cranberries (1.75 ounces) = 3 doughnuts (34 grams of sugar)

- Vitamin Water, 20 ounces = 3 doughnuts (33 grams of sugar)

- Naked Pomegranate Blueberry Juice = 3 doughnuts (32 grams of sugar)

- McDonald's Fruit and Maple Oatmeal = 3 doughnuts (32 grams of sugar)

- International House of Pancakes Whole Wheat Pancakes with banana, four pancakes without syrup = 3 doughnuts (32 grams of sugar)

- Pom Wonderful 100% Pomegranate Juice, 8 ounces = 3 doughnuts (31 grams of sugar)

- Starbucks Greek Yogurt and Honey Parfait = 3 doughnuts (30 grams of sugar)

- Starbucks Blueberry Muffin = 3 doughnuts (29 grams of sugar)

- Stonyfield Fat Free Blackberry Blend Yogurt = 3 doughnuts (28 grams of sugar)

- Can of Coca-Cola = 2.5 doughnuts (26.4 grams of sugar)

- Yoplait Blackberry Harvest Yogurt = 2.5 doughnuts (26 grams of sugar)

- Tropicana Orange Juice, 8 ounces = 2 doughnuts (22 grams of sugar)

- Nutella Spread, 2 tablespoons = 2 doughnuts (21 grams of sugar)

- Campbell's Classic Tomato Soup on the Go = 2 doughnuts (20 grams of sugar)

- Dole Mixed Fruit Cup = 1.5 doughnuts (17 grams of sugar)

- Subway 6" Sweet Onion Teriyaki Chicken Sandwich = 1.5 doughnuts (17 grams of sugar)

- Motts Applesauce (one cup) = 1.5 doughnuts (16 grams of sugar)

- Nature Valley Chewy Trail Mix Fruit and Nut Granola Bar = 1 doughnut (13 grams of sugar)

- Kellogg's Fruit Loops = 1 doughnut (12 grams of sugar)

- Prego Fresh Mushroom Italian Spaghetti Sauce = 1 doughnut (11 grams of sugar)

- Luna Bar = 1 doughnut (11 grams of sugar)

Doughnuts also contain trans fats, as do many processed foods.

Margarines are generally 40% trans fat and 45% vegetable oil. I call them liquid plastics. Do not eat. Avoid at all costs. Eat real butter from grass-fed animals or Ghee (clarified butter).

"Those who have failed to work toward the truth have missed the purpose of living." – Buddha

If a meat label says it's restructured or bonded, it's processed meat.

When zero doesn't equal zero. The FDA allows companies to list 0 grams of trans fat on labels, even if there's up to .5 grams of trans fat. This may not seem like much, but on the label below, there are 30 servings of 1 tbsp per container, so that's as much as 15 grams or 3 tsp/1 tbsp of trans fat that you and your family are consuming in that tub of margarine. Consuming even low levels of trans fat is a health risk, leading to cardiovascular disease, heart attack, stroke, and cancer.

Eighty-four percent of products labeled with 0 grams of trans fat still have some trans fat in the product. Look as the label below. The label lists 0 grams of trans fat, yet the ingredients list 3 hydrogenated oils. What does the FDA think trans fats are? Bottom line, read the labels. The fault for this lies with our politicians and lobbyists. Big Agra, Big Pharma, the USDA and FDA have been cozy bedfellows for many years.

Beware of the labeling on protein bars or health bars. They contain alcohol sugars (glycerin, glycerol), and even though they do not affect blood sugar the same way, they are still carbs. These bars are usually loaded with carbs and calories and can stall weight loss. Nutrition labeling does not require sugar alcohols to be listed as sugar grams and are not sugar-free. You must read labels to find the total net carbs and hidden sugars.

General label rule of thumb: no more than 30% of total calories from fat.

BPA plastic containers are marked or etched with either 3 or 7.

If the label for a product has more than 3 ingredients or you can't pronounce them or don't know what they are, forget it and leave the item behind on the shelf or clean it out of your house.

Hydrogenated oils, partially hydrogenated oils and trans-fats are fats damaged through overheating, overuse or industrial processing. They wreak havoc on human health and should not be consumed. They are prevalent in fast foods, French fries, most margarines, virtually all commercially baked goods, cookies, cakes, crackers, potato chips, and even movie popcorn. These oils are to be completely avoided as they are associated with all modern, common, degenerative diseases.

Since 2006 manufacturers have been required to list these oils in the Nutritional Facts labels, but they skirt the intent of the law with the 0.5 gram per serving loophole and preposterously low serving-size portions, so "you can't eat just one" – you end up actually consuming a gram or two of trans-fats from alleged "zero trans-fat" foods. It's the old hidden label trick.

If hydrogenated or partially-hydrogenated oils are listed in "other Ingredients," it means there are trans fats, no matter what the main label or package marketing says. Beware of deceptive labeling.

Plastic water bottles are dangerous to your health. The plastic used to make water bottles is full of chemicals. Most plastic bottles contain BPA: bisphenol-A. It's a toxic chemical that is linked to major health problems, including cancer. Plastic water bottles also contain phthalates; they mimic hormones in your body. If left in the sun or exposed to heat, these chemicals are leached into the water.

In "BPA-free" containers, the BPA is replaced with BPS, which is perhaps just as bad. Do not eat or drink from plastic bottles or containers that have been heated. If you leave a bottle of water in your car and it was heated up from the sun, throw it out because the plastic may have leached into the water and made the water unhealthful to drink.

CHAPTER 13:
Eliminating Sugar, Wheat, and Grains

Sugar is not a nutrient, so don't pretend that it is. Consider sugar a recreational drug. It's more addicting than cocaine and just as toxic to your body and brain.

Your health and likely your lifespan will be determined by the proportion of sugar versus fat you burn over a lifetime.

Fat was the food villain these past few decades but sugar is quickly muscling in to take its place. As rates of sugar-related disorders such as diabetes, obesity, and heart disease climb, many experts believe that when Americans rid their diets of fat, they simply replaced it with sugar in all its forms.

The real demons of the American diet are sugar, wheat, dairy, refined flour, refined cereals, soft drinks, vegetable oils, and any high-glycemic processed carbs.

Virtually all processed foods are loaded with high fructose corn syrup (HFCS). Of the 600,000 items in the US food supply, 80 percent of them contain HFCS and other added sugars. And the reason for this is because the food industry knows that when they add sugar, you eat and buy more of it, becoming fat, sick and dying.

120 calories of fructose results in 40 calories being stored as fat. Fructose is turned into free fatty acids (FFAs), very-low-density lipoprotein (VLDL, the damaging form of cholesterol), and triglycerides, which are then stored as body fat.

The higher your fructose intake, the faster chemical reactions within your body take place and the faster you age.

Fructose over consumption damages your pancreas, liver and brain much like alcohol does, yet, despite its similarities, alcohol is regulated and fructose is not. You'd never consider giving your kid a beer, but you wouldn't think twice about giving him a soda, yet they do the same thing. That's the major problem!

The metabolism of fructose by your liver creates a long list of waste products and toxins, including a large amount of uric acid, which drives up blood pressure.

In short, fructose (HFCS) tricks your body into gaining weight by turning off your body's natural appetite-control system. The end result is overeating, increased visceral fat, insulin resistance, metabolic syndrome and the long list of chronic diseases that result from it.

Here are some important facts to keep in mind:

- A high sugar diet is a high fat diet. A low-fat diet turns out to be a high-fat diet if the fat is replaced with sugar.

- There are no healthy sugary beverages, including sport drinks.

- Fructose should be eaten with fiber, as in fruit.

- A beer belly and a soda belly are the same biochemical process. We don't hesitate to feed our children sodas (but not beer) but they cause the same bodily results.

- Childhood obesity is an epidemic.

- HFCS is classified by the government as GRAS so it's in nearly everything.

- Sugar and HFCS are toxins. Toxins are poisons.

- Too much sugar can affect the brain and cognitive health. It is no coincidence that diabetics have twice the risk for Alzheimer's, dementia, and cognitive impairment.

- Wheat and sugar are addictive appetite stimulants. They shift the diet from net alkaline to net acidic and cancer feeds off acidic environments.

- The average US per capita consumption of HFCS and sugars is about 150 pounds per year, and higher in those who have a high level consumption of sodas. We only need 1-2 teaspoons of sugar in our system at any one time to survive.

- Cardiovascular disease is predicted by hypertension, high triglycerides, and a high ratio of triglycerides to HDL cholesterol. Sugar raises every one of those markers, causes inflammation, spikes insulin levels, and damages cholesterol particles, starting the cascade of endothelial dysfunction, atherosclerosis, cardiovascular disease, and obesity.

- LDL is damaged in two ways: oxidation and glycation. Keep inflammation, hypertension, oxidation, glycation, and atherosclerosis under control by eliminating sugar and wheat. A low-carb diet goes a long way toward preventing stroke, heart attack, and many cancers.

- Sugar depresses the immune system. It makes the blood acidic. Cancer thrives on sugar and an acidic environment. Sugar has no nutrients of its own and gobbles up mineral reserves, resulting in mineral and nutrient deficiencies. Sugar also reduces HDL, adding another risk factor to cardiovascular disease.

- High fructose corn syrup (HFCS) is an artificial sugar manufactured from corn, usually GMO corn, containing toxic levels of mercury. Because of its unbalanced ratio of glucose to fructose, it is absorbed directly by the liver and stored as fat. This leads to weight gain, especially around the belly area. HFCS is linked to system-wide inflammation, which causes many chronic health diseases including heart attack, stroke, autoimmune diseases, and cancer.

- Artificial coloring, especially Yellow #5, is manufactured from coal tar and crude oil runoff, which contains benzene, a known carcinogen. If the label says "artificial coloring," leave it on the shelf. Caramel coloring is a hidden sugar.

- Eliminate sugar from your diet, and anything that turns into sugar or transports sugar, such as wheat.

Some foods are addictive in their chemistry and cause cravings. If we don't consume and introduce them into our system in the first place, the psychology of willpower is eliminated. That's one of the reasons for eliminating sugars and wheat, because they are addictive. They cause you to crave, binge, and overeat, thereby causing weight gain. "Bet you can't eat just one" is a slogan for a reason.

Think of sugar consumption the same way you think of fat consumption. It is metabolized into triglycerides or goes into the bloodstream, raising insulin levels, the fat storing hormone. Either way, the result is fat. Calories from fat in the American diet have gone down at the same time high fructose corn syrup consumption has skyrocketed, along with rates of cardiovascular disease, diabetes, obesity, and hypertension. It's not a coincidence.

Sugar is our enemy. It's actually more important to know what not to eat than what to eat. If it comes in a box, package, jar, or can and has a barcode, it is probably toxic to your body and brain. Don't eat it. An enlightened mind can move a body to take action. You can turn back the clock or have greater longevity and quality of life, with proper nutrition, diet, exercise, vitamins, supplements and hormone balance.

Sugar suppresses your immune system for up to 5 hours after consumption. Cancer feeds on sugar and acid, which the SAD (Standard American Diet) is full of. Processed foods devitalize your body and your immune system.

Sugar at a glance:

- The average US adult consumes 152 pounds of sugar per year.

- Sugar is 8 times more addictive than cocaine.

- Gluten is like sugar: addictive, toxic, and poison.

- The more sweet you eat, the more sweet you crave. The same goes for wheat.

- Retrain your taste buds.

- Use trade downs and food swaps. Watch the magic happen.

- Don't make your salad into a dessert. The dressing can do that. Balsamic is a sugar.

- Learn to read food ingredient labels.

- Like tobacco and alcohol, sugar is addictive, toxic, and has a detrimental impact on society and public health.

- 80% of US healthcare dollars are spent on diet-induced diseases.

Eating fermented vegetables such as sauerkraut and kimchi will reduce your cravings for sugar.

Is bread the staff of life or the stuff of disease?

The truth is there is nothing "essential" about whole grains and there is no such thing as "healthy grains." In fact, they are among the most unhealthful foods you can consume. According to research published in the *American Journal of Clinical Nutrition*, eating two slices of whole wheat bread spikes your blood sugar more than a can of soda, eating a candy bar or 6 teaspoons of table sugar. The glycemic index of whole wheat is among the highest of all foods.

Like sugar, wheat is addictive. Gluten is not just a fad. It is a toxin and a poison. It disrupts your hormonal system, weakens the immune system, causes digestive problems, and promotes systemic inflammation, the cornerstone of all degenerative diseases.

One thing people in all long-lived societies have in common is they have limited or no consumption of refined sugars and other processed foods. When Americanized or Western-style fast food creeps into their societies it always has a negative impact on their health and longevity.

Sodas and other sweetened drinks (liquid candy) likely cause at least 184,000 premature deaths each year, primarily by fueling chronic diseases such as diabetes, heart disease, and cancer. Artificial sweeteners have overwhelmingly been shown to promote weight gain rather than curb it.

Always read the labels for added sugars.

- Many meat packers feed sugar to animals prior to slaughter improving flavor and color to cured meats.

- Sugar in the form of corn syrup or dehydrated molasses is added to hamburgers sold in restaurants to reduce shrinkage.

- Breading on many prepared and fried foods contain sugar.

- Before some salmon is canned it's glazed with a sugar solution.

- Some fast-food establishments and restaurants serve chicken that has been injected with a flavorful processed honey solution.

- Sugar is added to lunch meats, bacon and canned meats.

- Pharmaceutical-grade sucrose is manufactured for use in some prescriptions drugs, vitamins, nutritional supplements, and cold remedies. (Read the labels under "other ingredients.")

- Sugar is found in soups, bouillon cubes, and dry-roasted nuts.

- Some iodized salt contains sugar in the form of dextrose.

- Some brands of vanilla extract contain sugar or corn syrup.

- Seasoning mixes such as taco seasoning, sauce mixes, and salad dressing mixes often contain some form of sugar.

- Condiments such as ketchup, mustard, and mayonnaise contain sugar.

- Nearly all fat-free salad dressings contain more sugar than regular versions.

Sugars are found in crackers, tortillas, bread, canned goods, canned fruits and vegetables, frozen entrees, pickles, peanut butter, macaroni and cheese, spaghetti sauces, breakfast cereals, jams, jellies, pork and beans, relishes, flavored yogurts, milks, and of course in an endless assortment of desserts. Milk contains lactose, which is a sugar.

The healthy eating strategy outlined in this book promotes eliminating sugars (simple carbohydrates) and starches, (complex carbohydrates). Only consume carbohydrates that are nutritionally dense and fiber- rich (in vegetables, fruits, seeds and nuts).

There are no such things as healthy grains. If you must eat bread, eat sprouted wheat bread. If you must eat rice, eat brown or wild rice. Don't eat white bread or white rice.

Eight cereal grains – wheat, corn, rice, oats, barley, rye, sorghum, and millet – now provide 56 percent of the calories and 50 percent of the protein consumed on earth.

First, many of these grains are GMO. Second, they are processed. Third, there is added sugar. And last but not least, they rapidly metabolize to sugar when eaten, causing blood sugar and insulin to spike and the body to store fat. Add table sugar and milk and we have a bowl of dietary nightmare.

Humans can digest leafy green plants but are unable to digest the seed heads of plants, from which grains are derived. These disruptive proteins cause an inflammatory response and inflammatory mediators remain in your digestive tract. Since 70% of your immune system is located in your digestive tract, this can result in disruption of your immune system and can contribute to diseases like colon cancer, irritable bowel syndrome, celiac disease and the inflammation leading to system-wide chaos.

Sugar, wheat, soy, and corn are GMOs. Processed foods are all micronutrient-depleting and health-robbing foods and ingredients that must be eliminated from a healthy eating strategy.

Refined carbohydrates promote chronic inflammation in your body, elevate low-density LDL cholesterol and ultimately lead to insulin and leptin resistance, which are at the heart of obesity and many chronic diseases, including diabetes, heart disease, stroke, cancer, and Alzheimer's, the top killers in the US.

Contrary to popular belief, you do not get fat from eating fat. You get fat from eating too much sugar and grains. It's difficult to calculate how many Americans have succumbed to chronic poor health and death from following the FDA food pyramid conventional low-fat, high-carb recommendations, but the number is staggering. It is the worst dietary guide and human health experiment in US history. False premises lead to false conclusions.

The American food pyramid should literally be turned upside-down, eliminating sugars and grains and dramatically increasing fat intake, thereby reducing risk factors for heart disease to near zero. Regardless of your genetic predisposition (DNA), your diet is ultimately the determining factor in the expression of your genes. You are stuck with your genes but you determine their destiny by your nutrition or lack thereof.

To reverse insulin and leptin resistance you must avoid refined sugar, processed fructose and grains, and all processed foods, as they are full of chemicals that wreak metabolic havoc.

There are over 10,000 chemicals registered with the US government that are in our food supply that do not have to be listed on the label and are considered GRAS.

Eat a healthful diet of whole, real, organic foods and replace the grain carbs you restrict or eliminate with:

- Moderate amounts of high-quality protein from organic, grass-fed or pastured animals (this is to ensure that you're not ingesting antibiotics, genetically engineered organisms, and altered nutritional fat profile associated with factory farmed animals).

- High amounts of high-quality healthful fat, including saturated and monounsaturated fats. Many health experts now believe that if you are insulin or leptin resistant, as 85% of the US population is, you likely need anywhere from 50 to 85 percent of your daily calories in the form of healthful fats. Good sources include olive oil, coconut and coconut oil, avocados, butter (ghee), nuts (particularly macadamia, pistachios, walnuts and almonds), and animal fats. Avoid all trans-fats and processed vegetable oils, such as canola and soy oil. Also take a high-quality source of animal-based omega-3 fat, such as fish or krill oil.

- Eat as many vegetables as you can consume from the food list in this handbook. Juicing your vegetables is a good way to boost your vegetable intake. Eating raw vegetables is a good eating strategy. Shoot for 9-13 servings of vegetables and fruits daily.

Another suggestion is to start intermittent fasting, or "IF," which will be described in more detail later. IF will dramatically improve your ability to burn fat as your primary fuel. IF will help restore your insulin and leptin signaling.

Even if a high-fat, low-carb diet raises your total cholesterol and LDL, it doesn't automatically mean that your diet is increasing your risk factors for heart disease. You need to test your LDL particle size and number, as described later. Large-sized LDL particles are good, while the smaller, denser LDL particles can penetrate the lining of your arteries and exacerbate the plaque formation associated with heart disease. The former does not increase your heart disease risk; the latter one does.

Sugars and whole grains are the main culprits in GERD (acid reflux: gastroesophageal reflux disease). The medical costs associated with GERD in the US are in excess of $9 billion annually. By eliminating sugars, wheat, and starches and restricting carbohydrates to healthy vegetables and fruit, the burning sensation from GERD improves or completely goes away. Say goodbye to heartburn products such as Rolaids, Tums and Nexium, save money and get relief, all by making dietary changes.

Five grams, 1 teaspoon ("tsp") of sugar, is all that's needed in the adult bloodstream at one time to function. One teaspoon equals five grams, and half a bagel has approximately 10 grams of carbs, so from that one food you are consuming twice the sugar needed in your body. Add a glass of orange juice to that and no wonder blood glucose and insulin levels go through the roof. All the while you think you're eating a healthy breakfast, but keep gaining weight despite working out harder.

Each glass of wine has approximately 1 tsp of sugar. Since sugar raises insulin and excess insulin stores as fat, no wonder you need to stop alcohol consumption if you want to lose weight. Plus, alcohol is burned first before your body burns sugar or fat. Alcohol is a toxin that is not readily recognized by the body.

Essential nutrients for humans are water, vitamins, minerals, protein, and fat. Carbohydrates are not essential, do not have an RDA, and are not necessary for human life. The best carbohydrate sources are vegetables, fruits, seed and nuts. There is no such thing as a healthy source of grains. Eat healthy protein and healthy fat to eliminate cravings for carbs.

Fat has no effect on insulin and protein has only a minimal effect. Fiber isn't digested so it has no effect on insulin. The thousand-pound gorilla in the room is carbohydrates, especially sugar, wheat, cereals, bread, rice, pasta, potatoes, high glycemic load carbs and starchy carbs. It's not weight loss we are striving for – it's fat loss.

Choose dark chocolates with at least 72% cacao content. The higher the percentage of cacao, the lower the percentage of sugar.

Glycemic load is more important than Glycemic Index.

Example: Carrots vs. pasta.

- Carrots have a GI of 47, whole wheat pasta 32, so you'd think pasta is healthier than carrots.

- When examining the Glycemic Load, which is net carbs/effective carbs, (carbohydrates minus dietary fiber) multiplied by glycemic index equals carb load.

- The carb load (GI times net carbs): carrots 47 X 6=282; spaghetti 32 X 48=1,536.

- Therefore, spaghetti has more than 500% more glycemic load than carrots.

The Glycemic Index (GI) scale is:

- GI of 70 or more = high

- GI of 56-69 = medium

- GI of 55 or less = low

The Glycemic Load (GL) scale:

- GL of 20 or more = high

- GL of 11-19 = medium

- GL of 10 or less = low

Not only do grains contribute to an expanding waistline, but certain grains, wheat and corn in particular, can lead to and worsen many health conditions. Not only are they GMO, but are high glycemic and cause blood sugar spikes, insulin resistance, diabetes, and weight gain. If breads, pastas, rice, cereal, cakes, muffins, and pastries are your comfort foods of choice, you crave them for a reason. They feed the fat-promoting gut bacteria. These are found in almost all processed foods.

(1/2 cup = 4.1 tsp.)

- 1 cup of cooked brown rice contains a whopping 8.2 tsp of sugar.

- Quinoa: 3.4 tsp

- Banana: Total carbs: 27g-3g dietary fiber÷5 = 4.8 tsp sugar

- Blackberries: total carbs-7g-4g dietary fiber÷5 = 1.4 tsp sugar

- Spinach: Total carbs-7g-4g dietary fiber÷5 = 0.6 tsp sugar.

Studies show that what expectant mothers are eating during pregnancy will transfer to the baby's taste preferences after birth. If the mother ate fruits and vegetables the baby will have an inborn taste for fruits and vegetables, but if the mother ate junk foods, fast foods, processed foods and sugar, guess what, a new generation of junk food dependency is born and on the cycle goes. Sugar and wheat become an addiction.

"To food manufacturers, wheat is like nicotine in cigarettes, the best insurance they have to encourage continued consumption." – Dr. William Davis, MD, "Wheat Belly"

The average American consumes 55 pounds of wheat flour every year, making refined flour the #1 source of calories in the American Diet, contributing to a public health catastrophe.

Go against the grain. There is no such thing as a healthy grain. Eliminate them and you will not only lose weight, you will be on your way to optimal health, wellness and longevity.

When your omega-3 to omega-6 fatty-acid ratio is turned upside-down, favoring omega-6s like the Standard American Diet does, it is a major driver of diet-induced chronic inflammation.

Some irresponsible authors have claimed that the only problem with wheat is its content of glyphosate which, of course, is not true. If that were true, all the problems of wheat would disappear just by choosing organic wheat products. There would be no high blood sugars, no weight gain, no acid reflux, no bowel urgency, no brain fade, no behavioral/emotional effects, no iron deficiency anemia, no celiac disease, as long as you choose organic wheat. This is absolutely not the case. Glyphosate is indeed yet another aspect of the wheat and grain issue for humans, as it may be one of the more crucial reasons underlying the epidemic of disrupted microbiome. Glyphosate is something you need to avoid to have a healthy gut microbiome. This is science-based biochemistry.

Humans can digest leafy green plants but are unable to digest the seed heads of plants that grains are derived from. Since these disruptive proteins are not actually digestible, cause an inflammatory response, and inflammatory mediators remain in your digestive tract, and since 70% of your immune system is located in your digestive tract, this can result in disruption of your immune system, contributing to diseases, like colon cancer, irritable bowel syndrome, celiac disease, and the inflammation leading to system-wide chaos.

Just because you eat gluten-free, you are not off the hook, as the ingredients in most gluten-free products will send your blood sugar soaring, as well. Read the labels.

Examples are:

In place of wheat flour, most gluten-free products and many online recipes use flours with glycemic values that are off the charts, including:

- Corn Starch

- Rice Flour

- Potato Starch

- Tapioca Starch

- Sorghum flour

- Millet

"These powdered starches are among the few foods that increase blood sugar higher than even whole wheat. It means these foods trigger weight gain in the abdomen, increased blood sugars, insulin resistance, diabetes, cataracts, and arthritis. They are NOT healthy replacements for wheat." – Dr. William Davis, MD, "Wheat Belly"

The medical establishment has greatly exaggerated the role of cholesterol in heart disease. But, there is one type of cholesterol closely linked to this killer: Small dense LDL particles.

A study published in the Journal of the American Medical Association showed that people with high levels of small dense LDL have a 300% greater risk of heart attack!

Many doctors believe this is the number one risk factor for heart disease in the U.S.

And guess what triggers these dangerous compounds to form more than any other food?

It is the amylopectin A found in wheat!

Now that you know the problems with sugar and high fructose corn syrup, with the excess empty calories, the massive blood sugar spikes, and the resulting insulin surges this creates in your body, that not only promotes fat gain, but also stimulates your appetite further, making cravings even worse. These massive blood sugar spikes also contribute to glycation in the cells of your body, which basically makes you age faster (AGE's).

So, what about artificial sweeteners?

Artificial sweeteners may save calories, but there's growing evidence that they increase your appetite for sweets and other carbohydrates causing you to eat more as the day progresses. As a result, you don't really save any calories at all.

Artificial sweeteners trigger "sweet receptors" in your stomach that tell your body to produce insulin, even though you didn't actually consume sugar. These high insulin levels from artificial sweeteners promote fat storage and trigger cravings, just like sugar itself.

Studies show people who drink "diet" soft drinks often gain even MORE weight than those who drink regular soft drinks. They theorized that people drinking "diet drinks" eat more calories because they have fooled themselves with the calories they thought they had saved from the diet drink, so they eat more.

The four artificial sweeteners listed below are nasty chemicals that the human body was simply not meant to ingest. Humans historically would never have ingested these in nature.

Just to clarify, some of the most popular artificial sweeteners on the market today are:

- Splenda (sucralose)

- Aspartame

- Saccharine

- Acesulfame Potassium (aka - acesulfame K)

Sucralose (aka, splenda) is probably one of the worst offenders of claiming to be "healthy" as they say that it's "made from real sugar." Don't be fooled! It's still an artificial substance, and a fairly nasty chemical at that.

What they don't tell you is that Splenda is actually a chemically modified substance where chlorine is added to the chemical structure, making it more similar to a chlorinated pesticide than something we should be eating or drinking.

If the product says "diet" anywhere on it, avoid it. "Diet" is a code word for chemicals.

Avoid all artificial sweeteners like the plaque and the products they are found in for optimal health.

Since calorie counting, weighing and measuring are not part of my diet guidelines, your primary goal will be to avoid the modern foods that our bodies can't digest efficiently. Replace them with nutrient-rich, whole, real foods. Eliminate sugars and grains to control blood sugar/insulin levels, and allow good foods to be absorbed into our cells and tissues efficiently for optimal health and wellness. It's pretty simple.

CHAPTER 14:
Inflammation

Inflammation is our enemy. It is the root cause of virtually all modern degenerative diseases known to mankind, including our leading causes of death and disability in the U.S.: cardiovascular disease, heart attack, stroke, cancer, Type 2 Diabetes, obesity, cognitive decline and Alzheimer's disease and a wide range of additional health problems, including but not limited to chronic pain, ADD/ADHD, peripheral neuropathy, migraines, thyroid issues, dental issues and cancer are all rooted in inflammation, all the diseases of aging.

The good news is, most (80%) can be reversed, eliminated or prevented through lifestyle change, nutrition, diet, supplementation and exercise. Since diet-induced inflammation is the cause of most of these modern diseases, it makes sense to change what you are eating, not only for your heart, but also in the long-term for cancer, your brain and Alzheimer's.

Diseases are not causes, but effects. Americans are becoming sicker, fatter and more demented, primarily due to increased dietary-induced inflammation. Eat Clean. Food is one of life's greatest pleasures. Changing the way you eat is a huge proponent in fighting diet-induced inflammation.

The majority of inflammatory diseases start in the gut with an autoimmune reaction which progresses into systemic inflammation. To be truly effective at managing or hopefully overcoming a disease, it needs to be addressed on all levels, including diet-induced inflammation. What you put in your mouth.

Simply put, inflammation results when the body is unable to keep up with the process of healing itself from toxins in the bloodstream and the major culprit is diet-induced inflammation.

The #1 source of inflammation in the body is a poor diet. Low-carb diets reduce inflammation by controlling your insulin. Inflammation is a fire and you need to treat the fire and not the smoke by treating the cause, not the symptom.

There are two types of inflammation: acute and chronic. Acute inflammation hurts. Chronic inflammation kills slowly over time. Most of us are walking around in a state of chronic inflammation, a silent killer.

So, that makes two silent killers lurking: hypertension (high blood pressure) and chronic inflammation and we can eliminate both through proper nutrition and exercise.

When you see a wrinkle on your face or skin it hurts your vanity but we are actually rusting, wrinkling from the inside out where we can't see it. When it happens to your heart or vascular system it will shorten your life.

The very foods that are loaded with anti-inflammatories tend to be loaded with antioxidants, so you get a double dose of healing. The true heart-healthy diet is not necessarily low in cholesterol, but high in anti-inflammatories and antioxidants

Bread, pasta, potatoes and rice not only cause weight gain and high blood sugar, but these carbs also cause increased hunger cravings and most importantly, inflammation. Increased insulin is caused by eating too many carbohydrates or too many calories. The average American does both. Diet-induced inflammation is most likely the cause of insulin resistance.

One of the consequences of increased dietary inflammation is the development of insulin resistance, which results in chronically elevated insulin levels, eventually ending up in fat storage, making you fat and keeping you fat, for a lifetime. Belly fat is associated with inflammation, so eating too many processed foods will hinder your ability to lose belly fat.

The fact that your immune system drives the inflammatory process in disease is well established. Unfortunately, Western medicine offers little in the way of actual answers as to managing or overcoming the autoimmune process. The typical approach to therapy is generally to suppress the immune response with immune suppressive agents or sometimes steroids. Both approaches are designed to reduce inflammation but neither stops the underlying disease processes or allows for damaged tissues to regenerate.

Unless you turn off the actual cause of inflammation, all you have done is postponed the inevitable by allowing the inflammation to continue in a sub-clinical fashion.

The more fat cells you have the higher your level of inflammation is likely to be. Inflammation is the reason we get sick, gain weight and age faster. By reducing inflammation we maintain wellness, lose and maintain weight, and most importantly, we slow the aging process. Eliminate all dietary inflammation. The beauty is, we can control inflammation through our nutrition.

The gene-supportive environment you create for your arteries by what you eat, can determine whether you are going to have cardiovascular disease or not.

Omega 6's are pro-inflammatory. Omega 3's are anti-inflammatory. Your genes don't dictate inflammation, the environment and what you eat do. Eat an anti-inflammatory diet. Avoid and eliminate toxins.

The SAD (Standard American Diet), is packed full of excess Omega-6s. When excess Omega-6s interact with excess insulin, the result is dietary inflammation and very powerful inflammatory hormones known as eicosanoids. This becomes a real health-care crisis.

When your Omega 3/Omega 6 fatty-acid ratio is turned upside down, favoring Omega 6s like the Standard American Diet does, it becomes a major driver of diet-induced chronic inflammation.

Unless you treat the underlying cause of diet-induced inflammation, losing weight is going to be very difficult. By adapting a nutrition-rich eating strategy of low carbs, moderate healthy proteins and higher healthy fats you will extinguish the flames of diet-induced inflammation. The higher healthy fats will not hurt you as long as you consume low glycemic load net-carbs, fresh whole food, vegetables and fruits.

Diet induced nutritional deficiencies and diet induced inflammation are powerful disease producers related to most all modern diseases that accumulate over time, as a result of these nutritional deficiencies and the accompanying chronic inflammation. Polyphenols, which help control dietary-induced inflammation, are found in colorful fruits and vegetables and are a powerful antioxidant.

The more visceral fat you have, the more chronic or silent inflammation you generate, increasing your risk of cardiovascular disease, heart attack, stroke, cancer and Alzheimer's disease. Anything that increases inflammation is going to be bad for your future. Remember, chronic inflammation is cumulative. It doesn't build up overnight, it accumulates over years.

Controlling or slowing the aging process is a process of controlling diet-induced inflammation; creating and maintaining cellular rejuvenation and not cellular degradation, as a result of long-term chronic inflammation caused by a diet high in carbohydrates, sugars and grains.

You cannot be in a state of wellness if your cortisol levels are too high. Cortisol is produced by long-term stress. The end result is an increase in inflammation and our goal is to eliminate chronic inflammation. Reduce visceral fat around your internal organs, reduce your CRP and IL-6 levels, and you'll reduce the primary source of silent and chronic inflammation in your body, thereby eliminating many of these degenerative illnesses and diseases.

By the time you get sick and head to the doctor, he treats the symptom, not the cause. He writes you a prescription and sends you on your way but didn't treat the imbalance in your nutrition, the underlying cause. These imbalances build up over years or decades.

If you had an 80% batting average in the major leagues you'd be in the Hall of Fame. Wouldn't you like to have your health in the hall of fame? I do. That's why I treated my causes, not just their symptoms. I didn't take medications, but changed my nutrition, my fuel, my life. Let food be your medicine and medicine be your food. Eliminate chronic inflammation. Eliminate disease.

Is it a coincidence that statins such as Lipitor, which lowers cholesterol and is the world's #1 selling drug, coincides with an increase in Alzheimer's cases? I think not. In addition, in cutting cholesterol, statins diminish testosterone levels. Testosterone needs cholesterol to be produced. So, low T causes ED. Is it another coincidence that Pfizer is the manufacturer of both Viagra and Lipitor? Think again.

As your weight increases your brain atrophies and shrinks. It is no wonder, as obesity and Type 2 Diabetes have risen, so has Alzheimer's disease. Your waist measurement needs to be half of less than your height.

Omega 6s become rancid inside the body due to oxidation and cause inflammation. Oxidized LDL leads to accelerated heart disease, heart attack and stroke. The dietary target is to decrease Omega 6s while increasing polyphenols, powerful antioxidants, by increasing consumption of vegetables and fruits.

You must have adequate levels of Omega-3 fatty acids and polyphenols to control and extinguish diet-induced inflammation. This is best achieved by a proper nutritional balance of low-glycemic carbs, protein, reduced consumption of Omega 6s, and a significant increase of Omega 3s and polyphenols. By reducing diet induced cellular inflammation, you will lose and maintain desirable weight, lose excess body fat, decrease the risk of modern chronic diseases, and retard the aging process. You will become more efficient at metabolizing food for energy and burning fat, not sugar. You won't have hunger cravings for junk foods, as your body will actually start craving healthy foods.

CHAPTER 15:
Toxins

Toxins can get into our bodies through eating any meat, poultry, fish, or diary, because by definition that animal drank water, and that water most likely contained toxins.

Toxins scar arteries. When arteries are scarred, LDL cholesterol attaches to the arterial wall, causing atherosclerosis. Chemical toxins such as chlorine and fluoride are in our tap water. Processed, manufactured and man-made foods are full of toxins and chemicals. We control what we put in our mouths, so we can control our disease destiny. Dinner is not DNA: it's destiny.

Toxins can lead to cancer by damaging DNA. Damage to DNA is a major initiating factor in cellular transformation into cancer. Such damage can induce mutations in the DNA that cause cancer. That's why nutrients that prevent DNA damage and ones that promote cellular and DNA repair are so potent in protecting against cancer. Given the role of oxidative stress in causing such damage, nutrients that reduce DNA damage such as vitamin C, vitamin E, vitamin D, the mineral selenium and probiotics that are effective in reducing DNA damage in the colon are all considered a first line of defense in preventing cancer.

A new study reveals that air pollution is responsible for as many as one-third of all strokes. That's because it contributes to high blood pressure and hardening of the arteries, which can lead to stroke.

Daily detoxification is a preventative lifestyle measure.

When you rid your body of toxins, pollutants and diet-induced inflammation by no longer eating the chemical pollutants found in processed foods and start eating organic, real, and whole foods, your improved skin, hair, and nails will be an automatic by-product of a healthier you, as will your weight loss and management. You will have an overall glow and radiance.

Detoxify:

- Do not use aluminum cookware or utensils. Excessive amounts of aluminum have been associated and implicated with Alzheimer's disease

- Eliminate fluoride toothpaste

- Eliminate fluoride in tap water

- Eliminate mercury in fish

- Eliminate mercury in teeth (filings and crowns)

- Eliminate aluminum (alcohol-free deodorant.)

- Avoid air pollution

- Practice grounding

- Practice oil pulling (coconut oil)

- Eliminates obesity

- Reverses metabolic syndrome

- Reverses atherosclerosis

- Reverses hypertension, the silent killer

Trash your non-stick, Teflon or Gore-Tex pots and pans, which contain PFCs.

We are routinely exposed to chemical additives and preservatives, many of which are banned in other countries. We face constant exposure to unlabeled genetically-modified organisms (GMOs), pesticide and herbicide residues, and perhaps the biggest threat of all that you've probably never even heard of – mycotoxins.

6 Common Toxins You Want to Avoid since they are considered the worst mycotoxic offenders, according to a 2011 study published in the Journal of Saudi Chemical Society:

- Aflatoxins (AF), a family of fungal-based mycotoxins often found in maize (corn), peanuts, cottonseed, and tree nuts

- Ochratoxins (OT), often found in cereal grains, coffee, dried fruits, wine, beer, cocoa, nuts, beans, peas, bread, and rice

- Trichothecenes, a protein-inhibiting mycotoxin often found in cereal-based foods

- Zearalenone (ZEN), a mycotoxic xenoestrogen found in many food crops grown in glyphosate-treated soils

- Fumonisins (F), often found in corn

- Tremorgenic toxins, often found in spoiled food products

Mycotoxins seem to be most often found in conventional grains, including wheat, corn, barley, and oats. Processed, non-organic foods in general tend to be prone to mycotoxin formation. Chemical Food Additives: Banned elsewhere but legal in the US? Ouch!

Most standard American fare, as you'll probably notice, doesn't even come close to fitting the bill for a mycotoxin-free diet. Not only is American food a mycotoxic nightmare, but it's also a chemical nightmare. This is because of all the additives, preservatives, and colorful food dyes used in much of what you'll find on grocery store shelves today.

These toxins found in food aren't visible to the naked eye and don't have a distinctive flavor, so you probably don't even know you're consuming them. But your body sure does, and the culmination of this perpetual toxic exposure could spell chronic disease or even early death.

Mycotoxins form from yeast and fungi that develop on foods grown in microbe-deficient soils, which are more the norm than the exception these days. Mycotoxins can lead to nervous system damage, hormone imbalances, and cancer.

FDA approved or not, these chemicals don't in any way contribute to your health or well-being. They only feed the bottom lines of large food corporations that use them to extend the shelf lives of their products and decrease manufacturing costs. There's a whole slew of chemicals used in the U.S. food supply that the FDA considers GRAS and as a result not required to be listed on the label. Crime? You decide.

Our increasingly tainted food supply is taking a major toll on public health.

- No animal byproducts

- No gluten or wheat

- No GMOs

Omega-3 fatty acids, found in oily fish, nuts, and flaxseeds, are resistant to oxidation (antioxidant) shielding LDL from being readily oxidized, reducing the risk of atherosclerosis, heart disease, heart attack, and stroke.

We live in a toxic world. According to Environmental Protection Agency (EPA) estimates, more than 6 trillion pounds of chemicals are released into the environment each year. This includes air emissions from factories and vehicles, as well as agricultural and industrial chemicals discharged into the ground and water.

Some of these pollutants inevitably make their way into our bodies through the air we breathe, the food we eat and the water we drink. Couple this with exposure to noxious elements in household cleaners, building materials in your home, personal care products and the like, and we're talking toxic overload. That's why it's so important to detoxify your body.

Your body's primary toxin-removal organ is the liver. It filters your blood (two quarts a minute), removes toxins, and converts them into nontoxic substances for elimination. You might be one of the millions of Americans suffering from the effects of toxin accumulation. Fortunately, you can safely and naturally detoxify your body. I believe that you should take daily measures to detoxify your body of toxins as well as parasites.

Food and environmental toxins are everywhere and when they enter your body they are stored in your fat cells. You may have trouble losing weight because your body holds onto that fat, because releasing it into your bloodstream would put your body at risk for disease. So as these toxins accumulate and fat is not released or mobilized, your fat cells become bigger and you get fatter. Combine this with a diet high in processed foods, sugar, and carbohydrates, triggering insulin stores as fat and insulin resistance, and it's no wonder America is obese.

Eating whole, real foods and organic vegetables and fruits will help on both fronts, by cutting toxins, detoxifying and insulin secretion all at the same time, along with proper hydration from water. I like alkaline water for detoxifying.

Environmental or external toxins that affect us include tap water, smog, alcohol, sugar, artificial sweeteners, food preservatives, food additives, artificial colors, artificial flavorings, tobacco, secondhand smoke, pesticides, herbicides, petrochemicals, animal steroids, animal antibiotics, heavy metals, viruses, bacteria, prescription and over-the-counter medications. All these contaminants lead to toxic accumulation and organ and tissue overload, resulting in an ideal environment for illness and disease to proliferate.

Every day our modern world assaults us with harmful substances, air pollution, smog, industrial toxins, secondhand cigarette smoke, additives and chemicals in our food and water, radiation, pharmaceuticals, and free radicals from oxidative stress. It's important to rid the body of toxins, oxidative stress, and inflammation, which cause many of our degenerative diseases. Much can be accomplished with a nutrient-rich diet and eliminating certain products can help somewhat, but it is wise to take daily antioxidant supplements.

Keep your insides healthy, then your health will manifest on your outside, and you will look and feel younger.

When you rid your body of toxins, pollutants, and diet-induced inflammation by no longer eating the chemicals used in processed foods and start eating organic, real, and whole foods, your improved skin, hair, and nails will be an automatic byproduct of a healthier you, as will your weight loss and management.

When your gut is out of balance and the "bad" bacteria overpowers the "good" bacteria from too much sugar and wheat and suffers toxic overload from poor nutrition and environmental chemicals, then your liver, which is the body's filter, gets clogged. It starts a domino effect: spreading and backing up to the kidneys, bladder, pancreas, spleen, and lymphatic system. Your immune system is compromised, your stomach is not sending the correct messages to your brain and your brain is nor sending correct messages to your thyroid. Now your hormones are out if balance. Throw in heavy metal contamination and no wonder you feel fat, sick tired and are dying. By this time, you need a heavy rescue, a lifestyle and diet change – a cleanse and detox, for starters.

Eat a healthy diet with plenty of fiber-rich vegetables, beans, and other plant foods. This will help to ensure that you have regular bowel movements, which, obviously, are required for proper elimination. For good measure, take a fiber supplement, such as psyllium, glucomannan, or my favorite: flaxseed. One of the easiest ways to use flax is to sprinkle a quarter cup of freshly ground seeds over salads, soups or other dishes every day.

Get into the habit of drinking at least eight glasses of clean, filtered water daily. The kidneys filter metabolic waste products and excrete them in the urine. Water is so important that if you don't drink enough, your body will divert limited resources to life-sustaining functions, such as maintaining blood pressure – at the expense of flushing out toxins.

Exercise and sweat. The lungs and lymph system are also involved in detoxification. Exercise encourages deep breathing and gets the lymph moving. Make sure you exert yourself enough to build up a sweat. Sweating mobilizes and excretes stored toxins, detoxifying your body.

Replenish the "good guys" that protect your health. Friendly bacteria, or probiotics, are the front-line soldiers of your immune system. They help crowd out the bad bacteria we're all exposed to in food and water, before they can add to your toxic load. They also help to support regular bowel function.

Take supplements that support your liver such as:

- 100 mg of lipoic acid

- 500 mg of silymarin (milk thistle extract)

- 200 mcg of selenium

- 500 mg of n-acetyl-cysteine

- 1000 mg Chlorella

- Milk Thistle

- Chlorophyll (Liquid - 30 drops in glass of water / one dropper full)

We can't escape the toxicity of our world. But with the recommendations listed above, you can safeguard your health, by helping to naturally detoxify your body.

I also use, in tandem with a Chlorella supplement, an activated charcoal supplement. Together they will help detoxify your GI tract, which needs to be free to eliminate toxins through urine and feces. For best results, you should pulse or vary the frequency of supplementation. Do 4 days on and 3 days off to 7 days on and 7 days off. The reason for pulse or variation is because your system gets restrictive and resistant, so you have to vary the frequency to reach optimal absorption and maximum elimination of targeted toxins. There are toxins from the environment as well as from fish you consume, so detoxifying is central to optimal health. The least-toxic fish to eat are always wild caught and not farmed. The least toxic fish are wild caught Coho and Sockeye Salmon, Anchovies and Sardines. You could eat these fish in abundance every day and show no signs of mercury toxicity. Again, test, don't guess.

Be sure to drink extra water to flush the toxins out.

Toxin-free health includes taking into consideration choices about toothpaste, deodorant, non-stick pots and pans (your best and safest options for cookware are stainless steel, cast iron, ceramic, or glass), detergent, shampoo, body soap, dish soap, dryer sheets, BPA plastic containers, and microwave ovens.

Sugar is also a toxin, referred to as the White Devil, eight times more addictive than cocaine.

A toxin is a chemical or substance that brings imbalance to the body's cells, creating an adverse environment. Toxins are a poison; sometimes ordinary foods that act as poisons. For example, gluten is a poison from eating wheat, barley, or rye.

Personal care items also contain toxins. Toss traditional toothpaste and replace with fluoride-free products. Your mouth and the rest of your body will love you.

Fluoride is both an endocrine disruptor chemical that causes thyroid disease and dysfunction, as well as being a neurotoxin impacting memory, IQ, ADD, and ADHD in children. It has little or no benefit on teeth. It's in our municipal water supply. It can't be filtered out of tap water and should be eliminated from your daily consumption in both the water you drink and your toothpaste. It is clearly a toxic poison that you need to eliminate for you and your family's health.

Additional ingredients to eliminate are artificial flavors and colors, polysorbate-80, ethanol, titanium dioxide, benzoate, benzoic acid, and lauryl sulfate.

Replace your aerosol spray deodorant with a roll-on for environmental purposes, as well as allergies, skin irritations, and clothing stains. Choose a product that is aluminum-free; aluminum is estrogenic and can be carcinogenic. Have you ever noticed white spots or rings on your clothes near the armpits and you thought it was sweat stain and you couldn't get it clean? Well that wasn't a sweat stain – it was an aluminum stain. If it's doing that to your clothes, just think what it's doing to your body. Other unwanted ingredients to eliminate are parabens, triclosan, steareth, propylene glycol, and talc, all possible allergens.

Pitch your plastic storage containers and Tupperware. Buy glass storage containers or Pyrex and make sure all plastic, including lids, are BPA-free, lead-free, PVC-free and phthalate-free.

Don't be fooled by misleading marketing using terms such as "nontoxic," "biodegradable," "earth friendly," "natural," and even "organic," as there are no federal regulations to require advertisers to live up to those claims, leaving you with a false sense of safety. Read the labels, especially under "other ingredients." When in doubt, call the manufacturer and ask.

Pitch your non-stick, Teflon or Gore-Tex pots and pans, which contain PFCs (perfluorinated compounds). The harmful PFCs, which are found in the bloodstreams of 98% of the American population, remain in the body for 5-8 years, and research has been shown they increase the risk of cancer, ADHD, heart disease, infertility, and obesity. Safe cookware alternatives are made of glass, enamel, ceramic, stainless steel, or "Made in USA" cast iron.

Do not use aluminum or cooper cookware or utensils as both leech unsafe chemicals. Excessive amounts of aluminum have been associated and implicated with Alzheimer's disease.

If toxins are introduced into your system, your body will try to flush or remove them. In the process, your body will be depleted of nutrient sufficiency and it will negatively affect your health. For maximum health we are trying to eliminate all inflammation, toxins, and funguses.

The world we live in exposes us thousands of times each day to chemicals that science now shows have very dangerous and unwanted side effects. Today's children will be the first to live their entire lives in this toxic soup and murky bath. We must limit or eliminate these toxins from our lives and theirs. There are safer ingredients to purchase. You can and must eliminate all toxins.

There are many toxins, but here are a few of the most sickening ones: Growth hormones in meats, antibiotics, pesticides, refined and enriched flour, BPA in plastics, HFCS (high fructose corn syrup found in most sodas and many processed foods), artificial sweeteners, preservatives, trans fats, artificial and natural flavors, food dyes, dough conditioners (think donuts), carrageenan (a polysaccharide or sugar used as an emulsifier in processed foods that is often found in organic or "natural" foods, including almond milk and coconut milk), monosodium glutamate (MSG, in chips, canned foods, and junk foods) which you all must know by now is bad for you, and finally heavy metals and neurotoxins (from sugar and artificial sugars found in sugar-free products, gums, and drinks).

Facts about fluoride:

- Infants receiving baby formula mixed with fluorinated tap water receive up to 100 times the daily dose considered safe.

- 30% of 1-year-olds exceed safe dosages.

- 47% of 2- to 3-year-olds exceed the safe dose, as it builds up over time.

- The fluoride most water agencies use is not a pharmaceutical grade product that was once considered safe, but an industrial waste product of fluoride a byproduct of fertilizer contaminated with heavy metals, arsenic, mercury, cadmium, lead, and other toxins.

- Fluoride has never been approved as a drug by the FDA.

- More information at www.fluoridealert.org

Mercury in fish

Eat wild-caught Alaskan salmon such as Sockeye Salmon. Test your blood for mercury and if your numbers are high, detox with chlorella, liquid cilantro extract, and liquid chlorophyll. You may have excess mercury in your blood due to amalgam fillings. Consider removing and replacing with non-amalgam fillings or porcelain crowns. Use aluminum-free deodorant: a non-spray, or roll-on. Air pollution is hard to escape, so detox on a daily basis with supplements as stated above such as chlorella, chlorophyll, milk thistle, or cilantro extract.

Health problems from mercury toxicity include hypertension, coronary heart disease, myocardial infarction, cardiac arrhythmias, reduced heart rate variability, increased carotid intima-media thickness and carotid artery obstruction, cerebrovascular accident, generalized atherosclerosis and renal dysfunction.

The general effects on the blood vessels from mercury include increased oxidative stress and inflammation, reduced oxidative defense, thrombosis, dyslipidemia, and immune and mitochondrial dysfunction.

Mercury reduces the protective effect of fish oil and omega-3 fatty acids, which have value in the management of reducing high blood pressure and overall wellness.

Thirty-five million Americans suffer from toenail fungus. With all the serious health dangers in our lives like cancer, heart attack, strokes, and diabetes, having a discolored or yellowed toenail from fungus may seem pretty insignificant and merely cosmetic, since it is generally not painful and can be kept out of sight and out of mind.

However, left untreated or ignored, a toenail fungus could have health consequences beyond appearances, leading to wider infection, foot pain, and cracked skin where bacteria can get into your bloodstream, compromising your immune system and becoming deadly.

Lamisil 250 mg daily is an excellent toenail fungus fighter. It requires a doctor's prescription.

We are trying to rid our bodies of all inflammation, toxins and funguses.

Chlorine in Your Shower

Shower filters reduce or eliminate chlorine, dirt, sediment, odors, metals, sulfur, scale, and other chemicals and contaminants from your shower water.

Chlorine is universally used to chemically disinfect water. It kills germs, bacteria, and other living organisms. Chlorine readily passes through the cell wall and attaches to the fatty acids of the cell, disrupting life sustaining functions. The human body is composed of billions of cells. Most people are aware that the quality of their drinking water can be improved by filtering their tap water or buying bottled water. However, many do not realize that they are addressing only a part of the problem.

Around 50% of our daily chlorine exposure is from showering. Chlorine is not only absorbed through the skin, but vaporizes in the hot environment of the shower and is inhaled directly into the lungs, then transferred directly into the blood system. In fact, the chlorine exposure from one shower is equal to an entire day's amount of drinking the same water. Drinking filtered or bottled water only does half the job.

Documented scientific studies conclude that taking long hot showers is a health risk. To a lesser degree, dermal absorption also occurs. As chlorine is added to kill pathogenic microorganisms, such as bacteria, the highly reactive chlorine combines with fatty acids and carbon fragments to form a variety of toxic compounds.

Medical studies suggest a link between absorption and inhalation of chlorine in the shower environment with elevated risks for diseases and serious illnesses. Showering in chlorinated water may also cause pre-existing conditions, such as asthma and eczema, to become exacerbated.

In addition to health benefits of filtering shower water, there are cosmetic benefits. Symptoms of chlorine exposure are dry and/or flaking skin, dry, brittle hair and red, irritated eyes. Filtering the shower water reduces these symptoms. Skin and hair feel softer and eyes become less red and irritated.

Benefits of Using a Shower Filter:

- Using a shower filter is one of the easiest and most effective ways to reduce harmful exposure to chlorine, fluoride, and other toxic chemicals.

- More chlorine enters your body via inhalation while showering than through drinking tap water. Showering in filtered water results in greater respiratory health by reducing the risk of asthma and bronchitis from chlorine inhalation.

- Showering in chlorine-free, filtered water decreases the risks of bladder and breast cancer.

- Children, who are particularly at risk of the harmful effects of chlorine inhalation, benefit especially from the removal of chlorine from showering water.

- As chlorine is a leading cause of fatigue, showering in filtered, chlorine-free water results in higher energy levels and overall greater health.

- Removing chlorine from showering water results in better air quality throughout the house.

- Without the drying effects of chlorine, skin becomes softer, healthier, and younger looking.

- Removing chlorine from showering water reduces the presence of skin rashes and the appearance of wrinkles.

- Because the hair is able to preserve its natural moisturizing oils, it becomes softer and healthier when chlorine is removed from showering water.

- When the body is able to retain its natural moisturizers, the need for costly lotions and moisturizers is greatly reduced.

- Vaporized, inhaled chlorine damages lungs, as the chlorine turns into a gas. (Think hot shower.)

- Multiple studies reported by the CDC demonstrate that that there is a link between chlorinated water and bladder, kidney, and rectal cancer and it is known to cause asthma and allergy attacks.

- Exposure to vaporized chlorine is 100 times more damaging than drinking chlorinated tap water. (U.S Council of Environmental Quality.)

- In our modern day, industrialized society we are exposed to more than 75,000 toxic environmental chemical pollutants. Our public water supplies are known to contain 2,100 of these. Most, if not all of these toxins can be inhaled and absorbed while showering.

Reducing our exposure to toxins is critically important to our optimal health and wellbeing. A shower filter is a great and effective way to do so.

I use the Sprite Shower Filter model#: SL2-CM.

An enjoyable detoxifying method is taking an Epsom salt bath. Don't forget to reward yourself for all your hard work. Our skin is our biggest organ so you will absorb the magnesium from the Epsom salts while relaxing and soaking.

Filter your bath water just like your shower water, as you do not want to defeat the purpose by absorbing the same aforementioned tap water toxins through your skin while bathing.

Epsom salt bath benefits:

- Epsom salts have been used to treat a variety of health ailments by numerous cultures for centuries.

- Epsom salt baths have amazing health benefits and are an excellent way to relax, de-stress, and detoxify the whole body.

- Unlike other naturally occurring salts, Epsom salts are formed from a pure mineral compound containing magnesium and sulfate. These minerals are absorbed through your skin while taking an Epsom salt bath.

- More than 325 enzymes in the body require magnesium to function properly. Magnesium stimulates nerve and muscle function, limits inflammation, and improves oxygenation and blood flow through the body.

- Epsom salts have been shown to improve many conditions associated with inflammation and to provide pain relief by pulling out harmful toxins, and improving both mineral and sulfur balance in the body.

- Relieves migraine headaches.

- Schedule 40 minutes in the tub for an effective Epsom salts bath treatment. Within the first 20 minutes of treatment the salts pull toxins out of your body through the skin. The second 20 minutes allows for the absorption of minerals to occur.

- Use approximately 1/2 cup of Epsom salts for every 50 pounds of weight. (An individual weighing 150 lbs would use around 1.5 cups of Epsom salts for a bath treatment.)

- You should not take Epsom salt baths if you are pregnant, have exposed cuts or burns on your skin, or are severely dehydrated. People who suffer from cardiovascular disease should first consult a doctor before taking an Epsom salt bath.

Skin detox:

Daily skin brushing improves the functioning of your skin and lymphatic system and improves skin hygiene by keeping the skin free from dry, dead skin cells. Waste removal from the body is greatly enhanced, blood flow is increased, and buildup of bacteria is decreased.

I brush in the shower as part of my daily routine. Use a soft natural bristle brush. I brush from my forehead, face and neck to my arms and body, back, butt, down my legs to my toes. An invigorating, full-body scrub, that exfoliates my skin while stimulating my blood flow.

Daily bowel movements are one of your most natural and potent detoxifiers. By maintaining regularity, toxins will not build up in the colon and will be excreted from the body. Eat lots of fiber, fruits and vegetables; drink plenty of clean water, and sweat. Since our skin is our largest organ, toxins are removed through sweat: one more reason to move with purpose every day!

Most air "fresheners" that are on the market today are ironically polluting the air with harmful industrial chemicals and contain an array of toxic chemicals, most notably phthalates. Phthalates have been directly linked to cancer and hormone disruption. Not only that, but plug-in type fresheners coat your nasal passages with an oil film called methoxychlor, which will kill the nerves in your nose over time, inhibiting your ability to smell.

Wash new clothing at least once before wearing. New clothes are contaminated with chemicals and dyes that can lead to skin irritations and other health issue. Insects like lice and scabies can be transmitted as well. Someone contaminated may have tried the clothes on before you. If buying clothing mail order or online, these items may have been returned and repackaged. Most are made in a foreign country. In addition, most clothing is wrapped in plastic and from the heat of shipping, chemicals can leach onto the garment.

You might be surprised to learn that cotton is considered the world's dirtiest crop due to the cotton industry's heavy use of hazardous herbicides and insecticides, including some of the most hazardous insecticides on the market.

According to the Organic Trade Association, cotton is considered the world's 'dirtiest' crop due to its heavy use of insecticides, including the most hazardous pesticide to human and animal health. Cotton covers 2.5% of the world's cultivated land yet uses 16% of the world's insecticides, more than any other single major crop.

Producing a textile from the plants involves more chemicals in the process of bleaching, sizing, dying, straightening, shrink reduction, stain and odor resistance, fireproofing, mothproofing, and static- and wrinkle-reduction.

Unless the clothing you buy is organic, it also is likely made from genetically engineered (GE) cotton that is heavily treated with pesticides and other chemicals during production.

This information comes from the Organic Consumers Association (OCA).

What types of illnesses could you potentially get from trying on contaminated clothes? Organisms that cause hepatitis A, traveler's diarrhea, MRSA, salmonella, norovirus, yeast infections, and streptococcus are all fair game when it comes to clothing items tried on by multiple people.

Formaldehyde resins are also used in clothing to cut down on wrinkling and mildew. Not only is formaldehyde a known carcinogen, but the resins have been linked to eczema and may cause your skin to become flaky or erupt in a rash or hives, particularly if your immune system is not functioning well.

NO

Say NO to ALL these Chemicals and Toxins:

- No parabens

- No synthetic colors

- No synthetic fragrances

- No phthalates

- No Bisphenol A (BPA)

- No sodium lauryl sulfate (SLS)

- No Mono or Diethanolamine (MEA, DEA)

- No polyvinyl chlorides (PVCs)

- No polyethylene glycols (PEGs)

- No 1, 4 Dioxane

- No propylene glycol

- No formaldehyde

- No mineral oil

- No hydrated oils

- No animal byproducts

- No gluten or wheat

- No GMOs

CHAPTER 16:
Oxidative Stress

Unbeknownst to many people, oxygen is both a blessing and a curse. Humans need oxygen in order to live, yet the simple act of breathing in oxygen results in the formation of highly reactive molecules called free radicals. As the free radicals interact with other molecules in the body, they cause oxidative damage that can result in the development of a wide range of illnesses and diseases.

Oxidative stress occurs when our system is overwhelmed by an abundance of free radicals, damaging and destroying our cells, leading to chronic inflammation. Chronic inflammation contributes to most degenerative diseases, including heart attack, stroke, and cancer.

Sugar and its processing by the body cause oxidative stress. Additionally, oxidative stress occurs when the production of reactive oxygen is greater than the body's ability to detoxify the reactive intermediates. This imbalance leads to oxidative damage to proteins, molecules, and genes within the body. Since the body is incapable of keeping up with the detoxification of the free radicals, the damage continues to spread.

Free radicals occur naturally within the body, and for the most part, the body's natural antioxidants can manage their detoxification. But there are certain external factors that can trigger the production of these damaging free radicals, including:

- Excessive exposure to UV rays

- Pollution

- Smoking

- Eating an unhealthy diet

- Excessive exercise

- Certain medications and/or treatments

The body naturally produces antioxidants like superoxide dismutase, catalase, and an assortment of peroxidase enzymes, as a means of defending itself against free radicals. The antioxidants neutralize the free radicals, thereby rendering them harmless to other cells.

Unfortunately, the antioxidants produced naturally by the body are not enough to neutralize all of the free radicals in the body. Therefore, a constant supply of external sources of antioxidants should be a part of one's daily diet, in order to reduce oxidative stress and related damage

Antioxidants have the remarkable ability to repair damaged molecules by donating hydrogen atoms to the molecules. Some antioxidants even have a chelating effect on free radical production that's catalyzed by heavy metals. In this situation, the antioxidant contains the heavy metal molecules so strongly that the chemical reaction necessary to create a free radical never occurs. When the chelating antioxidant is water-soluble, it also causes the removal of the heavy metals from the body via the urine.

Flavenoid antioxidants actually attach themselves to your DNA, forming a barrier of protection against free radical attacks, while some antioxidants even have the ability to cause some types of cancer cells to self-destruct in a process called apoptosis (cell death).

Astaxanthin is one of the most complete antioxidant sources available, and one of the most effective against oxidative stress and free radicals. I take it, as well as R-Lipoic Acid and Glutathione: together they are the three most powerful antioxidants.

Good health and wellness is about creating a life that feels good on the inside, not just looks good on the outside. You can look skinny on the outside, but be fat on the inside, literally rusting (oxidizing) from the inside out. You may have visceral (dangerous) fat around your internal organs. Your blood and veins could be full of gunk and you wouldn't even know it until it's too late.

CHAPTER 17:
Calories

D on't fall for the calories in, calories out mantra. Burn more than you take in, as in a calorie deficit. Calories are not created equal: calorie quality is more important than calorie quantity.

It helps in losing weight to have a calorie deficit diet and burn fat, not sugar, but if you eat a nutrition-rich and low-carb diet, it is hard to not lose weight. Exercise has many benefits, one of which is burning calories to help accomplish a calorie deficit.

The wrong carbohydrates and refined carbs, including flour, cereal grains, starchy vegetables, sugars and high fructose corn syrup, literally make us accumulate fat, driving hunger, making us sedentary and obese, sick, tired and eventually, dead.

Calories are burned primarily in the muscle cells. Losing muscle means you lose calorie burning ability and gain fat much more easily.

Avoid alcohol. Alcohol is recognized as a toxic substance by the body and there is no place to store it, so it burns and disposes of it before anything else, so if you want to lose weight, you must eliminate alcohol. Once you have established your ideal weight and are in maintenance mode, then wine, vodka or tequila are the least harmful.

Larger portions mean more calories.

All calories aren't created equal. Sugar calories do more harm than fats, starches, and complex carbohydrates.

If reducing calories-in doesn't make us lose weight over the long term – since with most fad diets you lose weight to begin with for a short duration, but usually gain it back long term – and if increasing calories-out (burned) doesn't prevent us from gaining weight, then what does? Could it be the quality of our nutrition and not the quantity?

Some foods create body fat – other foods do not create body fat. A calorie is simply a measurement, like an inch, yard, or mile are measurements.

When humans starve themselves, they consume their muscles as food. That eventually includes the heart muscle, so calories-in, calories-out is not a good model, nor is simply eating less or burning more calories than we consume. The take-home message here is quality nutrition over quantity of calories. Simply cut out the sugar and wheat.

Eat low carbs, high-quality fats and moderate proteins, along with fiber, throw in the right kind of exercise and supplementation and you're on your way!

Scientific fact: We don't get fat because we overeat; we overeat because we're getting fat.

Published in the British journal The Lancet Diabetes & Endocrinology: Low-carbohydrate diets "led to significantly greater weight loss" than did low-fat ones. People assigned low-fat diets tended to lose a small amount of weight compared to no-change-in-diet control groups, but cutting carbs delivered better results than reducing dietary fat. "The science does not support low-fat diets as the optimal long-term weight loss strategy," lead author Deirdre Tobias of Brigham and Women's Hospital and Harvard Medical School said in a press release.

The study marks the latest indication that a fat-free diet habit is not likely doing you any favors by cutting your fat intake. But its sugary jolt may be doing more harm than you already realized. That's the suggestion of another new study, published in the journal *Obesity*, by a team led by longtime sugar critic Robert Lustig, a pediatric endocrinologist in at the University of California at San Francisco.

Lustig is a proponent of the idea that all calories aren't created equal, and specifically, that added sugars (in sodas, processed foods, etc.) do more harm than calorie-equivalent amounts of fats, starches, and complex carbohydrates. Both studies reinforce an emerging consensus that fat is not necessarily a dietary devil, while demonizing sugar at typical American levels. Sugar might just be the culprit.

Thermodynamics involves energy used up by the process of making nutrients available to your body. Calories are energy, so the idea is to feed your body nutrient-dense, real whole foods so your body burns efficiently, clean and high test, premium fuel. Get the best bang for your calorie buck.

Don't count calories. Count nutrition. If you're seeking to lose or maintain weight, counting calories is usually less than helpful. In fact, focusing on calories could easily divert you from the real answer, which lies in optimizing your nutrition.

As we age, we lose muscle mass every year. Muscle burns calories even at rest and while we sleep. So it's important to maintain our lean muscle mass. The only way to do that is with exercise: not cardio, but with resistance training. Whether you're doing calisthenics, like jumping jacks and pushups, weight training, or machine circuit training, which I prefer, add a program of resistance training, coupled with daily cardio by walking at least 20-30 minutes a day. Remember, weight maintenance is 80% nutrition and 20% exercise. You cannot overcome a poor diet on the treadmill.

To lose weight and improve your health, replace empty calories and denatured foods with nutrient-rich choices. According to the calorie myth, in order to lose weight, all you need to do is follow the equation of "eat less, move more." But we are finding that this simply isn't true.

CHAPTER 18:
Margarine

Margarines are generally 40% trans fat or 45% vegetable oil. Margarine is a fake fat, a liquid plastic. Do not eat. Avoid at all costs. Eat real butter from grass-fed animals or Ghee (clarified butter).

Margarine is not only liquid plastic, a fake food, but a heart attack in a tub, just waiting to wage war on your body, a Trojan horse disguised as butter, but loaded with trans fats and other chemical toxins. Trans fats contribute to cardiovascular disease, heart attack, stroke, cancer, bone problems, hormone imbalance, infertility, low birth weight, child growth problems, and learning disabilities.

CHAPTER 19:
Corn

Corn is not a vegetable. It is a high-carbohydrate grain used to fatten up livestock and the livers of ducks and geese for foie gras (which literally means fatty liver). Corn will fatten you, too. Ninety percent of corn grown in the US is GMO, high in toxins, and nutritionally inferior, containing glyphosate and Bt toxin and heavily processed, potentially causing a range of ill health consequences. Don't consume it.

Polyunsaturated vegetable oils, including corn, canola, and soybean oils, create oxidized cholesterol and inflict damage on your health.

Despite being generally less expensive than other vegetable oils, a huge factor for consumers to consider with corn oil is the staggering amount of subsidies in the US. Corn is the most heavily subsidized crop in the country, receiving over 77 billion dollars from the government between 1995 and 2010, which helps unhealthy foods, such as those containing corn oil and high-fructose corn syrup (HFCS) to easily undersell healthier alternatives.

Some of the worst foods you can consume are those cooked with polyunsaturated vegetable oils and corn oils. The introduction of oxidized cholesterol into your system is a big concern. It converts good cholesterol into bad cholesterol, which leads directly to vascular disease. Hydrogenated oils increase both breast cancer and heart disease risk.

Marketing ploy: Corn oil is erroneously referred to as vegetable oil when it is not.

The harm from using corn oil as well as vegetable oils for cooking is not just the oxidized cholesterol they create (which significantly increases your risk for coronary heart disease), but also their very high amount of omega-6 fats, which throws your omega-6 vs. omega-3 ratio in the body out of balance. Corn oil is reported to have an omega-6 to omega-3 ratio of 49:1, a very long leap from the ideal 1:1 ratio. The standard American diet already has far too much omega-6, and the serious distortion of the ratio increases your risk of many degenerative diseases, including obesity, type 2 diabetes, heart attack, stroke, and cancer.

CHAPTER 20:
Soy

Soy produced in the US is 95% GMO. Unfortunately, many Americans who are committed to healthy lifestyles have been duped and manipulated into believing that unfermented and processed soy products like soymilk, soy cheese, soy burgers, and soy ice cream are good for them.

Asian cultures have been consuming fermented soy products such as natto, tempeh, and soy sauce and enjoying the health benefits for years. Fermented soy does not wreak havoc on your body like unfermented soy products do.

From 1992 to 2006, soy food sales in the US increased from $300 million to nearly $4 billion. This growth came about due to a massive shift in attitudes about soy. This was no accident. It was the result of massive advertising by the soy industry. Soy is very big business. From 2000 to 2007, US food manufacturers introduced more than 2,700 new soy-based foods.

- As of 2007, 85% of consumers perceive soy products as healthful.

- 33% of Americans eat soy foods or beverages at least once a month.

- 70% of consumers believe soybean oil is good for them.84% of consumers agree with the FDA's claim that consuming 25 grams of soy protein daily reduces your risk of heart disease.

This is a tragic case of shrewd marketing and outright lies resulting in huge profits for the soy industry and impaired health of most consumers who have been deceived into using unfermented soy as a nutritional and health food. There are large amounts of scientific research showing that soy is not healthy, and is, in fact, detrimental to your health on a number of different levels.

Thousands of studies link soy to malnutrition, digestive distress, immune-system breakdown, thyroid dysfunction, cognitive decline, reproductive disorders and infertility, cancer and heart disease. A sampling of health effects linked to soy consumption include breast cancer, brain damage, infant abnormalities, thyroid disorders, kidney stones, immune system impairment, severe and potentially fatal food allergies, impaired fertility, and pregnancy and nursing dangers.

Soy supporters argue that soy-based foods (they deceptively lump the fermented soy with the unfermented) protects you from everything from colon, prostate, and breast cancer to strokes, osteoporosis, and asthma. However, these enthusiasts never mention the studies that illustrate soy's downside and all of the dangers posed to your health, which are based on thousands of studies and research.

You have to know what you're eating ate. Eighty percent of the world's soy is used in farm animal feed.

Some soy proponents recommend that all of us become vegetarians, a dangerous recommendation and total disregard for American's health and nutrition. Soy contains natural toxins known as "anti-nutrients," such as goitrogens and estrogens, which adversely affect thyroid function. Some of these anti-nutrient factors interfere with the enzymes you need to digest protein. The amount of soy that many Americans are eating is extremely high.

Soy contains hemagglutinin, a clot-promoting substance that causes your red blood cells to clump together, making them unable to properly absorb and distribute oxygen to your tissues.

Soy contains phytates. Phytic acid binds to metal ions and prevents the absorption of certain minerals, including calcium, magnesium, iron, and zinc, all of which impact your body's biochemistry. This is particularly problematic for vegetarians, because eating meat reduces the mineral-blocking effects of these phytates, so it's helpful, if you do eat soy, to also eat meat.

Soy is loaded with the isoflavones, a type of phytoestrogen, which is a compound resembling estrogen. These compounds mimic and block the estrogen hormone and have been found to have adverse effects on various human tissues and cells. Soy phytoestrogens are known to disrupt endocrine function, (thyroid) and may cause infertility and promote breast cancer in women.

Drinking as little as two glasses of soymilk daily for one month provides enough of these compounds to alter a menstrual cycle. Although the FDA regulates estrogen-containing products, there are no warnings on soy.

Soy contains toxic levels of aluminum and manganese. Soybeans are processed by acid washing in aluminum tanks, which can leach high levels of aluminum into the final soy product. Soy formula has up to 80 times higher manganese than is found in human breast milk. Soy infant formula puts your baby's health at risk.

Nearly 20 percent of US infants are now fed soy formula, but the estrogens in soy can irreversibly harm your baby's sexual development and reproductive health. Infants fed soy formula take in an estimated equivalent of five birth control pills daily. Infants fed soy formula have up to 20,000 times the amount of estrogen in circulation as those fed other formulas. Always breast feed if you can.

Soy is both heavily sprayed with pesticides and genetically modified. Since the introduction of GMO foods in 1996, we've had an increase in low birth weight babies, infertility, and other problems in the US population. Multiple studies and research have shown you may simply want to avoid soy products altogether, not only avoiding GMO foods and their potential health problems, but avoiding becoming a lab rat in this massive, uncontrolled, human experiment by the biotech and food industries.

We were already duped into one of the largest human experiments in history, the diet-heart experiment of a low-fat, high-carbohydrate diet for the last 50 years. This has led our healthcare system to the brink of collapse and has produced epidemic proportions of obesity, type 2 diabetes, cardiovascular disease, heart attack, stroke, and cancer.

Soy can be healthful, but only if it is organic and properly fermented. After a long fermentation process, the phytate and "anti-nutrient" levels of soybeans are reduced, and their beneficial properties become available to your digestive system. Japanese people live longer and have lower rates of cancer than Americans because they eat healthy fermented soy products:

- Tempeh a fermented soybean cake with a firm texture and nutty, mushroom-like flavor. Tempeh is referred to as "vegetarian cheese."

- Miso, a fermented soybean paste with a salty, buttery texture, commonly used in miso soup and served at Sushi restaurants.

- Natto, a fermented soybean with a sticky texture and strong, cheese-like flavor.

- Soy sauce, which is traditionally made by fermenting soybeans, salt and enzymes. However, read the label, as many varieties are made artificially using a chemical process.

- Tofu is not fermented and is not among the healthy soy foods you should consume.

Soy foods to avoid include tofu, texturized vegetable protein, and soy protein isolate, which contains a large amount of MSG, soybean oil, soymilk, soy cheese, soy ice cream, soy yogurt, soy "meat," meatless products made, of edamame, soy lecithin, and soy infant formula.

Eliminate all non-fermented soy from your diet by avoiding all processed foods. Purchase whole foods. Check the label on all packaged and processed foods to see if it soy is listed.

The Food Allergen Labeling and Consumer Protection Act, which took effect in January 2006, requires that food manufacturers list soy on the label, because it's one of the top eight food allergens. Even if soy is hidden in other ingredients it must be clearly listed on the label.

Educate yourself. Become knowledgeable about the research and read the labels. Soy is pervasive in more than food products. It can be found in vitamins, supplements and many personal, non-food products – over 2,700 in all. I recommend passing on all soy, except for the fermented soy listed above.

CHAPTER 21:
Omega 3s vs Omega 6s

You need adequate levels of omega-3 fatty acids and polyphenols to control and extinguish diet-induced inflammation with proper nutritional balance of low-glycemic carbs and protein, reduced consumption of omega-6s, and a significant increase of omega-3s and polyphenols. By reducing diet-induced cellular inflammation, you will lose excess body fat, maintain desirable weight, decrease your risk of modern chronic diseases, retard the aging process, become more efficient at metabolizing food for energy (burning fat instead of sugar), and you won't have hunger cravings for junk foods. Your body will actually start craving healthy foods.

Ninety-five percent of your cell membranes are made of fat, so if you don't feed your body a rich source of omega-3 fatty acids from wild-caught Alaskan Salmon such as Sockeye, your body will not thrive. Wild salmon eats what nature prescribed for them: a complete nutritional profile of macronutrients, fats, minerals magnesium, potassium and selenium, and all the B vitamins and antioxidants like astaxanthin.

Omega-3 fatty acids reign supreme in maintaining cell walls that keep the body's hormonal receptors in a positive position to best interact with their environment. omega-3 fatty acids are essential to the fat-loss process because of their effect on hormone sensitivity.

Omega-3s are anti-inflammatory. Omega-6s are pro-inflammatory. Omega-3 is used by every cell in your body.

Do not buy or consume fish packed in oil (because it drains the omega-3s), BPA canned, GMO fish, farmed fish, blue-fin tuna, swordfish, shark, orange roughy, marlin, Chilean sea bass, tilapia, Asian-imported fish, canned salmon or smoked salmon with added sugars or artificial colors.

Omega-6s are Pro-inflammatory, omega-3s are anti-inflammatory.

- 1:1-1:3 ratio is optimal

- 16:1 or higher is SAD.

- 25:1 to 50:1 is a Fast Foodie

Buy all canned fish packed in water. If it is packed in oil, rinse it thoroughly because you don't know the quality of oil. Water doesn't permeate or absorb into the fish like oil does. Oil is also usually accompanied by high sodium, which is another reason to rinse.

When poultry and cattle are raised in harmony with nature, consuming the foods they were meant to eat, the omega-3 to omega-6 ratio in their meat, eggs, and milk tends to balance out at or around 2:1 or 1:1, which is considered optimal. Feedlot animals, on the other hand, produce meat, eggs, and milk with abnormally high levels of omega-6 fats and very little omega-3 fats, creating conditions in the body favorable to cancer growth.

Our dual epidemics of obesity and diabetes are direct results of the SAD (Standard American Diet) with its imbalance of omega-6s (pro-inflammatory) vs omega-3s (anti-inflammatory), creating increased cellular inflammation and hence, increased diseases, CVD, heart attacks, strokes, and cancer.

Up to 80% of heart attacks and strokes, our top killers, are preventable through proper nutrition.

Omega-6s become rancid inside the body due to oxidation, causing inflammation. Oxidized LDL leads to accelerated heart disease and increased heart attacks and stroke. The dietary target is to decrease omega-6s while increasing polyphenols, powerful antioxidants, through nutrition by increasing vegetables and fruits consumption.

Where do omega-6 fatty acids come from: vegetable oils, corn oil, soybean oil, safflower oil, sunflower oil, grains, corn and wheat. To exacerbate the problem, most are GMOs. These products are prone to oxidation in the body which causes free radical damage.

Diet-induced inflammation is caused by increased insulin levels and increased omega-6 fatty acids. The combination of the two is an explosion of diet-induced inflammation, like a match to gasoline.

Americans having been eating a diet of increased insulin production for over 40 years

– a high-carbohydrate diet loaded with sugar, wheat, grains, and processed foods – an unprecedented increase in dietary omega-6s, well as too many calories. As insulin levels have increased, so has the incidence of obesity and chronic diseases. This diet-induced cellular inflammation lingers for years or even decades, until there is enough organ and vascular damage to generate chronic diseases, heart disease, stroke, cancer, diabetes, weight gain, premature aging, Alzheimer's, and death.

Atlantic salmon is 99% aqua-farmed and represents 90% of the salmon consumed in the US. Much of it farmed in China. It is fed grain, corn, and soy, most containing GMOs, to fatten and enlarge the fish, much like cattle, so the salmon loses its beneficial omega-3 fats.

Wild-caught salmon has a 6-10 to 1 omega-3 to omega-6 ratio, while Atlantic salmon is 3-4 to 1 omega-6 to omega-3. Aqua-farmed salmon is fed pellets containing pink dye to give it a pink color, but if you ever see it side-by-side at the store with wild caught Sockeye Salmon, which is rich in omega-3 and a deep, dark, healthy salmon color. Atlantic salmon looks pale, sick and unhealthy by comparison.

The average American diet today is a 10-20 to 1 omega-6 to omega-3 ratio, and some are as high as 30 to 1. That's 10-30 times higher than our evolutionary ancestors, who never died of inflammation-driven diseases such as heart disease, obesity, diabetes, or cancer.

The only dietary strategy shown to actually increase lifespan in laboratory animals has been calorie restriction. When humans try calorie restriction on the Standard American Diet – a high-carb, low-fat, omega-6 rich diet that's been preached for years – we fail miserably, because we're hungry all the time and overeat.

With a diet lower in carbs, moderate in protein, higher in fat and higher in fiber from vegetables and fruits, we're more satiated. Our appetite is under control. Insulin, the hunger hormone, is no longer out of control. Blood sugar is managed. Weight becomes stabilized and we eat fewer calories, thereby restricting calories naturally. It is an anti-aging recipe. Sound like a plan?

CHAPTER 22:
Eggs

E at pasture-raised, organic eggs and poultry – not cage-free or free-range. (If labeled as free-range, like at Trader Joe's, ask if free-range is pasture-raised or just a small outdoor pen, which is still a confined area.)

The $9-billion egg industry produces 96% of its eggs in barns full of stacked wire cages. Hardly cage-free, free-range or pasture-raised.

Cage-free and free-range are marketing slogans for the egg carton and is hyperbole to make you think the chickens were raised humanely, so you would buy them.

Cage-free means the chickens are able to maneuver outside their wire cages and walk around a barn or confinement shelter, but are still fed traditional grain-based feeds or pellets, and are still confined and not able to roam in a natural pasture and forage for their natural diet.

Free-range means the chickens are able to get out of their wire cages, walk around the confinement area and then have a small penned-in area outside the confinement area to walk around, but not forage for the natural food source on grass and pasture. Most industrial farm confinement shelters and pens have concrete floors and are not grass or pasture, and the chickens are walking around in their own muck.

So, when buying eggs, look for pasture-raised, organic eggs and poultry and ignore the marketing ploys of "Cage-Free" and "Free-Range."

Not only do you need to know where your food comes from and who made it – you need to know what you are eating and what you are eating ate.

Organic pasture-raised eggs contain superior nutrients to factory raised eggs:

- 2/3 more vitamin A

- 3 times more vitamin E

- 2 times more Omega 3s

- 7 times more beta carotene

CHAPTER 23:
Stop Smoking

"There is only one good, knowledge, and one evil, ignorance." – Socrates

If I were a smoker, I'd be dead from my stroke.

Stop smoking! Smoking is the leading cause of avoidable death. Tobacco smoke contains more than 7,000 chemicals, including carcinogens, toxic metals, and poisonous gases.

Smokers are 5 times more likely to have a heart attack or stroke than non-smokers and 10 times more likely to develop cancer. Non-smokers live an average of 9.7 years longer than smokers. Smoking harms nearly every organ in the body, causes many diseases, and reduces health in general.

Smoking depletes practically every known protective vitamin and mineral your body needs. It wreaks havoc on your cardiovascular system. Nicotine constricts blood vessels, which raises blood pressure. It increases the fats that circulate in your blood (like cholesterol). Cigarette smoke contains carbon monoxide, which decreases the blood's ability to carry oxygen, in turn forcing the heart to work harder. Quitting smoking can naturally lower blood pressure levels 5 to 10 points.

Smoking carries toxins and free radicals that oxidize LDL, triglycerides, and the arterial walls or endothelium, increasing homocysteine levels. As a result, it greatly increases the risk of cardiovascular disease, heart attack, stroke, and cancer.

If you smoke, stop. If you don't smoke, don't start. Nothing should be simpler to understand. It is one of the most important decisions in your life.

- Smokers are 5 times more likely to die from pneumonia.

- Smokers have a 48% increased colon cancer risk.

- Smokers have a 1.7-fold increased risk of Crohn's disease.

- Smokers have a 129% increased risk in developing fatty liver disease.

- Smokers have a 2-fold increase in risk of dying from ALS or Lou Gehrig's disease.

CHAPTER 24:
Metabolic Syndrome

High blood pressure (hypertension), high cholesterol, high triglycerides, endothelial dysfunction, (atherosclerosis), type 2 diabetes, and obesity are all preventable and reversible through lifestyle factors, diet, nutrition, exercise and supplementation.

Metabolic syndrome is not so much age-related as age-accelerating.

Metabolic syndrome: obesity, type 2 diabetes (elevated blood sugar), lipid disturbances (high cholesterol), and hypertension (high blood pressure). Inflammation, oxidative stress, glycation, atherosclerosis combined with high blood pressure is a deadly combination of markers that lead to strokes and heart attacks. Most are reversible with lifestyle changes and dietary therapies.

You have metabolic syndrome if at least 3 of the following are present:

- Waist circumference over 40" (men) or 35" (women). Waist should be half your height.

- Fasting triglycerides: 150 mg/dL or above.

- HDL-C: 40 mg/dL or below (men) or 50 mg/dL or below (women).

- Blood Pressure: 130/85mmHg or use blood pressure medication.

- Fasting glucose: 100 mg/dL or above or use hyperglycemia medications.

Sixty-four million American adults have metabolic syndrome. That's one-fourth of all Americans, one-third of all adults, and one-half of adults over age 60. These people have a whopping 74% increased risk of dying from a heart attack or stroke.

Eighty million Americans have high blood pressure and don't know it. Hypertension can lead to heart attacks, strokes, and kidney failure. The first symptom is often death.

Blood pressure increases with age due to atherosclerosis, hardening of the arteries, plaque, endothelial dysfunction and stenosis. This causes your heart to work harder, not only causing higher blood pressure, but weakening your heart muscle and causing premature death.

The good news is, this can be prevented, treated, and even reversed. You must monitor your BP on a regular basis. Like weighing yourself regularly, you must weigh your BP, so to speak. The BP scale is a cuff monitor you can buy at a pharmacy. (Details under Tools.) If you don't measure it, you can't improve it. This is true with not only weight, but blood pressure and blood tests. Your health depends on it.

When we're younger our body is able to compensate for our unhealthy choices. These unhealthy choices build up year after year in our veins and tissues, turning into metabolic syndrome. As we age and our waistlines expand, we lose control of blood sugar, our blood pressure increases, and we have a higher the risk of atherosclerosis, heart disease, heart attacks and strokes.

Excessive insulin secretion and insulin resistance cause metabolic syndrome. Elevated insulin and leptin levels are typically the cause of hypertension (high blood pressure, AKA "the silent killer"). Implementing strategies to normalize these levels are the first step to resolving hypertension and the cascade of metabolic syndrome.

High fructose corn syrup (HFCS), wreaks the most biochemical havoc by negatively affecting your leptin and insulin sensitivity, which results in metabolic syndrome.

CHAPTER 25:
Obesity

O besity is overtaking smoking as the principal cause of cancer. Look at obesity as the canary in the coal mine.

Obesity is a biochemical problem. Ultimately, obesity is a problem caused by a toxic and addictive food environment, not behavior.

More than 2.1 billion people, or close to 30 percent of the global population, are overweight or obese. Obesity is responsible for about five percent of all worldwide deaths each year. In the US, nearly one in five deaths is now associated with obesity.

The average adult with sustained obesity has less than a 1% chance of attaining and maintaining a healthy bodyweight. So prevention would seem the key. Obesity's consequences are type 2 diabetes, heart attack, stroke, and cancer. Stress causes obesity.

A recent study shows that 3/4 of men and 2/3 of women in the US are overweight or obese. That's more than a 10% increase since the 1990s. That translates to 67.6 million overweight 65.2 million obese Americans.

Of adults 20 and older, 68.8% are considered overweight and 35.7% are obese. If you are obese or overweight you most likely have type 2 diabetes and insulin resistance, leading to inflammation and inflammation is the leading cause of most degenerative diseases including heart attack, stroke, and cancer. By 2048, if the current rates were to continue, all American adults would be overweight or obese.

According to the CDC (Centers for Disease Control), in 2014, 29 million American adults had diabetes, with another 86 million at high risk of getting the chronic disease. If the current trends continue, federal health officials predicted that one in five Americans could have diabetes by 2025 – one in three by 2050. The CDC said more than 12 percent of US adults had diabetes as of 2012.

Once obesity becomes a way of life, free-radicals slow our metabolism and decreasing amounts of hormones prevent us from efficiently burning the calories we consume.

Subcutaneous fat vs. visceral fat. You may not be obese and still have dangerous visceral fat. SOFI stands for: *Skinny* on the *Outside* and *Fat* on the *Inside*. The beer belly or soda belly. Visceral fat is the worst kind. It wraps itself around your internal organs, putting you at risk for CVE and diabetes. I see SOFI's every day on the treadmill.

When you're insulin resistant, it means your cells have become seriously impaired in their ability to respond to the insulin your body makes. At the heart of this problem is a diet too high in sugar, especially processed high fructose corn syrup.

Insulin resistance = carbohydrate intolerance.

While you can be insulin resistant and lean, obesity places far greater stress on your cells, which makes insulin resistance more probable. Insulin resistance is at the core of nearly every chronic degenerative disease.

Obesity is actually malnutrition. Lifestyle and diet changes are better than drug prescriptions.

The chemical makeup of highly processed foods can trigger cravings for the same food, which leads to a vicious cycle of unhealthy eating, resulting in obesity, type 2 diabetes, heart disease, stroke, and cancer.

Research presented during the 2013 American Heart Association's Epidemiology and Prevention/Nutrition, Physical Activity, and Metabolism Scientific Sessions suggested sugary beverages are to blame for about 183,000 deaths worldwide each year, including 133,000 diabetes deaths, 44,000 heart disease deaths, and 6,000 cancer deaths. A 15-year-long study, which included data for 31,000 Americans, found that those who consumed 25 percent or more of their daily calories as sugar were more than twice as likely to die from heart disease.

In the US alone, an estimated 25,000 annual deaths are attributed to the consumption of sweetened beverages like soda. The world's population is estimated to be 8.1 billion people in 2030, so that means 1 in 8 people, or 12.5% of the world's population, is obese. What will that mean to our healthcare system? Big Pharma is salivating over the potential profits.

Eventually, I wouldn't be surprised if the soda industry ends up facing class-action lawsuits similar to those filed against the tobacco industry, as sodas and other sweetened beverages are now scientifically linked to the obesity and diabetes epidemic.

Nearly one in five US deaths is associated with obesity, and one in every three deaths is attributed to cardiovascular disease, which includes heart attacks and stroke. According to a 2013 report from the US Center for Disease Control and Prevention (CDC), of the 800,000 cardiovascular disease deaths occurring in the US each year, a quarter of them, about 200,000, could be prevented through simple lifestyle changes.

According to statistics found in the Credit Suisse Research Institute's 2013 study, sugar consumption accounts for up to 40 percent of US healthcare expenditures for diseases directly related to the over-consumption of sugar. We spend more than a trillion dollars each year fighting the damaging health effects of sugar.

The US has exported obesity around the world with its fast food chains and subsidized, cheap grains, corn, and soy. Obesity worldwide is now an epidemic.

"The American Way" in developing countries around the world is led by Coco-Cola, McDonald's, Subway, Kentucky Fried Chicken and the huge conglomerate of American commercial processed food companies and the US government with its cheap subsidized grains.

No country in the world has been able to replace hunger without obesity and the health issues resulting in death. Why? Importing the "American Way" includes a diet of processed or fast foods, rich in refined sugars, carbohydrates, trans fats, and cheap grains, a recipe for illness and premature death. Commercial food companies have fundamentally altered our traditional diets, impacting our food choices, our weight, and ultimately our health.

The human system only needs 5 grams or 1 teaspoon of sugar to function. An order of medium fries at McDonald's contains 47 grams of carbohydrates, which converts to 47 grams of sugar, which is almost 10 teaspoons. So, when you eat those fries you're putting 10 times more sugar into your blood than is required to maintain a normal blood sugar level. If you figure that one quarter of a teaspoon is all the difference between a normal blood sugar and a diabetic blood sugar, the 10 full teaspoons would be 40 times that amount.

Since your metabolic system has to work very hard to deal with the sugar overload from an order of fries, imagine what it has to do when you add a large soft drink, a hamburger, and maybe an apple turnover for dessert. When you see the long lines of cars in the drive-through window and the long lines of customers at the counter inside, you can see why the incidence of obesity and type 2 diabetes is skyrocketing and America is sick, tired, fat and dying.

Break the stereotype, beat obesity. Live longer and be happy.

CHAPTER 26:
Insulin/Insulin Resistance/Type 2 Diabetes

There are two basic ways to raise insulin levels: first is to eat too many carbohydrates; second is to eat too many calories. Americans do both.

Type 2 diabetes is the end result of years of dietary abuse and nutritional wear-and-tear leading to disease.

- As of 2011 there were 26 million American diabetics, 7 million undiagnosed.

- In 2012, 29.1 million, or 9.3% of the population, had diabetes, 8.1 million undiagnosed.

- Cardiovascular disease is present in 75% of diabetes-related deaths; 68.8% of adults 20 and older are considered overweight or obese, 35.7% obese.

- 80% of the 17 million Americans with diabetes are insulin-resistant. Insulin resistance is reversible and type 2 diabetes is curable.

- 26.9% of Americans 65 or older have diabetes.

If you are obese or overweight you most likely have type 2 diabetes and insulin resistance leading to inflammation, the leading cause of most degenerative diseases including heart attack, stroke, and cancer.

Excess insulin:

- Stimulates excess cholesterol production;

- Stimulates insulin resistance;

- Elevates blood pressure;

- Prompts kidneys to retain salt and fluids, which adds to blood volume, increasing blood pressure even more;

- Promotes thickness and rigidity of artery endothelium walls, making them less flexible;

- Constricts blood vessels, raising the heart rate;

- Plays several key roles in atherosclerosis, plaque and hardening of the arteries, obstructing blood flow; and

- Increases the liver's production of LDL cholesterol, promoting accumulation of cholesterol beneath the endothelium arterial lining, leading to cardiovascular disease, heart attack and stroke.

Because the heart has to work harder and requires greater pressure to force blood through the hardened narrow arteries throughout the body, elevated blood pressure is the result.

Excess insulin and insulin resistance are preventable, reversible, and curable by controlling what you do or don't put into your mouth. You are the boss, and you are in control. Simply give your body the proper nutritional tools and it will heal itself.

One-third of Americans are insulin-resistant. A low-carb diet helps reduce insulin resistance and increase insulin sensitivity, which is what you want. Insulin and its behavior are critically important to longevity. Insulin is the master hormone of metabolism and life, affecting virtually every cell in the body.

In addition to regulating blood sugar, insulin controls storage of fat, directs flow of amino acids, fatty acids and carbohydrates to muscles and tissues, regulates the liver's synthesis of cholesterol, functions as a growth hormone, controls appetite, and drives the kidneys to retain fluid. Excess insulin circulation not only creates systemic chronic inflammation; it also works to create new fat cells.

Regular eating stabilizes blood sugar and your body releases insulin to utilize food as fuel, rather than storing it as fat.

In short, insulin works to increase the fat we store and decrease the fat we burn. Insulin works to make us fatter. That's why it's called the "fat storage" hormone. If carbohydrates raise insulin secretion and insulin makes us fat, why eat the kind of carbs that increase insulin, like bread, pasta, potatoes, rice, and sugar? It would make sense to restrict, limit, manage or formulate the fuel that is making you sick and fat, right? The bottom line is if you want to lose fat and burn fat as fuel, you have to decrease the amount of insulin in your system. The more of the wrong carbs you eat, the more insulin you secrete, the more fat you store, and the fatter you become. Insulin, besides being the fat-storing hormone, causes hunger and cravings.

Insulin resistance does not develop overnight. It is a slow, silent, progressive process occurring over years or decades. Insulin resistance and inflammation are interrelated, setting up a vicious cycle fueled by repeated ingestion of insulin-inducing carbohydrates. Insulin increases LDL and excess sugar damages the LDL, ultimately leading to plaque.

It's a fact that 75 percent of your cholesterol is produced by your liver, which is influenced by your insulin levels. If you optimize your insulin levels, you will also regulate your cholesterol levels.

Foods that increase your insulin levels will also contribute to high cholesterol by making your liver produce more of it.

Most type 2 diabetics are overweight or obese. This is because their fat cells are constantly maintained in fat storage mode by high levels of insulin secreted from the pancreas. This is due to high blood sugar in the bloodstream, caused by a poor diet of excess sugar, wheat, and high glycemic carbs and starches.

When you control insulin, you hugely increase the odds that you will control your weight, and you also reduce the risks of cardiovascular disease, hypertension, diabetes, inflammation, and even some cancers.

If you must eat sugar or dairy products (milk, cottage cheese, ice cream, butter, cheese) eat the healthy whole fat variety, because fat is neutral and doesn't increase insulin or blood sugar. Only drink organic, raw, grass-fed- whole milk and not 1% or 2% low-fat, because lower-fat milk processing usually replaces the fat with added lactose (sugar). Read the labels and chose the products with the least amount of sugar.

People with vitamin D deficiency have higher risk for insulin resistance, type 2 diabetes and metabolic syndrome.

Research shows that an unhealthy or high triglycerides/HDL-C ratio is highly associated with a greater degree of insulin resistance and LDL Pattern B, (small, dense LDL) increasing your risk for cardiovascular disease.

Lipid abnormalities, low HDL, high triglycerides and small, dense LDL, are all triggered by insulin resistance and the elevated insulin secretion that accompanies it, as a result of dietary carbohydrate consumption, sugars, and high-fructose corn syrup in particular.

Insulin accelerates aging by stiffening arterial walls and causing accumulation of triglycerides and cholesterol, and the building up atherosclerotic plaques. Chronically elevated insulin levels and insulin resistance cause oxidative stress and create free radicals, leading to the creation of advanced glycation end products (AGE). These cause a wide range of health issues. One of the reasons to consume foods rich in antioxidants is to help combat and even prevent oxidative stress and free radical damage. Always maintain a constant flow of antioxidant-rich nutrients and supplements circulating through your body.

Type 2 diabetes occurs when the pancreas can no longer secrete enough insulin to compensate for insulin resistance.

Cortisol is another culprit that increases insulin resistance, hence, fat storage.

There are no medications that treat excess insulin. A properly formulated and structured low-carbohydrate, healthy fat, healthy moderate protein diet is the only means. The low-fat, high-complex carbohydrate diet of the past 50 years has just the opposite effect, causing cardiovascular disease, heart attack, stroke, high blood pressure and diabetes, killing more than twice as many people every year as the combined wars of Korea and Vietnam.

Once insulin resistance is reduced, insulin levels decrease, and your body will then burn body fat stores as energy, thereby allowing you to lose weight. The only way to achieve this is by cutting your carbohydrate intake, which causes your insulin to secrete and high levels of insulin leads to fat storage and weight gain. Simple fact: eliminate or restrict sugar, grains, and starches, eat 10-13 servings of vegetables and fruits per day and you will lose weight.

Born into fatness: the higher the blood sugar in pregnant women, the more insulin-secreting cells the child will develop. The child will be born with more fat and with a tendency to over-secrete insulin, becoming insulin resistant and predisposed to fatten as it grows, in essence being pre-programmed in the womb to be fat. So, if fatter mothers have fatter babies who become fatter mothers, where does it end? That is why we have an obesity epidemic and this vicious cycle, including type 2 diabetes and diseases of inflammation, cardiovascular disease, heart attack, stroke, and cancer. Thus, not only do we have our health to consider when we get fat and eat a poor diet, we have the responsibility of our children paying the price, as well as our children's children and successive generations caught in this vicious cycle.

CHAPTER 27:
Good Oral Health/Hygiene

About half of Americans over age 30, including 70 percent of those over 65, have some form of periodontal (gum) disease, according to the CDC, but many if not most don't know it. The culprits are an estimated 10 to 20 strains of bacteria in the mouth, along with poor dental hygiene. When these bacteria build up in plaque (which then hardens into tartar), they cause chronic inflammation of the gums; this is called gingivitis and is characterized by redness and swelling, as well as bleeding during brushing and flossing. Gingivitis is a mild form of gum disease that can usually be reversed with daily brushing and flossing and professional dental cleanings.

Left untreated, however, gingivitis can advance to periodontitis, in which the gums are damaged and detach from the teeth and form pockets that become infected with bacteria. Bacterial toxins, along with enzymes released as part of the body's natural response to the infection, further irritate and inflame the gums. The immune system increases its inflammatory response to the bacteria as plaque and tartar spread below the gum line. In advanced stages, gums, bones, and other tissues that support the teeth are gradually destroyed; teeth may eventually become loose and have to be removed. Largely as a result of periodontal disease, about one in four Americans over age 75 have lost all their natural teeth.

If you don't brush and floss regularly, you're likely to develop gum disease. But its progression depends on many factors besides your oral hygiene, including genetics and how well your immune system responds. Brushing alone can't remove bacteria in tartar, in pockets, or below the gum line—this is where flossing and professional cleanings are crucial. Often a deep-cleaning method is necessary, in which tartar is scraped off at and below the gum line.

In recent years observational studies have consistently found that people who have periodontal disease are at increased risk for cardiovascular disease (CVD) and its progression to heart attacks and strokes. This has led researchers and dentists to suggest that gum disease and the bacteria that cause it can contribute to CVD—and that good oral hygiene and treatment of gum disease can help protect the heart and arteries.

The idea that dental disease can play a role in systemic disorders like CVD is biologically plausible. For one thing, oral bacteria can enter the bloodstream and affect the heart and arteries. And the inflammation involved in gum disease could conceivably trigger the inflammation that plays an important role in atherosclerosis and other chronic diseases.

If you have periodontal disease and your teeth aren't strong as you age you will have to eat softer and mushier food because you can't chew the more nutrient- and fiber-dense foods that are required. It's logical that the softer and mushier your food becomes, the softer and mushier you will become. (Think assisted living diet.)

Take care of your mouth and it will take care of you. Develop a symbiotic relationship with both your mouth and your gut. Remember, your mouth is the gateway of your food's journey into your cells. Oral health is the first line of defense against disease. Scientific evidence links poor oral health with inflammation and oxidative stress throughout the body, particularly concerning arterial health and immune function.

You can prevent many diseases by not putting their causes in your mouth to begin with, like sugars. Eating a poor nutritional diet will not only cause atherosclerosis, but periodontal disease, which, working in combination, increases the risk of CVD.

Periodontal disease creates a twin threat of bacterial infection and inflammation, which feed on each other in a vicious cycle that has disastrous systemic effects on your entire body, not just cavities and gums.

When you have gum disease, your body is in a state of chronic inflammation. Bacteria gets into the bloodstream through the gums and infected teeth. These bacteria stick to plaque in coronary arteries, narrowing the arteries even more and worsening the inflammation and atherosclerosis and the likelihood that a rupture will occur, causing a blood clot that results in a heart attack or stroke.

Diet has a huge impact on your dental health. There is a 70 percent lower risk of cardiovascular disease with good oral health. Brush and floss to your heart's content. Think of a frequent brushing and flossing routine as like a daily spa treatment for your heart.

Your health starts on the farm and the ocean, then to your plate and next to your mouth, so it's of utmost importance to start your food's journey to your stomach and eventually to your cells with a healthy mouth.

Mouth bacteria are linked to an imbalance of beneficial versus pathogenic bacteria in your gut. The addition of fermented vegetables to your diet may also prove to be an essential missing ingredient to help you successfully address this problem.

A 2010 study found that those with the worst oral hygiene increased their risk of developing CVD by a whopping 70 percent, compared to those who brush their teeth twice a day. Improved gum health was shown to significantly slow down the progression of atherosclerosis. Results show a clear relationship between what is happening in the mouth and thickening of the carotid artery, even before the onset of full-fledged periodontal disease. This suggests that early signs of periodontal disease, such as bleeding gums, should not be ignored.

Forty percent of all Americans do not see a dentist regularly. Your body is like a symphony and for the orchestra to play beautiful music all components must be interacting in concert and hitting on all cylinders. If one component is off, synchronicity is off and no synergy will be generated.

You should check with your dentist about a deep cleaning and then have regular cleanings every 3 months. In addition, brush and floss at least twice a day, in the morning and at night before bed. A Waterpik-type flossing device is also a good oral health investment.

In addition, check with your dentist to rid your mouth of all dental mercury and fillings. Mercury is a toxin. We are trying to rid our bodies of all toxins and inflammation.

When you have dental X-rays, ask for the thyroid cover as well as the chest vest protector. You do not want your thyroid exposed to X-rays.

It's important to realize that periodontal disease involves both bone and the tissue that is in contact with that bone. Bacteria and toxic inflammatory compounds can easily enter your bloodstream, where these toxic compounds can harm the lining of your blood vessels. Reducing inflammation is of primary importance for your optimal health. Brushing and flossing your teeth regularly is one way to combat chronic inflammation in your body.

Research has linked gum disease to other chronic, systemic disorders, notably diabetes, respiratory and kidney disease and even certain cancers.

Plaque and inflammation in periodontal disease has also been associated with prostate inflammation and erectile dysfunction.

Oral health is much more than a cosmetic consideration. It is necessary for not only healthy teeth and gums, but for overall health, wellness, and longevity.

CHAPTER 28:

Gut Microbiome Health-the journey continues after the mouth/Immune System

Rather than being confined to a particular organ, about 80 percent of your immune system resides in your gastrointestinal tract in the form of receptor cells. Because of this prime location, what happens in your gut powerfully influences your immune function and your health.

Our digestive anatomy is a human tube, with two openings: the oral cavity on one end and the anus on the other. They are connected by 25 to 30 feet of tubing from the esophagus, stomach, small and large intestines (colon) to the other end. We are like a worms with arms and legs and will process 60,000 to 100,000 pounds of food during our lifetime. The tube turns food into nutrients and energy allowing the body to function, grow and repair itself. How we feed and nourish that tube however, determines its final shape and life span.

Gut health is 85% good bacteria and 15% bad bacteria. When your gut health is balanced, the "good" bacteria outnumber the "bad" bacteria, fungi, yeast, and protozoa by 5 to 1. We have 100 trillion bacteria in our stomachs, 10 times more than the number of cells in our bodies.

When your gut is healthy, you have a large, thriving community of beneficial or friendly bacteria, or probiotics, supporting your immune system receptor cells. They help form a protective barrier within your colon and intestines.

The gut is our second brain and is made from the same type of tissue as our brains. Our gut is a complete ecosystem that influences all aspects of health.

Research and studies have shown that taking a probiotic supplement restores the diverse balance of "good" and "bad" gut bacteria creating natural protection and prevention against multiple diseases and a healthy gut reduces chronic inflammation, the cause of most modern diseases. Probiotics boost antioxidant and detoxification enzymes that prevent the activation of dietary carcinogens, especially colon cancer.

"L's" and "B's" refer to Lactobacillus and Bifidobacteria probiotics. I recommend a minimum of 13 billion CFUs (colony forming units). Aging gradually shifts our bacterial makeup from a disease-preventing state to a disease-promoting state.

Foods and products that feed bad bacteria or kill good bacteria include:

- Sugar

- Wheat

- Artificial sweeteners

- Antibiotics

- Advil, Motrin, Midol

- Chlorine

- Non-organic meat, chicken and dairy, because they are full of antibiotics

- Cigarettes, tobacco, alcohol and junk food

- Stress

- Radiation and chemotherapy

Your gut balance and good gut health are instrumental in manufacturing key nutrients and helping you in weight loss maintenance.

Good bacteria:

- Supports the immune system.

- Stimulates the gut mucosa to produce antibodies to pathogens.

- Produces natural antifungal and antibiotic substances.

- Produces vitamin K, which is essential for the formation and repair of our bones.

- Produces B vitamins required to maintain the muscle tone in the gastrointestinal tract that regulates digestion.

- Reduces the low-grade inflammation that can contribute to obesity.

- Uses nutrients, including vitamins, minerals, proteins, fats, and carbohydrates, making it easier to digest foods properly and efficiently, so we store less energy and fat.

- Recycles hormones, including estrogen, thyroid hormones, and phytoestrogens.

Good bacteria are known to help prevent food allergies, decrease gas, bloating, indigestion, acne, eczema, psoriasis, bad breath, colds, flu, chronic fatigue, and high cholesterol levels. This is because they properly break down the remaining nutrients of your foods, control the acidity (pH level) of the intestines, and secrete acids that less friendly microbes cannot tolerate well.

What you eat and your level of stress have a huge impact on the balance of bacteria in your gut. Incorporating foods that will build and grow your gut flora, while supporting a balanced state of mind through yoga, meditation, and other relaxation techniques, will ensure that you're building and supporting healthy flora for a lifetime.

The SAD (Standard American Diet) is devoid of most essential vitamins, minerals and nutrients and loaded with unhealthy fats, sugar, wheat, and simple carbs. It is also lacking in fiber, necessary for proper elimination of waste and toxins, and naturally occurring enzymes necessary for proper GI tract digestion.

In 2010 American doctors prescribed 258 million courses of antibiotics, approximately 8.5 prescriptions per 10 people in the US. The rise of antibiotic-resistant super-bugs is a well-documented adverse effect of widespread use of antibiotics. However, more important and far less publicized is the impact of these drugs on our resident microbes, resulting in significant collateral damage to our microbiota and taking weeks or months to recover. This can adversely affect your immune system's ability to fight other pathogens, especially in cold and flu season. Another reason not to take an antibiotic for a cold, as a cold is viral, not bacterial.

Antibiotics can destroy your gut balance for months, so if you gain weight during and after antibiotic use, it may not be a coincidence.

Most European countries have banned the use of antibiotics in agribusiness.

After a lifetime of work, Hippocrates concluded, "all diseases begin in the gut."

Your digestive tract is your Highway of Life. If you don't understand how to drive on this highway, you may have a fatal crash or at least a long, bumpy, painful ride. So put yourself in the driver's seat and get ready to learn where the bulk of your immune system lives and where the fate of your health resides.

We are not individuals but an ecosystem of 100 trillion microbes living inside our gut.

The body is made up of 25 million genes and 100 trillion bacteria. The bacteria outnumber the genes 4000 to 1. Bacteria outnumber human cells 10 to 1. We are our bacteria. We all have a unique internal fingerprint of a human genome. Our DNA and our unique microbiome of gut bacteria control the way our food is metabolized and digested, then sent on to our cells and our brain. Food is information and our gut is our second brain. We are stuck with our DNA but not the way our genes express themselves through epigenetics. That's why it is so important to feed our unique "ecosystems" the proper nutrition.

Most people process only 20% of their food. However, with gentle daily cleansing, a whole plant-based diet, and healthy water, absorption is increased to 80% or more. This is because of the improved digestive capabilities and restored immune system through the proper assimilation of nutrients and the elimination of toxic waste. Thoroughly chew your food.

Do not make the mistake that many people make - to exchange 4 inches of pleasure (i.e., that slice of pizza) for 30 feet of hell (that slice going through your digestive tract). This can make for a very bumpy and painful highway.

The path of food in the tube (digestive system) is as follows:

- Mouth: Chewing and mixing of saliva

- Esophagus: Minor absorption

- Stomach: Protein breakdown (storage)

- Small Intestine: Absorption of major components into the bloodstream to cells from villi extraction

- Large Intestine (colon): Absorption of water (important to keep this area healthy and clean)

- Excretion

Gut bacteria and the way polyphenols modify their composition in the gut may be more valuable to optimal health and wellness than vitamins. Polyphenols are primarily used to manage our 100 trillion gut bacteria.

Polyphenols support beneficial bacteria, inhibit infectious pathogens, and further assist in maintaining long-term digestive health. Lactobacillus salivarius is very important for oral health. In fact, this unique strain has been proven through research to dramatically decrease the level of plaque-forming bacteria in the mouth while naturally freshening breath and reducing gum sensitivity.

Optimize the interaction between your internal and external environment. You have control of your internal environment, ecosystem, hormones, neurotransmitters, immune system, oral and gut health, and stress. About 90% of the feel good neurotransmitter, serotonin, is made in the gut

The gut is the seat of good health. Healthy gut bacteria are powerful weapons in the fight to improve immunity, resist infections and diseases, extend life, and shorten duration of any illnesses.

Both sugar and artificial sweeteners alter the gut bacteria balance, affecting vascular health, brain health, and oral health.

Have a symbiotic relationship with your gut. Feed it the right nutrition. You take care of your gut. It will take care of you. Your body will love you. You won't hate your guts.

Your microbiome or gut health determines your brain's destiny. The gut is considered your second brain, and since food is information as well as fuel, nutrition should be of the utmost importance to your body as well as your brain's future health. Alzheimer's disease is now becoming an epidemic in America, just as obesity, type 2 diabetes, cardiovascular diseases, and cancer are on the rise. All are related to our nutrition.

Fiber in your diet from complex carbs like green leafy vegetables may be the most important feeder of your gut microbiome to enhance and support your immune system.

If you have heartburn or acid reflux, try digestive enzymes before meals, as opposed to anti-acids after, as antacids can deplete your protective micronutrients and upset your system even more.

Research shows that opening a window and increasing natural airflow can improve the diversity and health of the microbes in your home, which in turn benefit you. Make the outside, part of your inside. Open windows for fresh air. Walk outside for sunshine, fresh air and to nurture nature.

CHAPTER 29:
Probiotics

Optimizing and supporting the beneficial bacteria in your gut is one of the most powerful things you can do for your health and well being, including your immune system health. By helping your body maintain an optimal balance of 85 percent beneficial to about 15 percent "other" microbes, you support the health-promoting benefits of probiotics and strategically, you're overall health.

Probiotics, or beneficial gut microbes, influence many functions in your body. In addition to your immune health, researchers have found they affect your body weight, energy and nutrition, and your brain, both psychologically and neurologically. In addition, your gut microflora impacts the expression of your genes, epigenetics, which has a powerful effect on your well-being.

Probiotics benefit your health from head to toe in so many ways. They're essential for a multitude of bodily functions that research suggests taking a probiotic supplement may be even more important than taking a daily multivitamin.

Probiotics provide a necessary ecosystem balance and healthy distribution of gut flora, good versus bad bacteria. Our systems are bombarded daily with environmental toxins, damaged soil and the resulting degradation of the food supply in non-organic products. Probiotics may be the most important supplement you can take, along with a well-formulated multi-vitamin.

Probiotics improve bone health by enhancing mineral absorption in the gut. An unbalanced gut microbiome with bad bacteria causes inflammation. A strong immune system protects your body against disease-causing pathogens. Probiotics also help reduce high cholesterol.

Prebiotics stimulate the growth of healthy, good bacteria. But healthy bacteria need to be in the gut before they can be stimulated to grow. Probiotic sources to build up the good guys and then support growth by consuming sources of prebiotics such as dandelion greens, spinach, kale, artichokes, legumes, onions, leeks, garlic, oatmeal and flaxseed.

Probiotic supplements should contain and deliver 5 to 30 billion or more living organisms with as many probiotic species as possible, spanning both Lactobacillus and Bifidobacterium families; the more "L's" and "B's" the better. If you are consuming sugars and wheat and are not taking a probiotic, or using antibiotics or microbial soaps, chances are your gut is unbalanced.

Good probiotic foods are unpasteurized sauerkraut, kimchi, tempeh, miso and kefir.

CHAPTER 30:
Fiber

The type and amount of fiber in your diet plays an important role in your health. Fiber positively affects your intestinal microflora, which is important for maintaining health and preventing chronic disease. When you eat a nutritional diet you eat less, consume fewer calories and you feel full, because you are eating more fiber.

Eat a diet that includes whole foods, rich in fresh, organic vegetables and fruits that provide good nutrients and fiber; most of your fiber should come from vegetables and not from grains.

Fiber does far more than just keep you "regular." Research suggests a high-fiber diet can help reduce your risk of premature death from any cause, likely because it helps to reduce your risk of some of the most common chronic diseases, including type 2 diabetes, heart disease, stroke, and cancer.

Studies have also linked a high-fiber diet to beneficial reductions in cholesterol and blood pressure, improved insulin sensitivity, and reduced inflammation, all of which can influence all-cause mortality.

A meta-analysis published in 2014 evaluated the impact of a high-fiber diet on mortality and found that each 10-gram per day increase in fiber corresponded to a 10 percent reduction in all-cause mortality. Another study showed for every 10 gram increase of fiber intake was associated with a 15% lower risk of mortality. Those eating the most fiber had a 25% reduction of dying from any cause within the next nine years, compared to those whose fiber intake was deficient.

Fiber:

- Helps normalize your blood sugar level, which calms food cravings and helps you to lose weight.

- Slows your body's conversion of carbohydrates to sugar and supports blood sugar stability, helping you to lose weight.

- Suppresses your appetite. Eliminates extra calories by promoting bowel movements.

- Keeps you regular.

- Promotes supports gut balance by supporting the amounts if beneficial or good gut bacteria. When your gut is balanced it will help you achieve your desired weight for your body type.

Certain microbes in your gut specialize in fermenting fiber found in legumes, fruits, and vegetables. The byproducts of this fermenting activity help nourish the cells lining your colon and help boost your immune system to prevent inflammatory disorders.

Fiber benefits your health is by providing beneficial bacteria in your gut with the composition they need to thrive. These "good" bacteria assist with digestion and absorption of your food and play a significant role in your immune function, as 80% of your immune system is in your digestive tract.

Detrimental dietary changes that have led to general fiber deficiency include switching from fermented and raw vegetables to processed cereal grains. Cereal grains may have been a good source of fiber in the past, but not anymore. Today, most grains are grown using agricultural chemicals such as glyphosate, which has now been identified as a "probable human carcinogen" and a promoter of antibiotic resistance.

A high-grain diet tends to promote insulin and leptin resistance, which is counterproductive. It actually promotes many chronic diseases that healthy fiber can help decrease, most notably type 2 diabetes, heart disease, stroke, and cancer.

To boost your fiber intake, focus on eating more vegetables, fruits, nuts, seeds, organic whole husk psyllium, flax seeds, chia seeds, sunflower sprouts, and fermented vegetables. All are great sources of fiber; the latter few of those named being essentially fiber preloaded with beneficial bacteria.

Fiber undoubtedly contributes to sustaining health and longevity. It has a positive influence on your disease risk by feeding and promoting the proliferation of healthy gut bacteria. Gut health is paramount in improving your health and preventing or treating disease.

Avoid relying on grain-based fiber sources, as they threaten your health by raising your insulin and leptin levels, increasing your risk of glyphosate exposure. Processed grains are particularly harmful, and are second only to refined sugar and fructose in promoting chronic diseases.

Avoid processed sugar from any source. Get your fiber from fresh, locally grown, organic vegetables, fruits, seeds and nuts. Organically grown vegetables and fruits are full of natural fiber. Fiber is important for detoxing through the colon.

CHAPTER 31:
Cholesterol

L ess than 25% of our cholesterol comes from food. Our body (liver) and cells make the other 75%-80%. Only 50% of the cholesterol we eat is absorbed by the body, so it's essential to have a healthy liver. I feed or detox my liver daily with three divided separate doses of Milk Thistle Extract supplement.

Your liver produces new cholesterol and eliminates old, worn-out cholesterol. An unhealthy liver can lead to elevated cholesterol levels. Constipation is a problem because if you don't have regular bowel movements your body can't excrete the cholesterol the liver is trying to eliminate; it gets reabsorbed through the intestines back into circulation, again raising cholesterol levels. In addition, healthy arteries are important because if you have diet-induced inflammation your liver sends cholesterol into your arteries and blood vessels to fight the inflammation as a healing mechanism, but results in plaque buildup.

So, if your concern is high cholesterol, avoid refined carbs, pamper your liver with at least eight 8 ounce glasses of water (64 ounces) per day, and eat lots of vegetables and fruits which are high in fiber to prevent constipation. They also add to your water content, helping to flush and detox your liver. Foods that lower cholesterol naturally include organic red apples, beets, and carrots, raw or juiced.

High levels of insulin continuously stimulate cholesterol production, leading to abundance of cholesterol in the cells. LDL receptors in the cells are not sent to retrieve more cholesterol from the bloodstream, so the amount of LDL in the blood rises and remains elevated.

Glucagon slows down the production of cholesterol, much the same as a statin does. For many people it is possible to control cholesterol and triglycerides levels through diet by balancing insulin and glucagons. That's precisely what a low-carb, healthy-fat, healthy moderate protein diet accomplishes.

As levels of insulin decrease, levels of HDL increase. Dietary fat increases HDL.

Ideal total cholesterol is 180 to 200. Lowering cholesterol below these levels is trading one serious health problem for another: all-cause mortality. Total cholesterol of less than 160 can weaken the immune system.

One reason HDL cholesterol is dubbed "good cholesterol" is because it removes LDL or "bad cholesterol" affixed to arterial walls and transports it back to the liver for safe disposal. HDL does more than just cleanse arterial walls of plaque. It protects LDL from oxidation, which contributes to the process of blood clots and leads to stroke and heart attack. It inhibits chronic inflammation, vascular adhesion molecules, and platelet activation, all factors that lead to atherosclerosis and eventually to heart disease, vascular disease, and stroke.

Aging and poor diet result in a marked decline and reduced ability of HDL to protect against cardiovascular disease and stroke. Low levels of protective HDL help explain why an aging person's healthy arteries accelerate atherosclerosis within a period of only a few years and rapidly occlude with plaque.

By keeping insulin levels low and glucagon levels high, LDL receptors in cells keep busy retrieving LDL from the blood and pulling it into the cell interior for use as energy production and repair, thus, removing it from the blood, where it can get trapped in the artery walls and do damage, leading to CVE (cardiovascular event), heart attacks and strokes. The more LDL receptors the better. The less time LDL circulates in the blood, the better. That's what a low-carb diet accomplishes by lowering and controlling insulin.

The answer to reducing the risks of atherosclerosis, heart disease, and stroke is to reduce the oxidative damage of LDL cholesterol and triglycerides to the arterial lining or endothelium, so that plaque does not form and the LDL does not rupture, causing thrombosis and CVEs.

If LDL cholesterol is not oxidized and not damaged it will not stick to your arterial walls, and thus will not rupture, resulting in thrombosis, heart attack, and stroke. It's not the LDL itself the causes the cardiovascular event; it's the condition of the LDL. If you have damaged LDL and high blood pressure, you are a stroke or heart attack waiting to happen.

LDL only becomes bad when it's damaged by oxidation and free radicals. The oxidized LDL sticks to the damaged arterial walls or endothelium and initiates the formation of plaque and atherosclerosis.

Sugars and carbs that convert to sugar attach themselves to a protein (a process called glycation), which then attach to our arteries. This makes them stiff, increases blood pressure, and can lead to an artery tearing, which permits bacteria to invade and causes endothelial damage. In response to an endothelial tear, followed by bacterial infection, the immune system dispatches white blood cells to combat the inflammation in the artery wall. LDL within the white blood cells attacks bacteria in the artery wall as an immune repair response. LDL surrounds the tear to kill the bacteria. This process causes plaque from dead bacteria, white blood cells, and LDL. The LDL is sent to repair the infection, bacteria, inflammation, and tissue damage within the artery and arterial wall (endothelium). As this process is repeated, the endothelial membrane swells. The artery becomes thicker and choked off. A thrombosis or blood clot breaks loose, and boom! You have a heart attack or stroke. LDL is vilified as bad cholesterol, when in fact the amount of oxidized LDL and LDL particle size, may be what matters the most, especially in concert with high blood pressure and atherosclerosis.

Cholesterol does not really clog arteries. Saturated fat does not cause heart disease. Most people will not live longer by lowering their cholesterol. A low-fat, high-carbohydrate, FDA Food Pyramid diet is a death sentence. It was the biggest experiment in human health ever perpetrated on the US population, resulting in untold death and suffering.

Carbohydrate-rich diets not only lower HDL and raise triglycerides, they also make LDL small and dense, the most dangerous kind for atherosclerosis. These three components all increase risk for cardiovascular disease.

The danger is the LDL particle itself, not the cholesterol. The LDL particle size and number are the most important measurements in cholesterol. Statins, while lowering LDL, are not known to increase LDL particle size.

Persons with LDL cholesterol pattern A have large, buoyant particles. Individuals with pattern A are more likely to have normal blood levels of LDL cholesterol, HDL cholesterol and triglycerides. Pattern A is usually not associated with atherosclerosis.

Persons with LDL pattern B have predominantly small and dense BB-like, cholesterol particles. Pattern B is frequently associated with low HDL cholesterol levels, elevated triglyceride levels and the tendency to develop high blood sugar levels, type 2 diabetes, and accelerated atherosclerosis.

Some scientists believe that smaller LDL-B particles are more dangerous than the larger LDL-A particles because they can more easily squeeze into the tiny gaps between cells in the endothelium into the artery walls and this, combined with oxidation, causes formation of plaques or hardening of the arteries (atherosclerosis).

When we combine a well-formulated low-carb, higher healthy fat, moderate healthy protein diet, HDL increases, triglycerides decrease and the LDL becomes larger and fluffier. Individually and synergistically together, these markers decrease our risk of CVD and type 2 diabetes, as well as lowering weight obesity, type 2 diabetes and chronic inflammation, thus lowering all-cause mortality.

Lowering cholesterol too low subjects you to higher all-cause mortality, like kidney and liver disease, as well as Alzheimer's disease, which many doctors consider type 3 diabetes. If you get rid of oxidative stress, cholesterol levels decrease automatically.

Scrambling eggs oxidizes cholesterol, which contributes to atherosclerosis and inflammation. I personally eat eggs that are soft boiled in a water pot steamer, leaving the eggs moist and preserving their nutrition – not oxidizing from high heat, but yet fully cooked - about 6 minutes after you see steam rising from the pot.

CHAPTER 32:
Carbohydrates

America's obesity epidemic has been fueled by an increase in consumption of carbohydrates and processed foods, rich in sugars, grains and starches. This has led to a deadly combination of diet-induced, excess insulin, insulin resistance, toxic fat and an out of balance ratio of omega-6s to omega-3s. This creates diet-induced inflammation resulting in obesity and its fellow travel mates, type 2 diabetes, cardiovascular disease, heart attack, stroke, cancer, and most likely, Alzheimer's disease. Eighty percent of these are preventable.

If 80% of all these diseases are preventable and 80% of all healthcare costs are associated with these same diseases, wouldn't this save the collapse of America's healthcare system? Simple lifestyle changes, one person at a time, will start a healthcare revolution, save lives and save America's healthcare system.

High triglycerides strongly correlate with dangerous high levels of LDL-B particles, and low levels of triglycerides correlate with higher levels of LDL-A. So, the higher your triglycerides, the greater chance your LDL is LDL-B and the greater risk for cardiovascular disease. Reduce your triglycerides and raise your HDL and you will reduce your risk of cardiovascular disease. A low-carb diet will do this for you, besides giving you the benefit of losing weight.

The more high glycemic-load carbohydrates you consume, the hungrier you become. With increased hunger comes increased calorie consumption, primarily in the America diet from fat-free carbohydrates and processed foods. No wonder the average American is sick, fat, tired, and dying. Crappy carbs.

Carbohydrates are driving insulin and insulin is driving fat. Insulin is the fat storage hormone. That is why we get fat.

Control your carbs = control your weight.

I don't believe in weighing food or counting calories. Portion sizes are as important as calories when you are overeating from the wrong side of nutrition. But when you eat from a nutrition-rich food selection and proportions from mostly vegetables, fruits, healthy fats, healthy proteins and healthy fiber, it is almost impossible to overeat. Sugar, wheat, cereals, chips, crackers, cookies, cakes, pies and ice cream are not part of that nutrition-rich strategy.

Another benefit of the nutrient rich, low-carb diet, is it's almost always naturally free of trans-fats.

Three good predictors of a long and healthy life are low triglycerides, high HDL and low fasting insulin. All of these variables can be improved by a lower-carb diet.

Those with a waistline greater than 40" for men and 35" for women are at risk for insulin resistance and are considered overweight or obese. Forty-seven million Americans have some sort of metabolic syndrome and virtually all of them would improve substantially on a low-carbohydrate diet.

A diet of lower-carbs, higher-fat and moderate-protein vs. a high-carb diet will increase glucose control, reduce insulin resistance, reduce weight, lower triglycerides and improve cholesterol. My own blood lab reports for more than a 3-year period of time show steady, significant improvements, reductions and reversal, eliminating all the markers contributing to most, if not all degenerative diseases including stroke, heart attack, and cancer.

Calorie counting is not as important as carb counting.

Low-carb or controlled carbs, does not mean no carbs. Just get your carbs from whole foods – fruits, vegetables, beans, legumes, seeds and nuts, and not sugar, wheat, junk foods, processed foods, or fast foods. Simple.

Even if the weight loss results were similar between low-carb and high-carb diets, if the low carb was marked by greater improvements in insulin and triglycerides, two markers for cardiovascular disease, wouldn't you chose the low-carb diet?

The primary reason most diets fail is hunger. Insulin, the hunger hormone, is elevated the most by high-carbohydrate diets. A low-fat, high-carb diet leaves you continually hungry and craving sweets. But if you eat a nutrient-rich, satiating, whole foods diet that doesn't leave you hungry and allows you to eat fewer calories, burn fat, and drop weight, why would you not make that choice?

I believe that you can even consume more calories on a low-carb diet than a high-carb diet and still lose weight, because you are able to reduce insulin levels and balance hormones.

A low-calorie dietary approach is generally low in fat and high in carbohydrates. This leads to weight cycling or yoyo-ing up and down and ultimately, higher body fat and weight gain. This leads to both physical and psychological damage, adding failure and guilt to the equation over supposed lack of willpower or self-control, when in fact it was due to addiction and dependence or intolerance of carbohydrates.

In view of the poor track record of low-fat/high-carbohydrate diets in controlling the current US epidemic in obesity and diabetes, plus an apparent of impact by both pharmaceutical and exercise interventions on metabolic syndrome, CVD, heart attack, strokes, and cancers, a well-formulated low carbohydrate diet strategy offers an effective plan for the millions of Americans suffering from these preventable and reversible diseases. All aboard!

A number of recent studies have shown that weight loss is actually greater on a low-carb diet than on a conventional low-fat diet that has the same number of calories. I believe that you can even consume more calories on a low-carb diet than a high-carb diet and still lose weight, because you are able to reduce insulin levels and balance hormones. Remember, insulin is the fat-storing hormone.

A diet lower in carbs is much more satiating and easier to maintain over the long-term as a lifestyle eating strategy than a diet that simply reduces fat. Long-term maintenance is the ultimate goal. Studies show that more weight is lost on low-carb diets than high-carb diets with the same number of calories, with the added benefit of better blood chemistry. Lowering fat in the diet is not the answer to obesity.

Virtually every low-carb diet, by definition, contains incredibly low amounts of trans fats. Saturated fats are not as much of a problem as trans fats.

Studies show that while the traditional high-carb, low-fat diet may in fact lower LDL, it raises the dangerous pattern B molecules and lowers protective HDL cholesterol, so while your total cholesterol may go down, your risk goes up, along with a rise in triglycerides in a high-carb to low-carb diet. The combination of high triglycerides and low HDL is a far better predictor of cardiovascular disease than elevated total cholesterol.

Who would benefit from a restricted carbohydrate diet? Currently, 2 in 3 US adults qualify as overweight, 1 in 3 as obese. Among certain ethnic groups, including Latinos, Mexican-American men and African-American women, 4 in 5 are overweight. More than 1 in 3 US adults have metabolic syndrome, 1 in 4 have impaired blood sugar and 1 in 10 have type 2 diabetes. Most, if not all, of these people have some degree of carbohydrate intolerance, so all would benefit immensely from a low-carb diet. This represents 100 million American adults.

We are now passing these traits and bad eating habits on to our children. Childhood obesity is now a major problem, as well as autism and ADHD. Our seniors are experiencing an epidemic of Alzheimer's. As we age we become more carbohydrate intolerant. Carbohydrate restriction is commonly practiced, but seldom taught and is becoming more and more popular as the evidence and science catches up.

"Tell me what you eat and I will tell you what you

are." - Savarin

Savarin's quote has been modified to "You are what you eat." However, it is more complicated than that. We all metabolize food differently and need a personalized diet strategy that works for you. So it is more of a "you are what you burn and store" concept — what you burn as energy and what you store as fat.

Carbohydrate intolerance is at the root, however, and most people (but not all) have a problem with burning and storing carbs. If you are on a low-fat, high-carbohydrate diet and are carbohydrate intolerant, most likely you are overweight, obese, type 2 diabetic, full of inflammation, suffering from chronic diseases and are sick and tired. Sound familiar? A well-formulated low-carbohydrate diet is empowering.

The amount of carbohydrates in your diet dictates your need for salt or sodium. A high-carbohydrate diet makes the kidneys retain salt. A low carb diet increases sodium excretion by the kidneys. A nice side effect of a low-carb diet is not only weight loss from fat, but less water retention from less sodium and less water weight as a result. A win-win.

Research shows low-carbohydrate diets outperform low-fat diets in improving triglycerides, HDL-C, LDL particle size, glucose (blood sugar) and insulin. Adding high healthy fats and moderate healthy proteins to a low-carb diet blows away the low-fat/high-carb diet that is causing millions of Americans to be sick, tired, and dying. The evidence is in, but few are practicing the low-carb, higher fat, moderate protein diet and even fewer are teaching it.

Carbohydrate intolerance, carbohydrate dependence, and carbohydrate addiction are synonymous. Yes, carbohydrate addiction is real. The treatment is the same for any dependency/addiction: restrict the foods that cause the addiction. Treat the cause, not the symptoms

Removing most carbs from the diet causes your kidneys to aggressively secrete sodium, and along with it, extra fluids and water weight. This is why many people experience a dramatic early weight loss with a carb restriction diet. I add a pinch of Himalayan pink rock salt to my daily Green Drink to compensate.

Surprisingly, it is not uncommon to find wide swings and unstable blood sugar in normal-weight people, and it negatively affects their lives just as it does for overweight and obese people. That's why a well-formulated low-carb diet strategy can benefit most people in the long-term.

All carbohydrates are basically sugar. Improving the quality of the carbohydrates you eat should make you leaner and will improve your health. Carbohydrate-rich diets not only lower HDL and raise triglycerides, they also make LDL small and dense, the most dangerous for atherosclerosis. These three components all increase risk for CVD.

A high-carbohydrate diet and subsequent insulin resistance promotes endothelial dysfunction and inhibits a potent vasodilator, nitric oxide, and at the same time stimulates a vasoconstrictor, causing a one-two punch that increases your risk for cardiovascular disease, heart attack, and stroke.

Studies using carbohydrate-restricted diets consistently show increased glucose and insulin control and increased insulin sensitivity, both in healthy populations and especially, in people with metabolic syndrome and type 2 diabetes. This is another reason why a low-carb strategy can benefit nearly all people, even those who metabolize carbs well.

When we combine a well-formulated low-carb, higher healthy fat, moderate healthy protein diet, HDL increases, triglycerides decrease and the LDL becomes larger and fluffier. Individually and synergistically together, these markers decrease our risk of CVD, type 2 diabetes, high blood pressure and chronic inflammation, thereby, lowering all-cause mortality.

A low-carb diet is anti-inflammatory as well. Remember, one of our goals for optimum health is to drive down inflammation, as it is present in all debilitating chronic diseases, such as heart attack, stroke, and cancer

Your body has no physiological requirement for carbohydrates. Carbohydrates are not required in a healthy human diet. If you want to lose weight and improve your health you should take in the vast majority of your carbs from vegetables, fruits and beans and not from pasta, rice, bread, baked goods, cereal, and sugar-laden desserts. Carbs from fruits and vegetables are loaded with vitamins, minerals, phytonutrients, fiber and all the good stuff your body thrives on. Add healthy protein and healthy fats and you have a blueprint for weight management, health, wellness, and longevity that will work for just about everyone.

Preconceived ideas or notions can be puzzling. There is NO minimum daily requirement for carbohydrates. The body has no physiological need for carbohydrates. You can live without them. But you can't live without proteins and fats.

Refined carbohydrates, starchy vegetables, and sugars are fattening and make us sick. Don't eat them, don't drink them. It's actually a pretty simple formula: the quality and quantity of carbohydrates we consume is what makes us fat and makes us sick. Get your carbohydrates from fruits and vegetables, not from sugar, wheat, starches, and grains. The low-fat, high-carb diet is killing us one bite at a time.

Once you accept the fact that it's the carbohydrates, and not gluttony or sloth, making you fat and sick, dieting will no longer be your goal. You'll want a lifestyle change. Selecting foods that best avoid the refined grains, starches, sugars and the other components outlined in this handbook.

If you follow a high-carb/low-fat diet that has been promoted for almost 50 years, based on a 2,200 calorie diet that is 60% carbohydrate, as was recommended, metabolically, your body will have to contend with nearly 2 cups of pure sugar, daily.

The human body can function extremely efficiently on 2 teaspoons of sugar at any given time. There are 48 teaspoons per cup, 96 in 2 cups, so where does that extra 94 teaspoons go? If you guessed fat and disease, you guessed right. And it is why obesity, diabetes, metabolic syndrome, inflammation, and diseases, such as cardiovascular disease, heart attack, stroke, cancer, and Alzheimer's are killing us at record levels.

A low-carb or carbohydrate restrictive diet increases the prevalence of larger, healthier LDL particles, whereas a low-fat/high-carbohydrate diet has the opposite and overtly harmful effect. By consuming a low-carb diet you will convert unhealthy pattern LDL-B to healthy pattern LDL-A, and thus decrease your risk of cardiovascular disease.

The higher the level of triglycerides circulating in your blood, the greater your risk of cardiovascular disease, heart attacks, and strokes. Carbohydrates elevate triglycerides levels. Low HDL cholesterol is also a risk factor for CVD. Carbohydrates lower HDL. If your HDL cholesterol is low, you're very likely eating a lot of carbohydrates. If your HDL is high, it's a good bet you're eating few carbohydrates. The higher your blood sugar level is, the more glucose enters your cells and the less vitamin C. When we eat carbohydrates we excrete vitamin C through our kidneys and urine rather than retaining or absorbing it.

Reducing carbohydrates creates an absence of insulin circulating in your blood stream, allowing fat cells to release fat and muscle cells to burn it.

Carbohydrates drive up insulin. Carbohydrates make us fat and obese, and cause diabetes. A low-carbohydrate, high fat diet improves every metabolic and hormonal abnormality of metabolic syndrome and the diseases it causes, including cardiovascular disease, heart attack, stroke, cancer, and dementia/Alzheimer's disease.

Recent studies show there is a cluster of risk factors for type 2 diabetes and vascular disease, including high blood sugar, obesity, high blood pressure, elevated triglycerides, insulin resistance. All these factors, individually, collectively and synergistically work to increase the risk of Alzheimer's disease: one more reason to eat a low-carb diet and age gracefully.

The more high glycemic-load carbohydrates you consume, the hungrier you become and with increased hunger comes increased calorie consumption, primarily in the American diet from fat-free carbohydrates and processed foods. No wonder the average American is sick, fat, tired, and dying.

Sugars and whole grains are the main culprits in GERD. The medical costs associated with GERD in the US are in excess of $9 billion annually. By eliminating sugars, wheat, and starches, and restricting carbohydrates to healthy vegetables and fruit carbs, the burning sensation from GERD improves or completely goes away. Say goodbye to heartburn products such as Rolaids, Tums, and Nexium, save money and get relief, all by making dietary changes.

Essential nutrients for humans are water, vitamins, minerals, protein, and fat. Carbohydrates are not essential, nor do they have an RDA, nor are they necessary for human life. The best carbohydrate sources are vegetables, fruits, seeds, and nuts. There are no such thing as healthy grains.

The fact is, eating carbohydrates makes you hungry. Speaking of making you hungry, combine alcohol with protein, not carbs.

Everyone is different and has different carb tolerance levels. Most people need 50g or less of carbs per day and those with metabolic syndrome should consume 30g or less per day to maintain a fat-burning target zone, as opposed to sugar or glucose-dependent zones.

One diet does not fit all because we have varying degrees of carbohydrate tolerance, which is part of the equation of individuality and customization. As an example, some people need to restrict their consumption of fruit to lose weight, while others don't. I was able to eat several pieces of fruit per day and lose weight, and still do to this day, but some may have to eliminate fruit or add it back gradually. By choosing from the food list and eating strategy contained in this handbook, you will be able to attain your ideal weight.

For 700,000 years, humans ate a diet mainly of meat, fat, nuts and berries. Around 8,000 years ago we learned to farm and as our consumption of grains increased, our health declined.

A diet heavy in carbohydrates sends our insulin levels soaring and signals the body to store calories, make cholesterol and conserve water, leading to weight-related health problems, type 2 diabetes, inflammation, CVD, heart attacks, strokes, and cancer.

To lose weight or maintain your ideal weight long-term, most people will need to manage their carbohydrate intake and definitely cut back or eliminate sugar, wheat, and starches. Get your carbs from vegetables, fruits, nuts, and seeds. If you are unable to lose weight, limit fruit intake, because the fructose may be the culprit. I was able to eat fruit during my weight loss period and now on my maintenance lifestyle, I eat several pieces of fruit a day, especially, bananas, apples, blueberries, blackberries, strawberries, and raspberries.

A standard high-carbohydrate, low-fat diet (or SAD) tends to lower total cholesterol and lower HDL at the same time, putting people at increased risk for CVD.

Not all carbohydrates are equally fattening. This is a critical point. The most fattening foods are the ones that have the greatest effect on blood sugar and insulin levels. Concentrated sources of carbohydrates, ones that we digest quickly, are refined flour, wheat, sugar, bread, cereal, pasta, beer, fruit juices, sodas, starches, potatoes, rice, and corn. Corn is not a vegetable – it's a grain. These foods quickly flood the bloodstream with glucose, blood sugar shoots up, insulin shoots up, and we get fatter. These foods are also the cheapest calories available, usually government subsidized. Unfortunately, the poorer we are, the fatter we"re likely to be. These populations are not fat because they eat too much or don't exercise enough – they are fat because the foods they live on are literally fattening them, making them obese.

On a high-carb diet, the body takes all the excess sugar and packages it into triglycerides, so less sugar in the diet means less triglycerides in the blood, and a lower risk for cardiovascular disease.

The ratio of triglycerides to HDL cholesterol is a much greater predictor of cardiovascular disease than cholesterol alone.

If a low-carb diet can reduce inflammation, triglycerides, LDL particle numbers and size, perhaps there's less need for drugs.

CHAPTER 33:
Fats

The idea that "If no fat touches my lips, then no fat will reach my hips," is a fallacy or myth. Removing fat from the diet does not solve the weight gain and obesity epidemic, as dietary fat has no impact on insulin, and excess insulin is what causes fat and keeps you fat and makes you fatter. Elevated insulin and insulin resistance, not eating healthy dietary fats, prevents the release of fat stores. Eating a healthy high-fat diet helps you burn fat. If you want your rocket to fly, you fuel it with rocket fuel.

Most of the fat that people eat is unhealthy and consists of processed omega-6 vegetable oil (and most of that fat is from soybean oil). In fact, the amount of soybean oil consumed in 2000 was more than 1,000 times higher than it was 100 years ago in 1900.

Ever since the surgeon general recommended in 1988 that Americans reduce their fat consumption, especially saturated fat, the race to reduced fat has been on; however, it doesn't work. The low-fat, high complex carbohydrate diet has proven a failure.

The low-fat/high-carbohydrate diet has been in practice since the 1970s. It has been a failure, causing near epidemic levels of obesity, type 2 diabetes, cardiovascular disease, heart attack, stroke, and cancer.

Fat has no impact on insulin, protein; some, carbohydrates; a huge response. A high-carbohydrate diet raises both triglycerides and cholesterol, LDL, and VLDL, all of which are bad. Sugar is our enemy and is far more damaging than fat. The liver is actually detoxifying sugar into triglycerides. The body sees sugar as a toxin, a poison. Lowering of triglycerides is a major benefit of a low-carb diet. High triglycerides are far more dangerous for cardiovascular disease than cholesterol.

There are two types of fats: saturated and unsaturated. Saturated fats come from animals, while unsaturated fats come from plants. There are two types of unsaturated fats, monounsaturated and polyunsaturated. There are two kinds of polyunsaturated fats, omega-3 and omega-6. In terms of priority of choices, a high priority should be given to monounsaturates, then saturates, and all sources rich in omega-6polyunsaturates, such as grains, should be avoided. Focus on foods sources rich in omega-3 polyunsaturates like fish. Eat at least 3 servings of fish per week. Wild-caught salmon, tuna, trout, mackerel, herring and sardines are good choices rich in omega-3s.

Olive oil, olives, walnut oil, avocados, seeds such as raw sunflower seeds and raw pumpkin seeds, and nuts like raw almonds, walnuts, macadamia and pistachios are all rich sources of healthy mono and polyunsaturated fats. Good sources of saturated fats are coconut oil and coconut meat; grass-fed beef; lamb and bison; pastured, free-range, organic chicken and eggs; and turkey.

We don't get fat because we overeat; we overeat because we're getting fat.

"Every man is the creature of the age in which he lives, very few are able to raise themselves above the ideas of the time." – Voltaire

Research shows that the brain and central nervous system run more efficiently on ketones (fat) than on glucose (sugar).

Training your body to burn fat as opposed to sugar for energy is infinitely healthier than ingesting and burning processed, nutrient-empty, high-carb foods. You will not only lose weight, but maintain your ideal weight, plus gain other health benefits in the process.

Many people have a fat phobia, not only in wearing it, but eating it. Once you start burning fat instead of sugar, you will actually be feeding your body its preferred high octane fuel.

"You are what you eat" is only applicable to what you digest, burn, or store. Most people think, and most diets suggest, that fat is not good for you, which is simply not true. Research shows that not only is fat good for you, the only time eating fat causes weight gain is when you eat too many carbohydrates or eat a low-fat/high-carbohydrate diet. High healthy fats paired with a well-formulated low-carb diet leads to weight loss and improved cardiovascular health. It makes sense to feed your body what it burns. Once you convert from burning sugar to burning fat, the fats you consume will burn as energy, which is what you want.

Good fat is not burned as sugar, as carbs and excess protein are, but burned as fat. Fat is your body's superior fuel for energy. Good fat stimulates the body to burn fat. The longer your body is in a calorie deficit, then the lower your leptin levels and metabolic rate become. What this means is your metabolism slows, and it will be extremely hard to lose that last bit of fat. Solution: Eat more healthy fats.

Leptin is the single most important hormone when it comes to understanding why we feel hungry or full. When present in high levels, it signals to our brain that we're full and can stop eating. When low, we feel hungry and crave food. It does this by stimulating receptors in our hypothalamus, the part of our brains which regulates the hormone system in our bodies. When leptin binds to receptors in this part of our brains, it stimulates the release of appetite-suppressing chemicals. People with leptin disorders eat uncontrollably.

Our bodies are hard-wired to burn sugar first. The trick is to retrain our bodies to burn fat, thereby losing unwanted fat and weight. That equates to limiting sugar and starchy carbs and eating more good fat. If you don't have sugar to burn, your body will burn fat. It's that simple.

Health and lifespan are determined by the proportion of fat versus sugar you burn throughout your lifetime. The more fat you burn as fuel, the healthier you are. The more sugar you burn as fuel, the fatter and more disease-ridden you will become and the shorter your life span will likely be.

By burning fat and not sugar, you will gain metabolic momentum, allowing you to lose weight permanently.

By controlling your insulin and leptin levels, you will control your IGF-1 hormones, instrumental in muscle development, growth and maintenance. Along with exercise, your lean muscle mass will be preserved, allowing you not to look thin and flabby.

Once you"ve adapted to a good fat burner, your consumption of saturated fat becomes less dangerous, because you are burning all fat as fuel. However, saturated fats (non-grass fed, non-pastured animal fat) should be kept to a minimum to moderate amount for all-cause mortality.

Most of the fat people eat is unhealthy and consists of processed omega-6 vegetable oil (most of that fat is from soybean oil). In fact, the amount of soybean oil consumed in 2000 was more than 1,000 times higher than it was 100 years ago in 1900.

Quality of fat trumps quantity of fat.

Saturated fat is not as much a problem with heart disease as we have been led to believe, but, the jury is still out on some long-term cancer effects, such as breast and ovarian cancers in women, PSA elevation and prostate cancer in men and may be an issue with weight loss and weight maintenance with some people. Again, everyone is different the way their body metabolizes and stores macronutrients. Healthy saturated fats, for optimal health; the benefits far outweigh any negatives long-term. It's more important to know what the animal ate and where it was raised. Organic and pastured raised to forage for its natural foodstuffs and not factory farmed, so the saturated fat is healthy. Moderation is the optimal word.

The problem may lie in combining unhealthy saturated fats with processed carbs, omega 6's and hydrogenated oils and fats, like margarine and corn oil, which are all found and consumed in the Standard American Diet (SAD.)

There are those proponents who advocate a plant based diet only for cancer prevention, as in vegetarian or vegan diets, however, I'm a proponet for all-cause mortality to include healthy animal fats as outlined in this handbook. If you smoke, all bets are off!

As a prime example, dark meats and the skin on chicken is among its most nutritious parts, but has been vilified by mainstream medicine. Like all fatty foods, chicken skin is a combination of saturated, mono-unsaturated, and polyunsaturated fats. For the skin of half a chicken, the breakdown is: 6.7g saturated fat, 10g mono-unsaturated fat, and 5g polyunsaturated fat. It's largely monounsaturated fat; that's the largest component, same as, olive oil. At 261 calories, the skin of half a chicken has 11g of protein and is rich in vitamins and minerals, especially Selenium which protects cells from free-radical damage. The skin also contains a complete amino acid profile, the building blocks of our cells and neurotransmitters. We should feel happy when we are eating the skin.

Dark meats also contain more saturated fats, along with omega-3 and omega-6 fats. The dark meat, while fattier (which isn't a bad thing), is more nutritionally robust than its whiter counterpart according to research from the NYU School of Medicine. White meat has about half the saturated fat of dark meat and for this reason alone it has been promoted as the healthier alternative. Dark meat gets its color from myoglobin, a compound that muscles use to transport oxygen to fuel activity. It's rich in a nutrient called taurine known to aid in anti-inflammation, blood pressure regulation, healthy nerve function, the production of bile acid (which breaks down fat), and other important functions. In addition to taurine in dark meat is far richer in minerals such as iron, zinc and selenium, as well as vitamins A, K and the B complex, B1 (thiamine), B2 (riboflavin), B3 (niacin), B6 (pyridoxine), B9 (folate) and B12 (cobalamin), riboflavin, niacin, thiamin and amino acids, than white meat.

Simply put, reconsider your choice of white meat versus dark meat, as it's a personal choice, but the numbers seem to favor dark meat. I have changed my preference and have added dark meat into my diet and actually find it delicious after years of white meat only.

Many ketogenic diet experts recommend dark meat chicken and turkey over breast or white meat because of its superior content of healthy fat. White meat is largely a protein delivery system; dark meat contains many more nutrients. Dark meat has been wrongly vilified for having a lot of saturated fat. Saturated fat is not as unhealthy as we have consistently been led to believe, and the public health guidelines that advise people to avoid all saturated fats will result in serious health consequences. (See bacon next.)

Another highly maligned saturated fat is bacon.

Bacon's primary asset is its fat, and that fat is primarily monounsaturated. Fifty percent of the fat in bacon is monounsaturated, mostly consisting of oleic acid, the type so valued in olive oil. About three percent of that is palmitoleic acid, a monounsaturate with valuable antimicrobial properties. About 40 percent of bacon fat is saturated. The remaining 10 percent is in the form of polyunsaturates.

Monounsaturated fat, the primary fat in bacon is widely lauded for reducing inflammation and lowering blood pressure, while the antimicrobial palmitoleic content in bacon fat can keep plaque at bay. Triglycerides too may improve because bacon fat is especially good at helping us achieve satiety and stable blood sugar

Bacon fat from pastured pigs also comes well-supplied with fat-soluble vitamin D, provided it's bacon from foraging pigs that frolic outdoors in the sun. Factory-farmed pigs kept indoors and fed rations from soy, casein, corn meal, and other grains, are likely to show low levels of Vitamin D.

Pork fat also contains a novel form of phosphatidylcholine that possesses antioxidant activity superior to Vitamin E.

Best to buy uncured-organic-pastured raised- bacon, as cured-bacon is generally cured with salt, sugar, phosphates, nitrates and nitrites.

Don't over-cook bacon to a crisp.

The Alzheimer's epidemic is possibly diet-related and attributable to a lifetime of eating processed foods full of sugar and no healthy fats. Our brains are made of 60% fat.

The average American has 10 years of stored omega-6s in their bodies. The ideal ratio of omega-6 to omega-3 is 1:1, at most 3:1, but the average American on a SAD is 25:1 and higher if they eat fast foods and processed foods.

Another way to look at calories: One gram of carbohydrate yields only 4 calories of energy, whereas, one gram of fat yields 9 calories of energy, so gram per gram, fat is a denser energy calorie and our body lives on energy.

Case in point: Not all fat calories are bad for you. We've been told for the last 30-50 years to eat a low-fat, high-carbohydrate diet. It has been one of the worst human experiments in US history and has caused an epidemic of diseases including obesity, type 2 diabetes, cardiovascular disease, heart attack, stroke, and cancer. You must however, choose healthy fats wisely as outlined in this handbook and in your well -formulated eating strategy.

Since there are 9 calories per gram of fat and only 4 calories per gram of carbohydrates, you get more energy per gram of fat, so in essence it's high-test fuel for your body and your brain. You feel more satiated with fat calories, suppressing your appetite, thus, consuming fewer calories and leading to weight loss.

Carbs are often empty, non-nutritional calories found in processed and fast foods and cause you to crave more and eat more and weight gain. Simply restrict carbs of sugar, wheat and starches, increase consumption of carbs from greens, vegetables, fruits and nuts, increase healthy fats and moderate healthy proteins. This is not a diet: diets don't work. This is a well-formulated eating strategy for a lifetime.

It was once thought that after adolescence we could not produce or grow more fat cells, but, not only do our fat cells get fatter, but as a result of adiopogenesis, we can grow more fat cells, all as a result of the SAD.

Do not mix sugars and fats together. It's a bad combination for weight gain, inflammation and overall health.

Fifty percent of all first-time heart attack patients have normal cholesterol levels. Our medical establishment, controlled by Big Pharma, still clings to the false theory that saturated animal fat and high cholesterol cause heart disease, so they can make bank on statin drugs. Inflammatory sugars, omega-6 vegetable oils, chemicals, and toxins in common foods cause heart disease, type 2 diabetes and obesity. Most cancers are caused by inflammatory sugars, bad fats, chemicals, and GMOs in our food chain.

The process of glycogenesis can make all the glucose the brain needs, once the body is keto-adapted, efficient at burning fat, not sugar, for fuel and energy.

Many heart attack victims have normal cholesterol, so there is more going on inside than meets the eye. If you don't measure it or test it, you can't improve it. Many times the first symptom of a heart attack or stroke is death.

Consider your body like a car. A car burns gas, so what do you feed it? Gas. If you want your body to burn fat, what should you feed it? Fat. Consume healthy fats from avocados, olive oil, coconut oil, nuts and seeds, omega-3 fatty acids from wild-caught fish, grass-fed beef, organic, pasture-raised chickens and eggs.

CHAPTER 34:
Protein

Protein is a macro-nutrient.

Excess protein that the body doesn't use to repair or make new cells is largely broken down into simple sugars, which increases blood sugar (insulin) and promotes insulin resistance and stores as fat. Furthermore, protein itself triggers insulin production, which worsens insulin resistance. So, diabetics should never go on a high-protein diet.

The primary difference between protein consumption from US dietary guidelines and optimal intake is that US guidelines do not take fat mass or lean body weight into account, which can vary widely from one person to the next, even if they are the same weight.

You're aiming for one-half gram of protein per pound of lean body mass, which would place most people in the range of 40 to 70 grams of protein per day.

Protein calculator: Weight – percent of body fat = adjusted net weight X .5 = daily protein consumption. (Example. Weight 180 lbs. per cent body fat = 10%.

180 – 18 = 162 X .5 = 81gm of protein daily.)

- Red meat, pork, and poultry average 6 to 9 grams of protein per ounce. An ideal amount for most people would be a 3-ounce serving of meat (not 9- or 12-ounce steaks!), which will provide about 18 to 27 grams of protein.

- Eggs contain about 6 to 8 grams of protein per egg. So, an omelet made from two eggs would give you about 12 to 16 grams of protein.

- Seeds and nuts contain on average 4 to 8 grams of protein per quarter cup.

- Cooked beans average about 7 to 8 grams per half cup.

- Most vegetables contain about 1 to 2 grams of protein per ounce.

Discerning the ideal amount of protein can be tricky business, with plenty of variables adding to the confusion. However, a good starting point is to calculate your need based on lean body weight. It would be quite rare for someone to need more than 0.5 gram of protein per pound of lean body weight, taking into account the fact that pregnant women, athletes, and seniors may need about 25 percent more in addition to that.

Substantial amounts of protein can be found in meat, fish, eggs, raw dairy products, legumes, and nuts.

Excessive protein can actually be worse than eating too many carbs. Excessive protein can stimulate two biochemical pathways that accelerate aging and cancer growth.

Excess protein can be metabolized as sugar leading to fat storage and your body burning sugar as fuel and not the preferred burn of fat.

People who get 20 percent or more of daily calories from protein have a 400 percent higher cancer rate, and a 75 percent higher mortality risk, compared to those who eat only 10 percent of daily calories from protein.

Most people would benefit from restricting their protein intake to 1 gram (gm) per kilogram (kg) of lean body mass.

CHAPTER 35:
Phytonutrients/Polyphenols/Antioxidants

Phytonutrients are defined as nutrients that have been scientifically proven to provide health benefits. "Phyto" in Greek means plants. Phytonutrients fall into their own category because they are not related to macronutrients (fats, carbohydrates, proteins, vitamins, or minerals). Phytonutrients work together in synergy like an orchestra. They allow cellular function and communication. When our cells communicate effectively, the proper sequence of enzymatic reactions takes place. This leads to biochemical reactions creating healthier tissues and organ systems, detoxification of foreign substances, a strong immune system, and lean muscle mass.

Polyphenols are a nutritional bonanza derived from vegetables, fruits, green tea, wine and cocoa. Polyphenols are powerful antioxidants and cellular anti-inflammatories. They reduce free radicals and oxidative stress and slow the rate of aging. I call it turning back the clock, literally. Grandma was right. Eat your vegetables before you go out to play

Vegetables and fruits (polyphenols) also aid in metabolic efficiency while reducing inflammation and reducing oxidative stress. Anything that decreases inflammation or increases metabolic efficiency extends longevity. Get rid of inflammation, increase metabolic efficiency, and live longer. It sounds like a pretty easy formula for lifestyle change.

Polyphenols deliver dual benefits for both heart and brain health. If you consume a diet rich in green and colorful vegetables and fruits, your likelihood of CVD (cardiovascular disease) and Alzheimer's should be reduced.

Polyphenols are anti-inflammatory and free-radical scavengers. Some have anticarcinogenic and cardioprotective effects. Polyphenols have beneficial effects on the endothelial lining of blood vessels by increasing the availibility of nitric oxide and preventing the oxidation of atherosclerosis.

Numerous studies suggest that polyphenols may work synergistically to protect against cardiovascular disease, cancer, diabetes, and endothelial dysfunction, osteoporosis, and neurodegenerative diseases without any known side effects.

The typical Western diet (SAD) lacks sufficient amounts and varieties of plant polyphenols to be of optimal benefit.

The fewer the calories you eat, the fewer free radicals your body produces. This is a paramount reason that calorie restriction slows the rate of aging. So restrict calories and add more polyphenol fruits and vegetables into your diet, and you'll live longer.

Maqui berries are 14 times more concentrated in beneficial nutrients than blueberries. I eat lots of blueberries and take a daily maqui berry supplement.

The average American consumes only 450 mg of polyphenols daily. We need 1g or 1,000 mg daily or more.

At low levels, polyphenols are powerful anti-bacterial gut agents. At higher levels, they act as powerful antioxidants and anti-inflammatory agents in the body. At the highest levels they become powerful anti-aging agents that can significantly increase your longevity with synergistic properties and profound benefits.

It is essential for good gut health to have a constant consumption of the proper low-glycemic load: non-starchy vegetables, fruits, and the polyphenols that are jam-packed, nutrient rich, and nutrient dense with proper carbohydrates.

Olive oil is rich in monounsaturated fats, but it also contains polyphenols that has many unique health benefits.

CHAPTER 36:
Pomegranates For Health

Studies over many years have extolled the age-fighting properties of pomegranates. Pomegranates are highly prized for their free radical-combating antioxidants. While both red wine and green tea contain high amounts, studies have found whole pomegranate fruit to have three times more antioxidant activity.

Antioxidants can decrease your risk of oxidative stress that exposes you to several serious diseases and chronic inflammation.

Research shows pomegranates help prevent atherosclerosis (hardening of the arteries.), decreased carotid artery thickness and improved cardiac blood flow.

Many grocery stores now have the nutrient rich pomegranate fruit packaged and separated from the rind for your convenience and eating pleasure. You can also purchase organic pomegranate extract powder to mix in your "green drinks" and smoothies.

One of my favorite recipes in a large mixing bowl is: Kale, 2-tbsp olive oil, 2-tbsp lemon juice, ¼-tsp Pink Himalayan rock salt, topped with pomegranates.

CHAPTER 37:
Cancer

Cancer is a cell imbalance, a metabolic disease and mitochondria disease, more so, than a genetic disease. It is a deficiency disease causing an abnormal growth of cells into tumors, and is correctable through proper nutrition, and control of environment. Contrary to conventional teaching, genetic defects do not cause cancer. Mitochondrial damage occurs first and this then triggers genetic mutation.

Most forms of cancer are almost entirely preventable. Not more than 10 per cent of cancer cases can be attributable to genetics. 90-95 percent are caused by lifestyle and environmental factors. Chronic inflammation is the most common cause of cancer.

Sugary processed foods may be cheap up front, but they exact a huge price tag on the back end, including obesity, diabetes, cancer and all cause mortality. Continuously eating more than your body really requires promotes insulin resistance. Your cells are stressed by the additional work-load placed on them by the excess nutrients. Insulin resistance in turn is at the heart of most chronic diseases, including cancer and sugar is a key contributor to cancer.

Obesity can promote cancer via a number of different mechanisms, including mitochondrial dysfunction, overeating, excess sugar in your diet, chronic inflammation and overproduction of certain proteins and hormones.

Cancers are preventable through proper nutrition. Avoiding toxic exposures, such as pesticides, is another important vector, one of the reasons to eat only organic foods, especially grass-fed or pasture-raised meats and animal products. Overall, insulin resistance is one of the key contributors to a heightened cancer risk and many studies have confirmed that type 2 diabetics are at a greater risk as elevated blood sugar sets the stage for cancer growth. Cancer feeds on sugar.

Cancer prevention, now in a convenient, easy to use package: vegetables and fruits. To prevent or treat cancer if you have insulin or leptin resistance, cut all forms of sugar/fructose and grain carbs from your diet.

Cancer doesn't typically develop overnight. You have a chance to make changes that can potentially prevent cancer from developing in the first place, through epigenetics, environment or lifestyle changes. Most people carry around microscopic cancer cell clusters in their bodies at any given time, before they mutate into tumors.

The reason why we all don't develop cancer is because as long as your body has the ability to balance angiogenesis properly, it will prevent blood vessels from forming to feed these microscopic tumors. Trouble arises if, and when, the cancer cells manage to get their own blood supply. Now, they can transform from harmless to deadly. It's much easier to prevent cancer than to treat it once it manifests itself.

There is an ongoing competition in your body between cellular damage and repair. As the damage becomes greater than your body's ability to repair, maintain and regenerate, deterioration starts, followed by illness, chronic disease and ultimately death. If we could repair damage as fast as it occurs we could live forever. If we can provide the body with enough raw materials through nutrition and supplementation, it will repair itself.

Cancer cannot survive on fat. Cancer cells need sugar to survive. Cancer develops over decades out of a condition of chronic body inflammation. The inflammation creates free radicals. The free radicals damage cell DNA. Cancer is nothing more than cells with damaged or lost DNA and mitochondrial energy (ATP). Typically, the malignant cells have lost their DNA-encoded instruction to die, and thus they replicate endlessly until they kill the host. Once started, cancer is fueled by inflammation and sugar.

The evidence is quite clear that if you want to avoid cancer, or if you currently have cancer, you absolutely MUST avoid all forms of sugar, especially fructose, which are dirty fuels generating excessive free radicals and secondary mitochondrial damage.

People with insulin resistance, type 2 diabetics and those with metabolic syndrome have high blood levels of both glucose and insulin. Many cancer cells have insulin receptors. Cancer avidly consumes glucose and insulin, enhancing and accelerating cancer growth. Fat cells secrete estradiol which acts like a fertilizer for cancer cells.

Leafy green vegetables contain a certain kind of sugar that feeds healthy gut bacteria, which in turn helps crowd out more harmful microbes. E. coli-derived enzymes allow the bacteria to metabolize the sugar. There is much research that eating leafy greens is a preventative for many forms of cancer as well.

I drink an 8oz glass of water with 30 drops of chlorophyll daily just to make sure I'm getting adequate "green sunshine." It is estimated that as many as 41% of people in the US will develop some form of cancer within the next 20 years. This translates to about 130 million individuals, a shocking statistic that, in spite of the cancer industry's best attempts to spin it, represents an increase in the rate of one of the leading causes of death over the past 50 years, and not a decrease as you may have been told.

Politics play a huge role in cancer treatment and cure. The standard of care in the US is basically surgery, chemotherapy treatment and radiation.

Cancer is a $50 billion business and there is a hidden economic agenda with those who dominate the medical establishment and medical industrial complex, from government, Big Pharma, Institutions, like ACI, AMA, medical schools, doctors and hospitals.

Federal regulatory agencies such as the US Food and Drug Administration (FDA) and Environmental Protection Agency (EPA), the very agencies designed to protect us, doesn't. They knowingly allow companies to use poisonous toxins in their products, and this is a major reason why cancer rates are soaring. There are over 10,000 registered chemicals with the US Government and many are categorized as GRAS (generally regarded as safe) and are allowed into our food supply and not even recorded on labels. They are silent killers, just like the hidden sugars on most all labels, as described in this book.

Many scientists, doctors and clinicians promote a low carb, ketogenic diet for cancer. The major argument is that unlike the majority of our body cells, cancer cells lack the ability to metabolize ketones, (fats) and require a significant amount of glucose (sugar) to survive and replicate. Since a ketogenic diet can keep blood sugar low, the theory is that cancer cells won't be able to survive and thus the cancer will not grow and metastasize. Some doctors have reported amazing results in the use of these diets to help their patients go into remission. There are a few studies that show potential benefits for some cancers, especially brain cancer, but not all cancers. Whether or not a ketogenic diet will make any difference in the outcome most likely depends and the type of cancer and severity of the cancer. None of these studies show any data that suggests a ketogenic diet would be helpful in preventing cancer, but ultimately, good blood sugar control is likely helpful in preventing cancer in the first place.

In a nutshell, we're no longer getting the nutrients we need from food to protect ourselves against diseases such as cancer and cardiovascular disease. On top of that, we're exposed to cancer-causing chemicals in our food supply – a one-two punch that, without the appropriate interventions, is a recipe for disease and premature death.

- Heart attack, cancer and stroke account for 60% of all deaths annually in the US

- The two biggest causes of cancer deaths are diet and tobacco.

- 35%-60% of cancer deaths are attributable to diet and lifestyle choices.

- Diet causes as many cancer deaths as smoking.

- Diebetes is the #6 killer in the US and we now have an epidemic of type 2 diabetes.

- Type 2 diabetes is nearly 100% preventable and reversible.

- 80% of all heart attacks and strokes are preventable.

The payoff in terms of extra healthy years of life is absolutely astounding when you look at the statistics and realize you can prevent or reverse many health risks leading to early death. You can live a happy, healthy life into your 10th decade.

Genetic predisposition is a factor with cancer, but you have an ability to control your metabolism through an anti-inflammatory diet, which makes it much more difficult for tumors to grow and metastasize. Tumors feed on glucose (sugar) and are driven by inflammation, so when your body has elevated blood glucose levels, accompanied by chronic dietary-induced inflammation, the lethal combination depresses the local inflammatory response from your immune system and then your body cannot fight off and destroy cancer cells. As a result cancer cells grow and metastasize. Only 5% of cancers are genetic or hereditary.

Cut the chemically enhanced junk food to reduce your risks of cancer and obesity.

"The truth is not for all men, only those who seek it." – Ayn Rand

- In the early 1900s: 1 in 20 people developed cancer

- 1940s: 1 in 16

- 1970s: 1 in 10

- 2013: 1 in 2 men, 1 in 3 women

- 1,660,000 new cancer diagnoses per year in US

- 500,000 Americans die from cancer annually

- World-wide 20,000 die every day, 8 million per year

- $50 billion is spent on cancer treatment in the US annually

- Over $100,000 average annual cost to fight cancer per patient

- Chemo and radiation cause cancer and are carcinogens

Chemotherapy is an invasive and toxic treatment intended to eliminate cancer cells. Unfortunately, its ferocious chemistry is unable to differentiate between cancer cells and healthy cells and surrounding healthy tissues. Simply put, chemotherapy is an intravenously administered poison that kills all living matter. Repeated chemotherapy and repeated radiation treatments kill the whole body by degrees. The immune system is hit particularly hard by chemotherapy and often does not recuperate enough to adequately protect against common illnesses which can then lead to death.

Two-thirds of cancer treatment patients die as a result of opportunistic infections arising as a direct result of the immune system failing because of the aggressive and toxic nature of the chemo. Eighty percent of all cancers are treated by chemotherapy. Many people develop another form of cancer as a result of being treated by chemotherapy and radiation. According to PreventDisease.com, studies show that chemotherapy fails to work 97% of the time and most patients will die within 5 years of treatment. (This number varies depending on the type and severity of the cancer, among other factors.)

"Insanity: doing the same thing over and over again and expecting different results." – Albert Einstein

Exercise reduces inflammatory chemicals, body fat and insulin resistance, all of which may fuel cancer progression and recurrence.

Both depression and chronic stress increase inflammatory chemicals that impair the immune system and may increase tumor development, while stress hormones can stimulate cancer proliferation by increasing blood supply to tumors.

Sleep is important in maximizing your immune system's functionality.

Diseases do not thrive in a clean body. You should detoxify daily by eating fiber and taking a liver supplement, such as milk thistle. Clean your cells through a systemic cleanse, not a deep cleanse (colonic).

A strong immune system is one of the keys to fighting and preventing cancer, as it promotes self-healing mechanisms and self-repairing, apoptosis, the regular schedule of cell death, as opposed to metastases.

Your body is amazingly engineered and will heal itself given nature's pharmacy and the right fuel, the right nutrition. Accentuate the positive, eliminate the negative. Learn the awesome power of food. You can harness this power by simply making the right food choices.

Your IGF-1 levels (see blood test section) should be low. If they are high it could be a predictor of cancer, as high means fast cell turnover. Cancer cells mutate, divide and grow faster.

Carcinogens initiate cancer, but diet can promote it. Fertilizers won't magically grow plants where there are no seeds, but will promote growth once seeds are planted.

Trans fatty acids, partially hydrogenated vegetables oils, margarine, all increase risk for cardiovascular disease and cancer.

Examples of cancer treatments that present alternatives to surgery, chemo, and radiation, the standard of care in the US, include:

- Dr. Stanislaw Burzynski, Houston, TX- Antineoplaston therapy.

- Hoxsey Bio Medical Clinic-Tijuana, Mexico

- Geson Therapy-Tijuana, Mexico

- RIGVIR-Republic of Latvia-EU

- Budwig Diet

- Vitamin B-17 Therapy

- Essiac Tea

- Bromaline

- Cannabis oil

Eat to starve cancer by eating foods that are anti-angiogenetic, starving the blood supply to cancerous (malignant) tumors and cells. Die with your tumors, not from them, the microscopic, hidden tumors that don't grow and metastasize, that we all have in our bodies. (See epigenetics.)

Cancer is not a death sentence. It's a revolution. As with any revolution, it goes against the norm. It takes guts to go against the norm. It requires tapping into your inner strength that comes from the conviction that you are willing to succeed against all odds. Once you tap into that inner strength and knowledge base you have confidence that you will succeed or you will die trying. Never give up. Life is worth living.

Alcohol and Cancer

A new study reported by The Guardian, a British national daily newspaper, states that alcohol causes seven forms of cancer, and people consuming even low to moderate amounts are at risk, according to new analysis. The study states alcohol causes cancer of the oropharynx, larynx, oesophagus, liver, colon, rectum and breasts.

Alcohol also increases your risk of heart and liver disease, strokes and pancreatitis. Smoking and drinking together increases your risk of developing throat and mouth cancer more than doing either on their own.

A growing body of evidence suggests that alcohol is likely to cause skin, prostate and pancreatic cancer. The study showed a drinker's risk increased in relation to the amount consumed, so there is a dose-response relationship equation.

Health experts endorsed the findings to tackle widespread public ignorance about how closely alcohol and cancer are connected. The study sparked renewed calls for regular drinkers to be encouraged to take alcohol-free days during each week and not binge on the weekends. Having some alcohol-free days each week is a good way to cut down on the amount you're drinking.

People drinking more than the recommended limits should cut down in order to safeguard their future health and well-being.

Alcohol-related deaths reached a 35-year high in 2014, when more than 30,700 Americans died from such causes as alcohol poisonings and cirrhosis of the liver. This amounted to about 9.6 deaths from alcohol-induced causes per 100,000 people in 2014, a 37 percent increase since 2002.

Alcohol is also a known toxin. Chronic alcohol consumption disturbs your healthy gut microbes and immune system.

Whether or not moderate alcohol consumption can be safe and even healthy is controversial, with studies showing mixed results. Research shows people who have one to two drinks a day may have a significantly reduced risk of death from heart disease and "all cause mortality," compared to those who never drink alcohol.

However, as reported in The New York Times and The Guardian above, alcohol consumption is now associated with an increased risk of cancer, even at moderate consumption levels.

Moderate alcohol intake is considered a 5-ounce glass of wine, a 12-ounce beer or 1.5 ounces (1-shot glass) of hard liquor, preferably with food, per day.

According to the Dietary Guidelines for Americans, moderate alcohol consumption for healthy adults, is defined as having up to one drink per day for women of all ages and men older than age 65, and up to two drinks per day for men age 65 and younger.

If you don't drink, don't start. If you do drink, drink red wine, vodka or Tequila, as they're all plant based.

To lose weight, you must abstain from alcohol use altogether. It's full of sugar, plus your body will burn the alcohol first, before it burns fat. Alcohol makes you crave carbohydrates, so you are hit with a weight-gain grand slam as a result, so you store even more fat. Ever hear of a beer belly?

If you're a chronic drinker, at least exercise, so you can sweat out some of the toxins.

CHAPTER 38:
Statins

I am not a big fan of statins. They are over-prescribed and unnecessary for most people. The people who do benefit from statins are those with familial hypercholesterolemia, and with total cholesterol over 300, which is a very small segment of the population. Some statin pharmaceutical manufacturers deceive consumers by using aggressive and deceptive marketing practices that stress the benefits of statins and exaggerate the need for them, while downplaying the known, serious, and adverse health side-effects. This is an example of failure to warn and the deceptive practice of relative versus absolute risk analysis.

Satins are an anti-inflammatory, but can increase neuro-inflammation. We are seeing a near-epidemic in Alzheimer's disease. Is there a cause or correlation, or is mere coincidence that as statin use has increased, so has Alzheimer's? Statins reduce cholesterol. The brain is 60% fat and uses 25% of the body's total cholesterol to function. I do NOT believe in using statins unless you have hypercholesterolemia. The ideal total cholesterol (TC) measurement should be 180-200 mg/dL for all-cause mortality health. However, if you can eliminate or reduce diet-induced inflammation, lower LDL and raise HDL through proper diet and nutrition, why take a drug with adverse health effects?

CHAPTER 39:
A Well-Formulated Eating Strategy - Where Science and Strategy Intersect

"If we could give every individual the right amount of nourishment and exercise, not too little and not too much, we would have found the safest way to health."

– Hippocrates

"Eat food, not too much, mostly plants."

– Michael Pollan

Green vegetables are especially important for getting healthy levels of iron, an essential component for the body to carry oxygen through to all organs and systems. Green vegetables also include lutein, an antioxidant that reinforces vision. There are so many other benefits for these green, tasty, nutrition-filled veggies.

"If man made it, don't eat it." – Jack LaLanne

We are not so much what we eat, but what we absorb.

J ust

E at

R eal

F oods

"You are what you eat." - Ludwig Feurerbach

We can exert incredible power over both the number of years in our life and the quality of those years by controlling what we put in our mouths.

An unhealthy diet is a proven cause of disease. In fact, three out of four Americans die every year from diet-related diseases such as cancer, heart disease, high blood pressure, stroke, and diabetes. So it's exciting to see scientific research proving what natural health practitioners have been telling us for the last 2,400 years. (Hippocrates)

Change your diet, change your life. Dinner, not DNA, is destiny. Eat fresh, whole, real foods, mostly plants (organic), whenever possible. Upgrade your nutrition to living fuels that sustain life.

Diets work because of their similarities, not their differences. The similarities are simply eating more plants, fruits, and vegetables.

"It's bizarre that the produce manager is more important to my children's health than the pediatrician." - Meryl Streep

It's the quality of carbs, fats, and proteins, more than the percentage or ratio.

Nature and culture intersect on our plates.

Moderate protein, low net carbs, high-quality fat. Mounting evidence and new research suggests that this eating strategy may be one of the most powerful ways to slow down the aging process and prevent most chronic degenerative diseases.

I look forward to fueling my body with life. I not only look forward to fueling my body with good nutrition, I look forward to creating it in my kitchen, from shopping to preparation to consumption, even looking at what comes out as proof of activities well done. You will too, as your body will crave healthy foods, not the junk foods and empty calories you have been eating.

Eating a nutritious diet is like hitting a reset button for your whole body. After a while, you will have cultivated a new approach to food and eating, a recalibration to more thoughtful, rational, and responsible choices, without even knowing you are doing it. It will become habit, a behavioral change, a lifestyle for life. Your mind will have changed. You will never look at food the same way again, almost like poison vs. health, death vs. life. You will look at unhealthy foods like you don't want them and not because you think you are denying yourself a treat, which takes willpower; but there will be no temptation, no expenditure of willpower. You will look and feel better for it, guaranteed.

95% of people don't fail diets; 95% of diets fail people.

A diet has to be something we can follow for life, a lifestyle program or strategy. By eating more greens and veggies or plant-based foods, you will actually eat more, but consume fewer calories, and feel full, getting healthy at the same time.

A low-carbohydrate diet can be done right. It's not a no-carb diet, just restricting or eliminating the wrong kinds of carbs like sugar and wheat and replacing or swapping with healthy, nutritious, rich, real, whole, fresh, fruits and vegetables, beans, legumes, seeds, and nuts. It's a simple swap.

Nutrition is a life skill. We live by our choices. We are not just what we eat. We need a personalized strategy. If we choose from the right food sources and restrict and manage carbohydrates, we will all be healthier for it.

There is no single magic food that makes for a nutritious diet, but a combination of low sugar, high antioxidants, high anti-inflammatories, high quality proteins, omega-3 fats and no trans fats, with a diet rich in whole foods, of plant based, vegetables and fruits will do the trick. Eat real, whole foods, with minimal processing, because these foods contain a virtual pharmacy of nutrients, phytonutrients, enzymes, vitamins, minerals, antioxidants, anti-inflammatories, and healthful fats and can keep you alive into your tenth decade.

Eating is like driving a car, paying attention actually makes a difference.

Humans have about 21,000 genes, of which 99.00% to 99.5% are the same from person to person. That tiny percentage makes the difference between how one person metabolizes food to the next, and how one person can eat the same thing and never gain weight, while the other person gains. Does either of these sound like you? That's why we need a personalized diet or strategy.

Become an alchemist in your kitchen. If you can fish it, hunt it, gather it, pick it, or pluck it, eat it. If it has a barcode, comes in a bag, box, jar, or container, beat it. Eat whole, real, fresh, organic foods when possible. No fast foods, no fried foods, no sodas, no processed foods, no sugar, and no wheat. Simple formula.

If you are on a low-carb diet and your body has converted from burning sugars or carbs to fat, then saturated fats (which we have been led to believe are bad for us) are actually burned as fuel and do not stay in our bodies. They become healthy components of your low-carb, higher healthy fat, higher healthy protein diet strategy. Energy is life, food is fuel for energy and therefore life, so food is life. Every time you put something in your mouth, it's about to affect your life, one way or another, good or bad, friend or foe, life or death. Ask yourself, am I taking a bite of life or am I taking a bite of death or poison?

Thirty thousand premature deaths a year are associated with trans-fats. Don't confuse saturated fat with trans-fats. The combination of saturated fats with trans-fats has a different effect than saturated fat alone.

Saturated fats from unhealthy sources such as fried foods, processed deli meats or hormone-treated beef are not good for you. Saturated fats from healthy whole foods, grass-fed animals like beef, lamb, and bison, and organic egg yolks are good for you, especially when these foods are part of a diet high in plant foods, antioxidants, fiber and all the nutrient-rich foods you eat on a controlled-carbohydrate eating strategy found in this handbook.

So, if carbs are low, insulin is low, saturated fat is handled more efficiently, you're burning the saturated fat as fuel, then your body makes and stores less fat. New research shows that healthy saturated fats are not a problem as long as people don't eat high amounts of carbohydrates, such as sugars, starches, grains, processed carbs, fast foods and high-calorie content foods.

Diet is Greek for "way of living." Food is information, food is energy, and food is fuel.

If given the right fuel, many people recover from chronic illnesses by giving their bodies the natural whole foods they need and leaving the rest to 10,000 years of internal healing.

We want homeostasis, or balance and equilibrium, in our bodies, finding a target zone that we can maintain for a lifetime, through correct nutrition and an individualized eating strategy so that it becomes a habitual lifestyle.

"The best way to predict your health future is to create it." – Abraham Lincoln

A low-carb diet simply selects foods that work with your metabolic biochemical machinery, instead of against it, controlling fat from within rather than trying to eliminate or restrict it from the diet, as low-fat diets attempt to do (but fail), because they replace fats with high doses of carbohydrates, which metabolically and biochemically produce fat and fat cells through the metabolic and biochemical mechanisms that produce insulin and hence, fat storage.

Changing the nutrient content of our diets has many beneficial effects throughout our body, including the brain.

All foods are composed of macronutrients, micronutrients, and water. The macronutrients are composed of protein, fat, and carbohydrates and provide energy to sustain life, known as calories. The micronutrients contain vitamins, minerals, and trace elements, which provide no caloric energy, but are essential to sustain life. Together, they perform a multitude of cellular functions, without which we would suffer malnutrition, starvation, diseases, declining health, and death. Simply put, the nutrients from both groups are necessary for life.

The human body is a complex, resilient, reactive, regenerative piece of biochemical machinery. It functions best when fed the correct nutritional fuel and can even heal itself from within.

A diet rich in omega-3 fatty acids and polyphenols and low in omega-6 fatty acids, refined carbohydrates and processed foods is the best medicine for a healthy now and a future of wellness.

A diet rich in omega-3s and polyphenols, combined with low-glycemic load carbs, will prevent excess insulin secretion levels and decrease diet-induced inflammation at the same time, decreasing risk of chronic disease and weight gain. Research shows there is a strong probability that constant insulin elevation levels, a product of insulin resistance, are caused by dietary-induced inflammation. The combination of elevated insulin levels and increased omega-6s not only increases cellular inflammation, but speeds up the development of chronic diseases, accelerates the aging process, shortens your life and affects the quality of your life.

When chronic cellular inflammation is maintained long-term due to a pro-inflammatory diet and lifestyle choices, the end result is that you become fatter, sicker, and more tired, and you age faster and die earlier. There is an epidemic of obesity, diabetes and soon-to-be Alzheimer's in our future, but it is preventable through a proper eating strategy.

You must have adequate levels of omega-3 fatty acids and polyphenols to control and extinguish diet-induced inflammation with a proper nutritional balance of low-glycemic carbs, protein, reduced consumption of omega-6s and significantly increased omega-3s and polyphenols. Flavanoids or bioflavanoids are plant-based, powerful antioxidants found in many fruits and vegetables and they provide medicinal benefits as an anti-inflammatory agent found in blueberries, green tea, and chocolate.

"The doctor of the future will no longer treat the human frame with drugs, but rather will cure and prevent disease with nutrition." - Thomas Edison

By reducing diet-induced cellular inflammation, you will lose weight and maintain a desirable weight, lose excess body fat, decrease the risk of modern chronic diseases, and retard the aging process. You will become more efficient at metabolizing food for energy and burning fat (not sugar), and you won't have hunger cravings for junk foods, as your body will actually start craving healthy foods.

Diet does not replace prescription drugs, but drugs, vitamins and supplements do work better, synergistically, with a well-designed eating strategy and the fewer prescription drugs you will need. In today's modern medicine, we over-medicate people to overcome diets that promote inflammation. We treat the symptoms, not the cause, and are running our healthcare system into insolvency. Paying for increasingly expensive drugs and medical procedures to treat symptoms is not sustainable healthcare and will bankrupt America and compromise our security. Hippocrates had it right 2,500 years ago: "Let food be your medicine, and let medicine be your food." Food is power.

"You have two choices for your health . . . life or death. Don't make the wrong choice. You have to eat, so why not eat smart?" – Unknown

A diet deficient in vitamins, minerals, and nutrients can cause malnutrition, even if a person consumes enough calories or eats more to compensate, leading to overeating, weight gain, and obesity.

Everyone's metabolism is unique, thanks largely to the genes we have inherited from our ancestors but also due to other external influences such as illness, stress, nutrient deficiencies, our lifestyles, and environment. As a result, everyone processes and utilizes food and nutrients differently.

Many researchers and studies recommend a balance of 40/30/30, discussed in detail below. That's a pretty middle-of-the-road template that will be healthy for many people; however, some people, especially athletes, want more fat or a ketogenic diet and have cut the carbs even further, as high as 80% fat/protein and 20% carbs. However, I believe a more balanced ratio is more sustainable long-term and healthier in the long-run.

I think as long as you get most of your carbs from vegetables and fruits, seeds and nuts, combined with 4-6 ounces of healthy protein, along with healthy fats, you will succeed in your health goals.

Minimize full-fat dairy products and saturated fats from non-grass fed, non-organic and non-pasture raised meats and eggs.

No dietary philosophy provides all the minimum daily requirements of micronutrients, vitamins, minerals, essential fatty acids, and amino acids to achieve nutrient sufficiency. This is another research fact and statistical-based reason to take supplements.

I don't recommend deli-meats, as they are generally processed, have added chemicals and preservatives to keep them fresh-looking and colorful, with a longer shelf life before rancidity. Additionally, sugars, salts and nitrates are routinely added, especially in packaged "deli-meats" from the grocery isle.

If you buy deli-meats be sure you ask them to slice your order in front of you, off the whole breast or whatever portion you are ordering, so you can see where it's coming from and be assured it is freshly sliced, not taken from a factory processed package and set out in a tray, having the same qualities of the unhealthy grocery aisle "deli-meats."

If your deli-meat has the skin on it, chances are it's real. Eat the skin, too. It's healthy fat and good for you. The sooner you start buying your meats and cooking them at home yourself and slicing them into proper portions, preparing in advance for a week's worth of food at work or on the go, the sooner you will be on your pathway to ideal health.

The healthiest people are those who eat and prepare their food at home using fresh, natural, whole food ingredients, and do not eat restaurant food, cafeteria food, or fast food. You not only have to know what you're eating, but what you're eating ate, and how your food was prepared.

Do a pantry purge. When in doubt, throw it out. If you don't have it in your pantry, you can't be tempted to eat it. When all you have in your pantry is healthy choices, you have no choice but to eat healthy. Avoid the "bad" stuff and take advantage of the "good" stuff.

Eat real food from a rainbow colors.

Healthy nutrition will not merely cause you to lose weight, but will prevent and reverse diseases.

Balance the ratios of carbohydrates, fats and proteins, individualized and customized for your metabolic and genetic type. The food list in this handbook is a great template for the majority of people who want to lose or maintain weight, or simply become healthier. If you really want to fine-tune and personalize, you must test to find your various blood profiles as outlined in the Blood Tests to Save Your Life section in this handbook, for long-term health and wellness.

When you eat more healthy vegetables and fruits, you are more satiated from the high fiber and water content derived from whole, natural foods, so you consume fewer calories, helping you to lose weight. By consuming fewer carbs, you control your insulin, thereby allowing even more weight loss. Control carbs, control insulin, control weight. Don't eat late at night after 8p.m. Simple formula.

Without adequate levels of polyphenols from a diet rich in vegetables and fruits, it's difficult to rid the body of excess free radicals, regardless of the amounts of supplemented antioxidants. I believe antioxidant supplements, like all supplements, are still a good insurance policy.

The goal of antioxidants is to move free radicals into the bloodstream and into the urine for excretion and elimination. Antioxidants either come from our food (from phytonutrients) or polyphenols (from fruits and vegetables). Grains and starches have relatively low levels of polyphenols.

The food we eat today becomes the cellular makeup of our human tissue tomorrow, from our plates to our forks to our cells. Replace bad foods with good foods.

Eat nutrient-rich, nutrient-dense, whole, organic foods as much as possible, avoiding or eliminating GMOs, global distribution foods, unnatural feeds, unnatural environments, processed foods and fast foods.

An effective state of a ketosis, or fat-burning as opposed to sugar-burning, is significantly anti-inflammatory, antioxidant, decreases free radicals and directly supports your immune system.

Non-irradiated foods spoil and are discarded while irradiated foods last longer and look fresh and vibrant but are far past their natural expiration or use-by dates. They entice us to buy products long after their nutritional value has faded, first from the depletion of nutrients from the irradiation process itself, then compounded by longer shelf life. The foods finally eaten contain little or no nutritional value and are little more than empty calories that add more potential damage to our health.

If it comes in a box, bag, bottle, can, jar, package, has a barcode, or has been pasteurized or irradiated, leave it on the grocery store shelf and don't eat it.

This includes cereals, chips, crackers, cookies, cakes, processed cheeses, sodas, fruit juices, candy, dried potatoes, dried fruits, pasta and most packaged deli meats, which all have been heavily processed and are not even real, whole foods, but manufactured pseudo-foods or Frankenfoods.

In 2010 President Obama signed into law the Food Safety Modernization Act, which allows irradiation of our food supply of fruits and vegetables to extend their shelf life. It exposes our food to radiation to supposedly destroy microorganisms, bacteria, viruses, and insects, while delivering the equivalent of 33 million to 150 million chest x-rays, altering a food's DNA, vitamins, minerals, and protein content, creating more Frankenfoods, far worse than microwaving your food.

Every time you touch food: slice it, dice it, peel it, sauté it, microwave it, steam it, fry it, process it, refine it, boil it, bake it, or expose it to heat, air or light, it reduces or depletes food's nutrients. Think of cutting an apple and watching it oxidize or brown. One more reason to eat locally grown, organic fruits and vegetables that haven't been trucked long distances or stored in warehouses: eat them in whole-food form, raw and fresh.

Europe has not allowed irradiation of foods since 2003.

People who eat a low-carb diet generally consume 1/3 fewer calories, naturally. The increase in fiber from vegetables and fruits makes you feel fuller and takes longer to digest, thereby limiting or restricting calories effortlessly, naturally, and automatically.

By following a lifestyle of a well-formulated nutritional diet, supplemented with vitamins and minerals, combined with proper exercise and a positive attitude, I believe one can live a healthier, longer, and happier life than by using any prescription medications produced by pharmaceutical companies, drug interventions, or drug therapies.

Excess glucose in the blood is a significant producer and driver of oxidative stress. That's why excess carbohydrates and excess omega-6s are dietary-induced factors that increase cellular inflammation, which we want to reduce or eliminate through the correct eating strategy.

Polyphenols from vegetables and fruits are powerful anti-oxidants and powerful anti-inflammatories.

Your eating strategy needs to be efficient in converting your food into energy. It's not the number of calories you eat, but the efficiency of those calories in producing energy in your body. If you eat fewer calories you will live longer, so it makes sense to eat efficient calories and not nutritionally empty calories such as sugar.

Prepare you vegetables either by steaming or lightly sautéing with olive oil, walnut oil, or coconut oil, avocado oil or macadamia nut oil, with a little water for moisture. I add garlic powder and black coarse ground pepper to taste. I eat many vegetables, fruits, and some meats and fish raw or seared.

Fiber and fat have no effect on insulin.

Good nutrition is the best way to unlock your body's natural healing energies.

"Success is when preparation meets opportunity." – Unknown

Don't count calories, make calories count.

The 40/30/30 balance combination of macronutrients is very similar to our Paleolithic ancestors and really hasn't changed for thousands of years, but agriculture and our food chain has.

- 40% carbohydrates, mostly from vegetables and fruits, nuts and seeds.

- 30% healthy fats (Some people may thrive on 50%-80% fats.)

- 30% healthy proteins

If you need a nighttime or before-bed snack, one of the best is a piece of turkey breast (not deli meat) and raw spinach. The turkey provides protein and tryptophan, which will accelerate production of your melatonin and serotonin release to help you sleep, while the spinach is a healthy carbohydrate.

However, it is not recommended to have nighttime or bedtime snacks. You should stop eating 2 hours before bedtime, preferably by 8p.m. Earlier would be even better. If you feel like you're hungry before bed, you probably have eaten too many carbohydrates and not enough fat. Reach for the coconut oil and eat a tablespoon full of that or a handful of Macadamia nuts.

Protein bars are often loaded with sugar and processed junk and are not as healthy as a good chocolate bar.

Good nutrition is the foundation of good health. We need macroronutrients, carbohydrates, fats, proteins, micronutrients, vitamins, minerals, water, and air to survive.

If we do not feed ourselves the proper nutrition, we impair the body's normal functions and cause ourselves great harm. Even though we may show no signs of illness, we may not necessarily be healthy. It's the TOFI syndrome (Thin on the Outside, Fat on the Inside.)

Grass-fed, grass-finished, not grass-fed, grain-finished.

If you must eat dairy, choose raw dairy products (non-homogenized and non-pasteurized, if possible). I'm not big on yogurt, especially since most are already pasteurized, killing all the good probiotics. However, as long as it is low in sugar (6 grams or less per serving) and loaded with probiotics, yogurt has good protein content, and if made from raw milk, may be well tolerated by many diets. Mix with fresh fruit, not with fruit already included which has too much added sugar. If you must, eat as a snack or a swap for ice cream.

Although not considered a favorite of the Western palate, organ meats such as liver are superfoods of the animal kingdom. Organic, grass-fed liver is one of the most nutritionally dense foods in existence and nature's most concentrated source of vitamin A. Liver is also abundant in iron, choline, copper, folic acid, B vitamins, purines, and natural cholesterol.

Dr. Weston Price, who has been called the Isaac Newton of nutrition, travelled the world studying diets of traditional cultures and found organ meats were nearly universally prized, primarily for their incomparable nutrient content.

Organ meats from grass-fed animals are safe and rich in high-quality amino acids, fat, B vitamins and B12, CoQ10, minerals, and "fat-soluble activators" (F A, D and K), important for mineral absorption.

Organ meats are extremely high in natural vitamin A, which is crucial for your health and may even prevent birth defects. Unlike synthetic vitamin A, natural vitamin A is not toxic.

While it's true that fresh fruits and veggies are full of vitamins and minerals, their micronutrient content doesn't always hold up to what is found in organ meats like liver.

A popular objection to eating liver is the belief that the liver is a storage organ for toxins in the body. While it is true that one of the liver's role is to neutralize toxins (such as drugs, chemical agents, and poisons), it does not store these toxins. Toxins the body cannot eliminate are likely to accumulate in the body's fatty tissues and nervous systems. On the other hand, the liver is a storage organ for many important nutrients (vitamins A, D, E, K, B12 and folic acid, and minerals such as copper and iron). These nutrients provide the body with some of the tools it needs to get rid of toxins.

The difference between products derived from grain-fed animals versus from grass-fed animals is that many grain-finished livers are "condemned," whereas this does not happen with grass-finished livers. Avoid meat and organs coming from animals that are grain-fed or grain-finished. Meats can be grass-fed, but then grain-finished, so you have to ask your meat provider or butcher. If they don't know, pass and go on to someone who does.

Your good health is at stake, so, know what was eaten by what you are eating. Restrict all of your meats to pastured, or at the very least, grass-finished animals. In the wake of mad cow disease, it is particularly important to consume animals raised on pasture and fed a biologically appropriate diet, which virtually eliminates their risk of mad cow disease, as well as many other dangerous contaminants.

Pasture-raised animal products are much higher in nutrients than animal products that come from commercial feedlot farming. For example, meat from pasture-raised animals has 2-4 times more omega-3 fatty acids than meat from commercially raised animals. And pasture-raised eggs have been shown to contain up to 19 times more omega-3 fatty acids than supermarket eggs. In addition to these nutritional advantages, pasture-raised animal products benefit farmers, local communities, and the environment.

The main objective of your lifestyle change is to make sure you're moving in the right direction and eating the right foods. This is not a calorie-counting or portion-size diet. You will not starve yourself to a good weight. Vegetables are virtually unlimited. You can fine-tune portion sizes once you've developed correct food choices and you're seeing and feeling the results. By focusing on the right carbs, healthy protein, healthy fats, fiber, and water, you will generally be satiated without overeating. Calories tend to self-regulate as you start to get lean and reconfigure your body.

Good nutrition is like building a foundation to support your body, one brick, one fork, one bite, one sip at a time – instead of killing yourself one fork, one bite, one sip, another nail in the coffin, at a time.

Eating combinations in a nutshell:

- Low fat and high carbs = obesity

- Low fat and low carbs = unhealthy

- High fat and high cabs = deadly

- Low carbs and higher healthy fat and moderate healthy protein = optimal health.

- Low-fat diets are by nature high-carb diets

The average American gets between 4 and 11 grams of fiber per day. Every major health organization recommends between 23 and 38 grams.

There's one other eating strategy that can yield good health results: "Eat breakfast like a king, lunch like a prince and dinner like a peasant." Studies show that if you front-load your day you will eat fewer calories and less junk food or empty calories throughout the day. Plus, you are setting the stage for your metabolism and thermal engines to be revved up and burning calories all day long.

I still like eating 5 times a day: 3 main meals and 2 snacks, with main meal plates mostly full of organic, green and colorful vegetables and fruits, topped with 4-6 ounces of grass-fed, pasture-raised or wild-caught protein, with snacks of an organic apple, banana and raw nuts or seeds.

A diet of protein from grass-fed meat, wild Salmon, organic free-range poultry and eggs, fats like olive and coconut oil, nuts, and avocados, with an occasional glass of red wine and a bite of dark chocolate, front-loaded with tons of organic fruits and vegetables, is light years ahead of the Standard American Diet. It is going to increase your energy and stabilize your weight, not to mention making you happy. Not bad, huh?

Eat smart, live strong, live long. A natural progression of healthy food choices, substitutes, swaps, transitioning into a lifelong practice of healthy eating habits, allows you to live, thrive, and feel alive. Practice a smart eating strategy daily. Do the wrong thing and you will experience disease, poor health and premature death. We live or die by the choices we make.

"If you don't design your own life plan, chances are you'll fall into someone else's plan and guess what they have planned for you? Not much." - Jim Rohn

CHAPTER 40:
The Healthy Plate

This food and nutrition journey is much more than a diet; it's a new way of eating and even a new way of looking at your food. It becomes simple: a habit and a way of life. Your body and mind will start craving healthy choices, making it easier than you think. Reestablish your relationship with your food.

The foods that we eat can have either an alkalizing or acidic effect on our bodies. Alkalizing foods are primarily leafy greens, vegetables, grasses, sprouts, herbs, and most seeds, nuts and fruits. Acidic foods are primarily meat, dairy, sugar, wheat, alcohol, and processed foods.

With consuming a nutritionally rich diet and controlling your insulin, you should notice increased luster and body in your hair, stronger nails, your skin should become more moist and supple, your endurance and energy should improve, you should sleep better and simply have a more radiant, vibrant, and energetic glow about you. Your system is like an assembly line, so getting those raw materials into the assembly line, blood and cells starts on your plate.

You are not going on a diet or starving yourself, you are simply adopting a new way of eating for the rest of your life. You and only you have complete control of what you put into your mouth. The results and rewards become the motivation.

Processed instant oatmeal is a bad choice because it's been pre-cooked via high-heat processing, robbing the oatmeal of many vitamins, minerals and nutrition, as well as added sugar. Go with steel cut, gluten-free, oats. I eat them raw with almond or coconut milk, blueberries, raw almond slices or raw walnuts and a sprinkle of cinnamon. It's packed with fiber and nutrition.

Beer is not good because of the yeast, but if you must drink beer, Miller Lite or Heineken are healthier choices because of their fermentation process and yeast content. Vodka generally is not good because of wheat and gluten, or potatoes and carbohydrates. Tequila is actually the best hard liquor because it is plant-based.

Wine, especially red wine, increases insulin sensitivity and decreases insulin levels, so it's a scenario to enjoy life, drinking 1-2 glasses with dinner. However, if you are trying to lose weight, you must stop all alcohol consumption, as your body recognizes alcohol as a toxin and burns it first before anything else.

Saving time isn't the only thing to consider with your food choices when it could take years off your life. Your everyday habits of nutrition, environment, and activities play a significant role in your health.

CHAPTER 41:
IF-Intermittent Fasting

Intermittent fasting (IF) is a term for an eating pattern which cycles between periods of fasting and eating. Humans have actually been fasting throughout evolution. Sometimes it was done because food was not available. It has also been a part of major religions, including Islam, Christianity, Judaism, and Buddhism. It is not a "diet" in the conventional sense. It is more accurately described as an "eating pattern."

With intermittent fasting your body burns fat, thus reducing the number of fats cells. This is important because the fewer fat cells a body has, the less likely it will experience insulin resistance or diabetes. Essentially, every aspect of your health will improve, including ideal weight management.

Intermittent Fasting has prolonged life in experimental models. It is a voluntary calorie restriction. It definitely will work for you as a weight-loss plateau buster (WLPB). Spontaneous intermittent fasting, if accomplished with no adverse side effects, is a very clear indicator and marker for optimum metabolic health. IF is not a diet: it's an eating pattern and a WLPB. I have developed a very specific IF protocol.

The idea is not to starve yourself. My IF protocol is simply a WLPB that works and still gives you not only your macronutrients, but 13.5 servings of vegetables and fruits, 69 grams of protein, 15 grams of fat and 60-oz of water. It's an amazing combination of nutrients and WLPB all rolled into one. It combines two traditional IF protocols, water fasting and juicing fasting, with calorie restriction. I have developed it into a WLPB as well as an IF protocol recipe. A winning formula!

Studies show that intermittent fasting and calorie restriction helps your cells regenerate and repair, clean out toxins and cellular debris, and permit natural apoptosis (or cell death) to occur, so that cancer cells cannot replicate, divide, and mutate into more dangerous cancer cells. Research suggests that fasting may be more powerful than drugs in preventing and reversing many modern diseases such as obesity, diabetes, cardiovascular disease, and cancer.

IF strengthens your mitochondrial network systems throughout your body. As long as your mitochondria remain healthy and functional, it's very unlikely that cancer will develop. You will see the best results with intermittent fasting when you combine a normal whole food, nutrient-rich diet, along with 20-30 minutes of cardio daily and some resistance training.

Intermittent fasting provides remarkable health benefits but it is just another tool and should not be confused with feast or famine, where the body assumes you are in starvation mode, so it starts storing fat. Quite the opposite, your body will burn fat, because for 36 hours you are not introducing any new sugars or carbohydrates to your system to store as fat or burn as sugar. It's simply a different method of assimilating food for 36 hours, during most of which you are asleep, while burning fat stores. It's a tool to get you through those stubborn plateaus on your way to your ideal maintenance weight. It also helps repair insulin/leptin resistance and helps re-teach your body to burn fat.

With intermittent fasting, cells focus on repair of damaged cells as well as cleaning up cellular debris, reducing inflammation and oxidative damage, allowing cells to stay healthy and vibrant. Cancer cells are known to divide and mutate. Apoptosis is the natural death of healthy cells. Our bodies use over 70% of its available energy towards digestion. We can harness that energy towards healing our bodies through intermittent fasting.

IF increases elimination of waste and detoxification. One of the secrets to good health, wellness, and longevity lies in internal cleanliness and regeneration. Traditionally, the longest-lived societies are those who have eaten the least number of calories. The long-lived people of Okinawa eat up to 40% fewer calories than Americans and suffer 80% fewer heart attacks, strokes, and cancers, and have a higher percentage of centenarians.

Research shows intermittent fasting helps brain function through neurogenesis, synapse strength and neurotransmission. In every species studied, calorie restriction extends life. I don't mean that you have to count every calorie or weigh your food, just be conscious of portion size and its nutrition value.

In America we are overfed and undernourished. The average American consumes 2,400-3,600 calories daily, with many eating more. Just eat 25-30% less than you normally would.

Target 1,500 to 1,800 calories daily, at the lower end for women. Intermittent fasting one day a week will help you cut calories and maintain desirable weight. Most food ingredient labels are based on 2,000 calories a day when referring to portion size. Obviously, the label information is irrelevant if you consume more calories and more portion sizes than the label recommends.

Intermittent fasting is an interesting concept. Fasting as a weight loss tool is difficult to sustain long-term, however, IF is a different story. The problem with long-term fasting is muscle loss. You work hard for that muscle gain and you don't want to lose it to a cannibal (your own body). You want to lose the fat, not muscle, plus you don't want to gain the weight that you lost back, plus more. So what you want is steady and sustainable weight loss and fat loss, without muscle loss.

IF is a way of cutting calories naturally without starving yourself as you do in traditional fasting or juicing. This is a hybrid that covers all the bases. Water, (hydration), carbohydrates from vegetables and fruits, protein, fat, fiber and omega-3s. You get 9-13.5 servings of fruits and vegetables 40-60 ounces of water, 3 tbsp fiber, omega-3 and 1-2 tbsp of fat. This is the only time I count calories, because the purpose of fasting is to restrict calories and elapsed time between meals. My Weight Loss Plateau Buster formula is as follows:

- 20-24 oz alkaline or filtered water in a shaker (breakfast 6-8 am)

- 1-scoop Green Vibrance (4.5 servings of vegetables and fruits per scoop)

- 1-scoop PlantFusion protein powder (plant based) (1/2 scoop for those who want less protein)

- 1-tbs ground Flax seeds

- 1-tbsp organic Chia seeds

- 1-tbsp organic whole Psyllium husk

- 1-tbsp organic Coconut Oil or 1 tbsp Olive Oil

A pinch of Himalayan pink rock salt. (When we are on a low-carbohydrate, ketogenic diet, we have lower insulin levels and therefore our kidneys excrete more sodium, which can lead to a lower sodium/potassium ratio and a greater need for sodium in the diet.)

Shake, pour, drink. Repeat (lunch and dinner)

First one in the morning for breakfast at 6-8 am; second one midday (lunch); third one (dinner) 6-8 p.m.

This "Green Drink" will be a little gooey at the bottom from all the fiber, so eat it with a spoon if necessary, as it's thick from all the fiber, but some of the most nutrient dense of the mixture, so don't throw it out. (For best results, stir with a spoon as you drink to keep fiber mixed, so it doesn't settle to the bottom.)

The fiber also feeds your gut microbiota, thereby helping to boost your immune system.

You had your last solid food and meal the night before at say 6-8 p.m., so you've gone 12 hours until your first WLPB the next morning at 6-8 am, so that's 12 hours of fasting.

Fast the whole day until 6-8 p.m., so that's 24 hours without a regular meal. Go to bed and wake up at 6-8a.m.the next morning. That's a total of 36 hours of Intermittent Fasting. You haven't starved yourself like you would with traditional water or juice fasting.

In fact, you have fueled yourself nutritionally throughout the day with a hybrid Intermittent Fast that I developed to break weight loss plateaus. Many people experience plateaus in their weight loss journey that are hard to overcome. They get frustrated because they can't reach their weight loss goals. so they cheat.

Try this method and you should lose 2-3 pounds. You can do a 6-1 or 5-2 IF protocol, meaning you can do 1 day of IF and 6 of your regular diet or 5 days on regular diet and 2 days of IF. However, I don't recommend 2 days of IF in succession, as it's too hard to sustain.

I have my last meal on Monday night 6-8 p.m. and do the WLPB IF starting on Tuesday mornings and then start my regular eating strategy on Wednesday 6-8 am, giving me those 36 hours of IF.

According to a 2016 study by the Public Library of Science, you will most likely weigh less on Wednesday first thing in the morning before eating or drinking anything than on any other day of the week. So you should experience a successful result from IF on Wednesday morning, not only for your weight number and busting through your weight loss plateau, but your blood pressure should be lower, your blood sugar should be lower, your diet-induced inflammation should be reduced, and cellular debris and toxins removed as well.

Now, if you want to do 5-2 IF, then do your next IF on Thursday, so your 5-2 would be Tuesday and Thursday of each week.

A modification or slight tweak to this formula, if you are famished and can't get through the night, when you have your last WLPB on any given night, add to a little snack of ½ apple, 1 strip chicken breast, 12-raw almonds and 1-celery stalk dipped in almond butter. Or you can substitute a strip of turkey breast and raw spinach if you like. It's very few calories, and a super healthy snack and will get you through the night to a date with the scale and weight loss plateau victory. (Watch the almond butter as it contains carbohydrates, especially if you're carb sensitive. Macadamia nuts are always a good substitute for almonds, as they contain more fat and less protein.)

This WLPB shake is also a good meal replacement shake/green drink whenever you're on the fly or have to skip a meal. Just mix it up, put it in a to-go cup and you're nourished nutritionally and won't feel guilty about skipping a meal and getting off your well-managed eating strategy.

You may also drink 12-16 ounces of Organic Turkey or Chicken Bone Broth. If you're going to the gym or walking in the morning you can add a cup of Organic Green Tea with caffeine, unless you're allergic or hyper-sensitive to caffeine: in that case, do de-caffeinated.

One of the keys to IF is staying hydrated. The first option, if done 3 times during the day, means consuming 60-70 ounces of water, plus if you drink 8-12 ounces of green tea, which is made from water, and then add organic bone broth, you have taken in 90 ounces of liquid for hydration.

I almost never count calories, but for the WLPB formula I did so to calibrate maximum efficiency for weight plateau busting. The calorie count for maximum effectiveness should be maintained between 500-600 calories. If you base this WLPB formula on a 2,000 calorie day, you are cutting or restricting calories by 1,500 on a 6/1 format or 3,000 fewer calories on a 5/2 format. Multiplied by 52 weeks, that's a calorie reduction of 78,000 to 156,000 per year.

Statistics show that a person must burn 3,500 calories to lose one pound, so theoretically, that equates to an average of 22 to 45 pounds that a person could keep off their body by following an IF protocol and reducing calorie consumption. Research shows you will live a longer, healthier life by cutting calories, not to mention all the other benefits outlined above, including weight loss and weight maintenance.

Another tweak to IF, although I don't like skipping meals, especially breakfast: there are those IF experts who simply recommend eating your food on an IF day in a window of 6-8 hours. You stop eating the night before at say 8p.m., you wake at say 8 a.m., so that's 12 hours without food. You drink water first thing in the morning, as well as coffee or tea and then don't have your first meal until noon, which still can be breakfast, then you continue your water intake to 6-8 p.m. when you have dinner, which is your second meal of the day, but you've eaten your food in a 6-8-hour window, so you've had 16-18 hours of fasting, little mini-fasts if you will. You can also add a little healthy snack or a green drink as outlined above between your two meals between 12-6/8 p.m. I like a green drink every day.

Intermittent fasting schedules:

- 8 a.m.-4 p.m. or 12 noon-8 p.m.

- 18, 24 and 36 hour fasts

- 6-8 hr windows of food intake

- Stop eating 3 hrs before bedtime.

Adding exercise to your IF day synergistically increases your results.

One additional IF technique is to eat a nutritious breakfast at 7-8a.m., then eat your second and final meal of the day at 3-4 p.m. By 7-8a.m.breakfast the next day you will have fasted for 16 hours. Each of these IF methods will work; it's just a matter of which one works best for you.

Cancer cannot survive on fat. Cancer cells need sugar and acid to survive. Intermittent fasting helps your body to become fat-burning as opposed to sugar-burning. Remember, calorie restriction is the only known modulator for longevity in animal models and is believed to work in humans.

Intermittent fasting lowers inflammation and oxidative stress. Oxidation damages cells promoting the development of cancers. IF helps to build neurons and synapses, challenges the brain, helps resist disease, builds stem cells, cleans and repairs damaged cells, and adds a multitude of healthful benefits.

I believe in eating 3 meals a day: breakfast, lunch and dinner, with a mid-morning and mid-afternoon snack; 5 eating sessions per day to keep your metabolism cranked and fire thermogenically burning. But IF does have many related health benefits. What I developed is a kind of hybrid between juicing, calorie restriction, and fasting. Try it and you will break through your weight loss plateaus. Remember to stay hydrated on your IF days. I drink two-12oz glasses of water upon waking on IF days. The water helps you to feel full.

CHAPTER 42:
Sinkers, Fluffy Floaters or Stinkers

Know your shit and get the scoop on your poop. Be #1 about #2.

Excrement is 75 percent water. The other 25 percent is fiber, bacteria, cells, and mucus. Soluble fiber in the diet is essential for healthy bowel movements. The fiber found in vegetables, fruit, beans, and nuts is ideal for creating the solid part of healthy poop. Insoluble fiber, on the other hand, as found in corn, carrots and oats, are difficult to digest and often show up in stools looking much the same as they did when they entered the body. It can take up to 72 hours to fully digest food and eliminate it out the other end.

Most of us try to suppress passing gas in public, but for the most part, passing gas is a sign of health. When your body breaks down nutrient-rich food, gas is released as a byproduct of your food being digested. The American College of Gastroenterology states that passing gas up to 18 times a day is normal and healthy.

Gas is good. It means your digestive tract is doing its job and the good gut bacteria is doing its job and since there's lots of gas, your poop is light, fluffy and floats, because the gas makes them lighter than water, so they float. Stinkers are also a sign of good health from the gases. Proper hydration and fiber will help with multiple bowel movements per day. Sinkers are heavy and full of nutrients that weren't absorbed and normally not long and fluffy, but small and dense, sinking and splashing.

Passing gas, or flatulence, is normal. It means your trillions of good gut bacteria are hard at work doing their jobs and your immune system is healthy.

One way to monitor your diet is to observe your bowel movement frequency and composition. With the increased fiber and water in your nutrition-dense food choices, there will be more water flow into your colon, loosening stools, determining whether they float or sink.

Increased water flow into the colon produces stools that are less dense and tend to float.

Ninety-five percent of your stools should be water. Another beneficial result of nutrition-rich food choices is you should not be constipated and should have frequent, healthy bowel movements three or more times per day.

Healthy bowel movements will be gaseous, which helps them float as well, but will make them stink. But it's a smell of health, so be proud of your floaters and stinkers and monitor often because knowing what goes into your body is just as important as knowing what comes out.

It's rare that we actually pause and consider that the green juice you drank an hour ago has already been absorbed by your GI tract, entered your bloodstream, been filtered by your kidneys, traveled down your urethra into your bladder and now passed freely into the toilet.

Mindful elimination (a consideration of what your body is doing every time you eliminate), creating calm, and eliminating stress, will encourage a feeling of gratitude that propels you to make healthier lifestyle choices every day. Bowel movements are our daily checkup to monitor our health. When you begin incorporating healthy choices and practices into your everyday life, pooping can go from a stressful experience to a truly pleasurable one, and few things are more satisfying than a good poop. Your poop knows best.

What you see in the toilet says something about your health. If you ignore what you deposit in your toilet you could be flushing your health down the drain.

The average person generates about 5 tons of stool in their lifetime, so you have a literal mountain of evidence to measure your overall health. Slow down and look down. It should be like a sausage or snake, smooth and soft. The ideal stool is smooth, soft and easy to pass and comes out in long snake-like pieces and floats. The lack of a splash means you are on the right track. You are shooting for frequency and ease, ideally at least three times daily.

If you are computer-literate you can relate to this term: GIGO (garbage in, garbage out.) So, floaters, stinkers (a pleasant aroma), and "poo perfection" are your goals. You will attain this by eating from the Food List in this handbook. Here's to "Poo Perfection."

CHAPTER 43:
Vitamins, Minerals & Supplements

"You take the healthiest diet in the world, if you gave those people vitamins, they would be twice as healthy. So vitamins are valuable."

– Robert Atkins

I strongly advocate supplemental vitamins, minerals, herbs and botanicals; however, it is still best to first get your nutritional value from organic, whole, real foods, vegetables and fruits, grass-fed and pasture raised meats, poultry and eggs that are outlined in this handbook.

In the US, sales of dietary supplements totaled nearly $37 billion in 2014, while the number of supplement users in the US reached a record high of 68 percent of the population.

Since 2008, the supplement industry has been required to report adverse events to the US Food and Drug Administration's (FDA) adverse effects reports (AER) system, pursuant to a 2006 Act.

Data from this reporting system shows there were 488 times as many adverse events reported from prescription drugs than from dietary supplements between 2008 and 2011. Adverse effects from drugs are far more likely to be deadly. In 2014, there was not one single death from a vitamin, supplement or herbal remedy.

Data also shows that adverse reactions to pharmaceutical drugs are 62,000 times more likely to kill you than food supplements and 7,750 times more likely to kill you than herbal remedies.

If you think drugs are safer than supplements because they're regulated by the FDA, consider these statistics:

At least 106,000 Americans die each year from the negative side effects of drugs taken as prescribed. People are taking more pharmaceutical drugs today, so the death toll is likely far higher

Prescription drugs kill more Americans each year than traffic accidents

Vioxx, killed 60,000 people before finally being withdrawn

Beta-blockers killed 800,000 in five years

Since 1999, more than 190,000 Americans have died from overdosing on opioid painkillers

Tylenol kills nearly 500 people annually. (Ironically the supplement NAC is used to save the lives of those poisoned.)

If you are buying your supplements at the same place you find powdered doughnuts and potato chips, you need to re-educate yourself and make better brand choices. (Gas station or grocery store syndrome.)

Big pharma is a US government approved drug dealer that leaves tax-payers and families to clean up after the avalanche of deaths and the messes of addictions they have caused.

Make sure all your vitamins and supplements are soy-free, gluten-free, dairy-free and rice-free. Gluten is a toxin and soy contains a number of problematic compounds, including:

- Goitrogens that can block synthesis of thyroid hormones and interfere with iodine metabolism and healthy thyroid function

- Isoflavones that resemble human estrogen and may disrupt your endocrine function

- Phytic acid, which bind to metal ions, preventing the absorption of certain beneficial minerals, including calcium, magnesium, iron and zinc

Vitamin A: Vitamin A and its building blocks, the carotenoids, support healthy eyesight, protect against heart disease and cancer, reduce sun sensitivity and promote healthy skin. Too much vitamin A can be toxic, unlike carotenoids. However, it's possible some people don't efficiently convert carotenoids to vitamin A. A multi-vitamin with both vitamin A and mixed carotenoids is a prudent choice. Labels may list vitamin A and beta-carotene at the top of the ingredients list and the mixed carotenoids separately in the Supplements Facts panel.

B Vitamins: Everyone needs adequate B vitamins for efficient conversion of carbs into energy and to break down fats and protein. Collectively known as B complex vitamins, they include the following:

- B-1 (Thiamine) Mega Benfotiamine (fat soluble, best)

- B-2 (Riboflavin)

- B-3 (Niacin)

- B-5 (Pantothenic acid)

- B-6 (Pyridoxine) 40 mg

- B-9 (Thiamine/Folate/Folic Acid)

- B-12-Methylcobalamin-sublingual-1000mcg minimum to 5,000mcg daily

- B-17 (Purported cancer prevention from Apricot seeds. AKA Amygladin or laetrile, illegal in the US.)

The B's support muscle tone in the digestive system and promote healthy eyes, skin, hair, and liver. They are also necessary for the proper function of the nervous system and help reduce stress. B12 is an energy booster and may help to alleviate depression and age-related memory issues. A deficiency in B12 contributes to anemia. A combo of B6, B12, and folic acid reduces levels of homocysteine, which is associated with endothelial dysfunction and atherosclerosis, a risk factor in heart attack and stroke. The same combination may reduce risk of macular degeneration.

B9, or folic acid, deserves a special mention, as it is associated with reduced heart disease, depression, and Alzheimer's disease. 800mcg.

Vitamin C: (from whole foods.) An antioxidant, C is especially important in times of life stress, recovering from injury or illness, and when physical activity is significantly increased. Our bodies require vitamin C for optimal wellness, healthy skin, heart function, cancer protection, and a healthy immune system. To absorb and utilize effectively, take vitamin C in split dosages throughout the day. Bioflavenoids, nutrients found in citrus fruits, are antioxidants and enhance the benefits of C. High-quality multi-vitamins contain bioflavanoids.

Vitamin D-3: (Not D-2) 5,000IUs to 10,000IUs daily. (cholecalciferol.)

Multi's will not contain adequate vitamin D. Once considered to be only a bone-building nutrient because it regulates calcium absorption, recent research suggests that vitamin D plays a much bigger role in overall health. Vitamin D is actually a hormone.

- 50-70ng/ml - normal range

- 80 - Optimal range

- 70-100ng/ml – fighting heart disease or cancer

- >100-ng/ml-Excessive

More than 3 out of 4 Americans have suboptimal levels of vitamin D. A recent 2008 study showed that people with low levels of vitamin D are significantly more a risk of dying from all-cause mortality and those with low D showed an increased risk of cancer. Your vitamin D optimal level should be between 60-70 and you should take 5,000 to 10,000 IU daily.

People with vitamin D deficiency have higher risk for insulin resistance, type 2 diabetes, and metabolic syndrome.

Vitamin E: (Tocotrienols-best, Gamma-mixed Tocopherol, next best) 400IUs daily.

Vitamin E has been shown to have a protective effect against heart disease, cancer, diabetes, skin sun damage, brain disorders, pancreatitis, pollution damage, premature aging, anemia, and scarring.

Studies have found that low vitamin E levels tend to be associated with a higher risk of cancer and heart disease. Vitamin E is fat-soluble, so be sure to eat an avocado or some coconut oil to help with absorption.

Tocopherols and Tocotrienols in vitamin E both have Alpha, Beta, Gamma and Delta molecules. It's best to have a mixture of all. Tocotrienols may have more cancer fighting properties,

Synthetic versions of E are typically identified by the "dl" at the beginning (dl-alpha-tocopherol), while non-synthetic uses a "d" (d-alpha-tocopherol.)

You want E from a natural or whole food sources and not a synthetic source.

Calcium: In addition to being a key component of healthy bones, calcium is required for breaking up fats, for normal transmission of nervous system signals, for transport of nutrients across cell membranes, for muscle contractions and heart rhythm, and for blood clotting and functioning of enzymes and hormones. (Be cautious when taking calcium as a supplement as it can lead to hardening of the arteries and possible kidney stones.)

Magnesium: Research estimates that at least 75% of Americans are deficient in magnesium. Plant foods are the main dietary food source. Magnesium keeps bones from becoming brittle and is important in the function of muscles, kidneys, heart, and other organs. It regulates levels of calcium, vitamin D, and other essential nutrients. Magnesium has a relaxing effect, alleviating muscle cramps and PMS symptoms, while improving sleep. Vitamin B6 is necessary to maximize magnesium efficiently. The mineral enables the heart and blood vessels to relax and pump blood optimally. Deficient amounts contribute to high blood pressure and heart disease. Risks for diabetes, osteoporosis, and possibly cancer increase with deficient levels. Stress causes magnesium to be excreted. Magnesium is a known laxative. Glycinate, citrate and threonate are best. (Theronate may support heart palpitations.)

Chromium: chromium is recognized for its beneficial effects on blood-sugar levels. It has been associated with weight loss. (I take chromium complex in tandem with L-carnitine for weight loss and maintenance.) Chromium increases cell sensitivity to insulin. Muscle cells refusing to accept blood sugar triggers hormonal disruption, contributing to weight gain. Chromium plays a key role in balancing hormones. By stabilizing blood sugar, it alleviates cravings for sugary and starchy foods, helping to control appetite. Chromium complex is best, followed by Picolinate.

Selenium: a trace mineral, acts as an antioxidant. Required for proper thyroid function and overall wellness. Low levels are associated with higher risk for thyroid malfunction, cancer, heart disease, infections, asthma, infertility, miscarriage, depression and rheumatoid arthritis. May solve acne and other skin conditions. Works synergistically with Vitamin E.

Zinc: a trace mineral, zinc is found in every cell of the body and is required by more than 300 enzymes for optimum function. Zinc helps insulin, critical in hormone balance, to do its job. Zinc is an antioxidant and necessary for healthy immune function, healthy eyes, skin, fertility, wound healing and overall wellness. American diets are zinc-deficient; however, too much can create a copper deficiency and can be toxic. Zinc lozenges are known to reduce duration and severity of colds, while topical zinc can help heal cold sores.

Iodine: a trace mineral necessary for proper thyroid function. (I do not generally recommend a separate iodine supplement, although it may benefit some people with thyroid disorders, it is best to get your iodine through nutrition from shellfish and seaweed.)

Omega-3: Omega-3 fatty acids are found in fish oil and reduce inflammation, protect the heart, reduce risk of disease from premature aging, and helps mitigate hormone balance. Studies show relief from PMS and menstrual pain. It reduces depression and mood swings among women in menopause. May help with weight loss. Helps balance hormones.

Fish oil is our richest source of EPA and DHA. EPA is viewed as a key anti-inflammatory component, while DHA is vital to brain health and function. EPA and DHA are classified as essential nutrients because our bodies don't make them, so diet or supplementation is the only source. Studies show a long list of fish oil benefits including: relief from chronic pain; reduced risk of diabetes; mood improvement; relief from depression, bipolar disorder, schizophrenia, and ADHD; reduction of aggressive behavior and healthy skin; and prevention or alleviation of arthritis, osteoporosis, eating disorders, inflammatory bowel disease, asthma, and macular degeneration. (I take Lovaza 4,000 mg daily.)

CoQ10: (Ubiquinol, not ubiquione.) It is found in every cell in the body and is essential for energy production (ATP), fuel for the mitochondria that keep cells alive. Levels of CoQ10 start declining at age 35, paralleling the aging process and contributing to the development of heart disease and other chronic and debilitating diseases, including cancer. An antioxidant, CoQ10 is used in cell growth and protects against cellular damage leading to cancer. Studies have found links between low levels of Co Q10 with cancers of the breast, prostate, lung, colon, kidney, head, and neck. Helps reduce blood pressure, improves blood sugar control. Aids in heart attack recovery. If you are post-menopausal or on a statin you should be on this supplement, as statins, used to lower cholesterol, deplete CoQ10 and with it all these wonderful health benefits. Take CoQ10 in the morning. 200mg daily or split dose: 100mg in the morning and 100mg in the afternoon.

75% of US adults over age 50 are deficient in CoQ10. Without enough CoQ10, the heart does not circulate blood efficiently, setting you up for congestive heart failure. Statins deplete CoQ10, so anyone on statins should supplement CoQ10. I recommend 200mg daily in 2 dosages of 100mg each, one in the morning, one at night.

CoQ10 has been shown to prevent underlying pathological disorders including reducing atherosclerosis risk factors, improving endothelial function and protecting against strokes or heart attacks, as atherosclerosis is the underlying cause of virtually all strokes, heart attacks and other blood vessel diseases. There are numerous other risk factors that are associated with the onset of atherosclerosis, including chronic inflammation, LDL oxidation, elevated blood sugar or type 2 diabetes, elevated cholesterol and triglycerides, and high blood pressure.

CoQ10 helps prevent oxidized LDL.

Flaxseed: It is rich source of omega-3, however it's ALA (alpha-linolenic acid), a precursor to EPA/DHA, which requires the body to convert ALA to DHA/EPA, so ALA is not as potent a source as fish or krill oil.

Chia seed: The reason Chia seeds are so beneficial is because they are rich in fiber, omega-3 fats, protein, vitamins, and minerals. Chia also contains essential fatty acids alpha-linolenic and linoleic acid, mucin, strontium, Vitamins A, B, E, and D, and minerals including sulphur, iron, iodine, magnesium, manganese, niacin, thiamine. They are also a rich source of anti-oxidants.

Psyllium: Research shows that taking psyllium is beneficial to many parts of the human body, including the heart and the pancreas. It has a great fiber component.

Vitamin K-2: (Not K-1) It drives calcium out of arteries and into bones and teeth, where it belongs. The type derived from MK-7 is best. (Jarrow brand.) K2 helps protect heart function. Helps prevent, reduce and even reverse atherosclerosis. Works synergistically with Vitamin D. Many Americans are deficient in K2. Brie/Gouda cheese good source of K2. 90-150mcg daily.

Probiotics: (Ls and B's) 13 billion minimum, the more the better. Immune system booster.

- Lactobacillus acidophilus
- Bifidobacterium

Essential Enzymes: Help digestion.

Minerals:

- Calcium
- Magnesium
- Chromium
- Selenium
- Zinc (No more than 50mg daily)

Flaxseed: Fiber. (1-Tbsp green drink daily.)

Chia Seed: Fiber. (1-Tbsp green drink daily.)

Psyllium: Fiber. (1-Tbsp green drink daily.)

Himalayan Pink Rock Salt: 80+ minerals and elements packed health benefits

Wild Green Oat Extract: 900mg daily-smoking cessation

Lauricidin: (Immune system booster, especially if you have been on antibiotics.)

Studies suggest that people who take supplements typically have a better quality of life, a lower risk of heart attack and diabetes, lower blood pressure, and live an average of 9.8 years longer. Oxidation and disease can be effectively controlled and managed with the use of vitamins, minerals, antioxidants, and other supplements.

The health of your body is dependent on the health of your cells. The body is dependent on 74 minerals. Vitamins are useless without minerals. You cannot receive all the vitamins and minerals a body needs with today's mineral-depleted soil, even if you eat all organic foods. If it's not in the soil, it's not in the plant! Supplement with high-quality vitamins and minerals, take the proper dosages, and achieve proper absorption and delivery to your cells, for optimal health, wellness, and longevity.

There are enormous benefits to increasing your dietary intake of vitamins and minerals through supplementation. So when it comes to making sure you're covering all the bases, quality supplements can be your daily backup for optimal health.

You cannot treat a nutritional deficiency with a drug.

How can you build a building that you expect to last 100 years if you put poor building materials in it? Same thing with your body, how can you expect your body to last for a long and enjoyable lifetime if you don't put the proper building blocks in it? Nothing will replace a diet rich in vitamins and minerals from whole, natural foods. However, supplementing helps to make sure we're getting the nutrition we need, each and every day, no matter what life throws at us.

The World Health Organization estimates that nutrition plays a role in 85% of disease.

If we are lucky, 40% of the nutrition from our food is delivered into our system, however, unless you are eating organic, you are nutritionally deficient and toxic. Supplementation is the only way to insure you will achieve optimal heath, wellness, and longevity.

Good health makes a lot of sense, but not a lot of dollars when it comes to fresh. Most food is a week old by the time it reaches the grocery store, not to mention the heat, trucking and time. Farmers markets or locally farmed raised may be the solution.

Although supplements are necessary for optimal health, wellness, and longevity, if you are not eating correctly, it's like running a race with one leg or running in opposite directions at the same time. Proper supplementation will offset some of the adverse influences of the bad foods you are consuming, but for optimal health results, high quality supplements, in concert with optimal dosages, combined with a well-managed eating strategy is your best pathway to overall good health. Supplements are health-protective, and therapeutic amounts are simply not available in our food supply (or not in the optimal amount or dosage requirement to make a difference in your good health, well-being and longevity).

- A recent report in 2015 reveals that proper use of certain nutritional supplements in protective doses from quality sources could save the American healthcare system BILLIONS of dollars each year in avoided hospitalizations.

- Researchers did not evaluate the full impact of vitamin D on chronic disease. If they had, the annual savings in the US alone would have been in the trillions of dollars!

- Use of omega-3 supplements among adults aged 55 and over who have been diagnosed with coronary heart disease could reduce annual hospital costs by more than $2 billion annually.

- If every person over the age of 55 with age-related eye disease were to take lutein and Astaxanthin at preventive dosage levels, medical savings would average $57.4 million annually.

- According to the 2013 GAO Dietary Supplements report, there were 488 times as many adverse reactions reported for prescription drugs as from supplements.

- Data from the EU indicate that pharmaceutical drugs are 62,000 times more likely to kill you as dietary supplements, but the average underreporting rate of adverse drug reactions (ADRs) is 94 percent, which means that risk may be even greater!

- Mass action. The recipe or quality of vitamins, minerals and supplements, plus the correct dosage and delivery systems, are vital to your supplementation success and allow absorption into your cells and blood stream where they belong. Otherwise, they could be needlessly excreted through urine and stool; however, just because it's in urine doesn't mean it didn't work on the way through!

- Our body needs 90 essential nutrients, so supplementation not only is a good insurance policy against gaps in our diet, but appears to be a fail-safe way to optimal health, wellness, and longevity.

The report titled "Smart Prevention—Health Care Cost Savings Resulting from the Targeted Use of Dietary Supplements" was produced through a grant from the Council for Responsible Nutrition Foundation. As reported by Drug Store News. The report examined four different chronic diseases and the potential for healthcare cost savings when US adults 55 years and older, diagnosed with these chronic diseases, used one of eight different dietary supplement regimens.

It demonstrated that supplementation at preventive intake levels in high-risk populations can reduce the number of disease-associated medical events, representing the potential for hundreds of millions, and in some cases, billions of dollars in savings!

Remember, the US healthcare system is almost bankrupt, but yet Big Pharma and the Medical Institution have a stranglehold on this debacle!

- Pharmaceutical drugs are 62,000 times more likely to kill you than vitamins and supplements.

- 106,000 deaths as a result of pharmaceutical drugs annually.

- 0 deaths as a result of vitamins or supplements.

- Iatrogenics, (Death by doctor), now #3 cause of death in the US.

Like exercise, no amount of nutritional supplements will counter the damaging effects of a poor diet. Nutritional supplements are like insurance; they cut your risk and add to an overall healthy portfolio!

"By the proper intakes of nutrients and by following a few other healthful practices from youth or middle age on, you can, I believe, extend your life and years of well-being by twenty-five or even thirty-five years." – Linus Pauling

RDAs levels for vitamins, minerals and supplements are generally woefully inadequate to ensure optimal peak performance, health, wellness and longevity.

When someone says taking vitamins and supplements just causes expensive urine, use logic, if it's found in the urine that means it was metabolized, so that doesn't mean it didn't work on the way down! You have health insurance coverage, using vitamins and supplementation is simply good health insurance. I want expensive urine, it's that simple! The key word is assimilation and absorption. If it's in your urine, it's highly likely it worked on the way down!

Disease is a result or an expression of an underlying imbalance of nutrition. If that's the case and you are not getting all your nutritional requirements from your food, why not supplement for insurance? Supplementation works for optimal health, wellness, longevity, and illness prevention. Studies show that people who take supplements on a regular basis have a better quality of life, lower blood pressure and a lower risk of heart attacks, strokes, cancers, and diabetes compared to those who do not take supplements. An extra health insurance policy.

Your pharmacist is your best source of drugs, vitamins, and supplement interactions or contraindications. Pharmacies have computer-assisted drug interaction programs that produce red flags. doctors don't, but you must use only one pharmacy. Remember, the #3 cause of death in the US is iatrogenics, death by doctor.

Supplements support a nutrition-rich diet; they are like an insurance policy that underwrites your good health, which along with exercise will synergistically combine into an overall lifestyle strategy for optimal health, wellness, and longevity.

Synergy: cooperative action between vitamins and minerals, which work as catalysts, promoting the absorption and assimilation. One nutrient aids the other in increased absorption. When taking supplements with food, food stimulates the natural digestive process and contains nutrients to help with the digestive and absorption process. Most supplements should be taken with food to allow for maximum absorption, however, there are some that should be taken on an empty stomach, per label instructions. Always split your dosages throughout the day for maximum absorption. Multivitamins should be taken in two dosages, a.m. and p.m. By spreading dosages throughout the day, you are eliminating or reducing competition among the nutrients for the pathways and receptor sites, thereby increasing absorption. Enhanced absorption and utilization into the bloodstream and cells is the key for optimal health. A well-formulated vitamin and supplement program simply covers the gaps of what nutrients your diet failed to deliver. Nutritional insurance, not expensive urine . . . and even if so, I want expensive urine!

We have soil that is no longer the mineral-rich dirt of our earlier generations, producing plants with reduced and inferior nutrient content. No diet supplies enough nutrients to meet minimum RDAs.

RDA, or recommended daily allowance, was established in 1941 by the National Academy of Sciences, US Food and Nutrition Board and adopted by the FDA as a standard for daily amounts of vitamins and minerals for a healthy person. Since 1994 product labels refer to RDAs as DVs (daily value), DRV (daily reference values) or RDIs (Reference Daily Intakes). RDVs are a set of daily references that apply to macronutrients, carbohydrates, fats, and proteins, as well as saturated fat, cholesterol, fiber, sodium, and potassium. RDIs are a set of dietary references based on RDAs for essential vitamins and minerals or micronutrients. The term RDI replaces RDA. Remember, the FDA is the same government agency that brought you the food pyramid, that may have been the largest human experiment in the US, responsible for the deaths of millions of people over the last 50 years on a high-carbohydrate, low-fat diet. The diet is responsible for our current epidemic of obesity, type 2 diabetes, cardiovascular disease, heart attacks, strokes, and cancer. These DRVs and RDIs do not account for optimal health, but rather borderline or minimum health. Again, the average American is fat, sick, tired, and dying!

Give your heart and cardiovascular system a helping hand by supplementing strategically. Supplements won't fix a bad diet, but they're a great way to help fill in nutritional gaps and provide additional support and protection, particularly for the heart.

Fish oil supplements help protect the heart by tamping down inflammation throughout the body.

A next-generation coenzyme is being introduced called pyrroloquinoline quinone (or PQQ) that has been shown to induce mitochondrial biogenesis—the growth of new mitochondria in aging cells. While CoQ10 optimizes mitochondrial function, PQQ activates genes that govern mitochondrial reproduction, protection, and repair. I use them in tandem.

Magnesium helps keep blood pressure in check by relaxing the blood vessels and promoting blood flow. You must be micronutrient sufficient for optimal health. Over 75% of the adult US population is magnesium deficient.

Chromium deficiency effects 90% of the American population, because the SAD is high in starches and sugars and exerts a heavy demand on the insulin system to handle the carbohydrate load, and that depletes chromium. One more reason not to carb-load before heavy exercise. Chromium not only helps you burn fat, but helps you build lean muscle mass. Chromium deficiency also causes sugar cravings and sugar consumption depletes chromium, so it creates a vicious cycle. Supplement with 200mcg daily.

Most people are unaware of the tremendous health benefits obtained from a high quality nutritional supplement program of vitamins, minerals, antioxidants, essential fatty acids, and even herbs and spices, and the importance of knowing the optimal dosages and synergistic combinations. You will never go another day without supplementing your body with the health promoting nutrients outlined in this handbook .

The greatest promise of vitamins and supplements is in prevention! Metabolic equilibrium and biochemical stimulation, coupled with synergistic effect can help correct lifestyle deficiencies, especially from our environmental toxins.

Look at supplements like a high-tech delivery system for your nutrients, a nutritional insurance if you will. We don't get the needed dosage or quality of some of the nutrients we need for true health and longevity from modern foods.

Vitamin and supplements working in the right dosage and high qualities work synergistically to enhance to optimal levels the nutrition that working independently cannot provide alone. Why not lower the risk, increase the odds and err on the side good judgment? An ounce of prevention equals a pound of cure! You have insurance on your car, your house, your health, and your life. Nutrition insurance trumps them all, because if you don't have your health, you have nothing!

The ideal ratio of omega-3 to omega-6 is 1:1, however, the average American is 16:1 to 25:1, or even up to 50-1, if consuming a lot of fast foods.

If you're deficient in vitamin D, your arteries are likely stiffer than they should be and not flexible, so your blood pressure may run high as a result.

The basic recommended minimum daily supplementation: (The Daily Dozen + 2)

- Multi-Raw One for Men & Women-1 per day

- Omega-3-EPA/DHA: the higher the DHA ratio the more you are feeding your brain. 2,500-4000mg daily. (Prescription Lovaza recommended.)

- CoQ10-200mg daily. (Ubiquinol not Ubiquinone, especially, if on statins.)

- B-complex, B6, B9 (folate) and B12-lower homocysteine levels, a known marker in coronary heart disease and stroke.

- B-12-sublingual-methylcolbalamin-500mgm-daily (best bio-available)

- C-1000mg daily-split doses-Raw Vitamin Code-Garden of Life (from whole food source, best bio-available). 1000-2000mg daily. No ascorbic acid from grocery store shelves.

- Vitamin D-3 (Not D-2) (Cholecaliferol-best bio-available) 5000-10000 IUs daily. (Test: 50-80 optimal range.)

- Vitamin E (High Gamma Tocotrienol (Best),Tocopherol-GAMMA mixed next. Natural vitamin E is listed as "d" forms as in d-alpha-tocopherol or d-beta-tocopherol. Synthetic vitamin E is listed as "dl" forms. The natural "d" and tocopherol form is what you want and not the synthetic "dl" forms.

- K2 (Not K1) (K2 from MK-7-best bio-available) (Drives calcium out of arteries and into bones and teeth where it belongs.)

- Astaxanthin-4mg-(Antioxidant)

- Glutathione (Antioxidant)

- R-Lipoic Acid (Antioxidant)

- Probiotic (Minimum 13 Billion)

- Essential Enzyme

A daily regime of these vital 12 vitamins, minerals, and supplements, plus a daily probiotic and essential enzyme for gut balance and gut health, will cover most of your bases, combined with a well-formulated nutritional eating strategy and exercise program, you will be well on a pathway to optimal health, wellness, and longevity! (All vitamins, minerals and supplements should be gluten-free, soy-free, dairy-free, nut-free.)

"You'll always miss 100% of the shots you don't take" – Wayne Gretzky

Healthy people are not the same as unhealthy people. They respond differently to medications, foods, exercise regimens, and antioxidants. If you are unhealthy, overweight, or obese, you may need higher doses for longer periods of time with all supplements.

However, if you are healthy, exercise, and have your weight under control, you may benefit from pulsing your frequency which may help with absorption and efficacy, especially with detox and chelator supplements like chlorella and charcoal, as well as mega doses of antioxidants.

Additional Vitamins, Minerals and Supplements to consider:

- **D-ribose:** A simple sugar molecule, D-ribose, is one of the key components of ATP. The more D-ribose that is available, the faster ATP levels return to normal. D-ribose supplementation has been shown to boost heart muscle function following heart attacks, and to improve blood pumping in people with congestive heart failure. 5 grams twice daily.

- **L-carnitine:** fat loss. If you are looking to get lean, then this is the amino acid you need. L-carnitine transfers long-chain fatty acids, such as triglycerides into mitochondria, where they may be oxidized to produce energy. It is synthesized in the liver and kidneys and concentrated in the body's most metabolically active organs: the brain, heart, and muscles. Carnitine has also been shown to reduce fatigue and serve as an appetite suppressant. (1,000 to 1,500 mg daily-Liquid in your green drink.)

- **S.O.D.:** superoxide dismutase. Power enzyme and antioxidant. Scavenges for and dismantles one of the body's most deadly free radical toxins, superoxide.

- **Super Chlorella:** Studies have shown that chlorella benefits the entire body by supporting healthy hormonal function, promoting cardiovascular health, helping to negate the effects of chemotherapy and radiation, lowering blood pressure and cholesterol, and aiding in the detoxification of our bodies. 1000mg (broken cell wall.)

- **Activated charcoal:** detoxifier. 2 caps daily. Use in tandem with chlorella for detox. Pulse dosage. 4 days on, 3 days off for maximum efficacy.

- **Serrapeptase:** plant-based proteolytic (protein-destroying) enzyme from bacteria native to the digestive system of silkworms. It is the enzyme responsible for dissolving a silkworm's cocoon. Traditionally, serrapeptase has been used for its anti-inflammatory properties. Atherosclerostic aid.

- **L-carnosine:** discovered in 1900, an abundant non-protein nitrogen-containing di-peptide (beta-alanyl-L-Histidine) found in meat. Battles oxidative stress (antioxidant.) L-carnosine is a potent amino acid compound antioxidant and is the most effective protective substance against the binding of sugars and proteins that cause free radicals, protecting against development of atherosclerosis and improving insulin resistance.

- **Pantethine**: Coenzyme A Precursor. Supports lipid metabolism. Pantethine, the metabolically active form of vitamin B5 (or pantothenic acid), offers a host of benefits. It is vital for dozens of enzymatic reactions that require coenzyme A, including those involved with processing fats and carbohydrates.

- **French Maritime Pine Bark Extract:** (Pycnogenol). Nature's super antioxidant for heart health. Helps to increase HDL cholesterol and metabolic syndrome. Improves endothelial function and arterial blood flow. 150mg daily.

- **Maqui Berry:** One of the most powerful polyphenols on the planet.

- **Fucoidan:** Brown seaweed extract. Wakame is a rich source of eicosapentaenoic acid, an omega-3 fatty acid. Wakame is also a good natural source of magnesium and zinc.

- **PQQ:** (Pyrroloquinoline Quinone) promotes mitochondrial biovenesis, supports heart andbrain function. 20mg daily. Synergistic in tandem with CoQ10.

- **NAC: (**N-Aceytl Cysteine) antioxidant, immune system support. As supplements go, this one might be among the most important ones you could take. NAC has broad benefits to health. Because it contains both sulfur and the amino acid cysteine, NAC serves as a precursor to glutathione, a key antioxidant that provides protection against free radicals and toxins in the body.

- **Pomegranate extract:** antioxidant, promotes cellular and cardiovascular health. Studies show a proven link to reversing atherosclerosis. 250mg daily.

- **TMG:** (Trimethylglycine.) Cardiovascular. Helps to preserve cell structure and make the cell more resilient to stress. May lower plasma homocysteine levels; this is important since elevated homocysteine levels can lead to blood vessel inflammation, making it a risk for heart disease. 1000mg.

- **Men:** For prostate health. Saw Palmetto complex-prostate health. (Pygeum bark extract, Pumpkin seed oil, Lycopene.)

- **Milk thistle extract:** Liver health. The active ingredient, the one that protects the liver, is known as silymarin, a chemical extracted from the seeds. Silymarin is actually a group of flavonoids (silibinin, silidianin, and silicristin), which are thought to help repair liver cells damaged by alcohol and other toxic substances. If you drink alcohol, a must-have detox agent for a healthy liver. 2-4 caps daily in split dosages.

- **Melatonin:** Beyond Sleep. Other benefits of melatonin: melatonin, a hormone produced in the pineal gland, is an effective natural sleep aid, a potent antioxidant, a free radical scavenger that helps combat inflammation, and an anti-aging therapy that has been shown to help prevent or treat multiple medical conditions, immune system issues.1mg. (night.) This is one where less is best.

- **DHEA:** A number of studies have found that DHEA supplements may help people with depression, obesity, lupus, and adrenal insufficiency. DHEA may also improve skin in older people and help treat osteoporosis, vaginal atrophy, erectile dysfunction, and some psychological conditions. There is good evidence supporting the use of DHEA for adrenal insufficiency, a condition in which the adrenal glands do not make enough hormones. Studies suggest that DHEA may improve hormone levels, health, and quality of life in people with adrenal insufficiency. 25-50mg daily. (Test.)

- **Ferrochel iron:** Iron is an essential nutrient in human health, playing a role in immune function and anemia. Must lab test for levels. Do not take a multi-vitamin with iron in it.

- **Pregnenolone:** like DHEA, is a steroidal hormone manufactured in the body.

Pregnenolone is a precursor hormone synthesized from cholesterol, principally in the adrenal glands, but also in the liver, skin, brain, testicles, ovaries, and retina of the eyes. May help with prevention of the onset of Alzheimer's disease, arthritis, or coronary heart disease. An additional advantage of bioidentical hormones such as pregnenolone is that they go to work quickly in the body. 50mg.

- **Anastrozole:** Test. A must with testosterone replacement therapy. Take .125mg - .250mg.

- **Colostrum:** Immunity, intestinal and stomach health.

- **Green Vibrance:** Daily "green drink." 4.5 servings of greens per scoop. 1 scoop daily recommended. Also has probiotics.

- **PlantFusion:** Plant protein powder. (I'm not a big whey fan.)

- **Curcumin:** (tumeric.) Many, many health benefits, including fighting cancer. I include the powder extract in my "green" drink. ½ tsp.

- **Resveratrol:** (grape seed extract.) Resveratrol protects the endothelial lining of arteries, helping blood flow. May protect nerve cells from damage and the buildup of plaque that can lead to Alzheimer's. Reduces oxidative stress, which prevents premature aging of cells. Diabetes: Resveratrol helps prevent insulin resistance, a condition in which the body becomes less sensitive to the effects of the blood sugar-lowering hormone, insulin. I use in my "green" drink. ½ tsp.

- **Green Tea extract:** The various health benefits of regular green tea consumption may result in a prolonged life span. I use in my "green" drink. ½ tsp.

- **Olive leaf extract:** benefits cardiovascular health and brain function. The olive leaf was first used medicinally in ancient Egypt and it was a symbol of heavenly power. It is the leaf of the olive tree, called Olea europaea. Olive leaves have been used in the human diet as an extract, an herbal tea and a powder. Works against LDL oxidation and may also benefit glucose metabolism and skin health. Differs from olive oil. I use in my "green" drink. ½ tsp.

- **Organic virgin coconut oil (cold pressed):** A superfood with amazing health benefits. A healthy saturated fat with MCTs: medium chain triglycerides. 1 Tbsp 3 times per week. Also good for oil pulling. (Oral health)

- **Himalayan pink rock salt:** Contains the same 84 trace minerals and elements that are found in the human body; that alone is quite impressive! (A pinch in "green" drink.)

- **L-Citrulline powder:** blood flow, circulatory health.

- **Glutamine powder:** Amino acids are the building blocks of protein. Glutamine is produced in the muscles and is distributed by the blood to the organs that need it. Glutamine might help gut function, the immune system, and other essential processes in the body, especially in times of stress. Mix in with "green" drink.

- **Fulvic acid:** aids in the elimination of harmful toxins: In the body, fulvic acid and humic acid molecules release trace minerals, amino acids, and other nutrients required for optimal cell function.

- **Cilantro liquid (tincture):** Heavy metal cleanser, detoxifier.

I have tried and use many of these powders and extracts on a regular basis in my "green" drink. I do alternate them.

Avoid using chewable vitamin C as it damages tooth enamel.

- Demand for vitamin C increases 10 fold during times of stress.

- When we are stressed, our adrenal glands secrete cortisol into our bloodstream, which spikes appetite and results in eventual fat deposits in the belly region or belly fat.

- Make sure you are taking 1000-2000 mg of vitamin C per day in split dosages from whole food sources.

In addition, too much cortisol for extended periods of time weakens your immune system. Stress also affects your gut bacteria balance, leading to digestive upset and malabsorption of nutrients from food intake.

Omega-3 supplementation can reduce stress-induced production of cortisol by 22%.

A growing body of evidence shows that vitamin D plays a crucial role in disease prevention and maintaining optimal health. There are about 30,000 genes in your body, and vitamin D affects nearly 3,000 of them, as well as the vitamin D receptors located throughout your body.

According to one large-scale study, optimal vitamin D levels can slash your risk of cancer by as much as 60 percent. Keeping your levels optimized can help prevent at least 16 different types of cancer, including pancreatic, lung, ovarian, prostate, and skin cancers.

Vitamin D deficiency is pervasive among stroke victims and those with continued chronic low D levels have the poorest functional outcomes in stroke rehab.

Around 6.8 million Americans, or 2.8% of the entire adult population, are living post-stroke and most are disabled, debilitated, dependent, or living in institutional confinement! Up to 80% of strokes are preventable. I continually increased my D blood levels until they were in the optimal range, taking 5,000-10,000IUs daily. But, you have to test, don't guess.

- Vitamin D and K2 help drive calcium into bones and teeth for optimal health.

- Vitamin K2 is every bit as important as vitamin D for protecting your heart and bone health; it's essential for activating enzymes involved in transporting calcium from your arterial walls to your bone.

- A recent study found statins may increase calcification in the arteries, another found statins deplete your body of vitamin K2, suggesting this may be a mechanism by which statins harm your heart.

- The quartet of calcium, vitamin D, K2, and magnesium all work together synergistically, and should ideally be taken in combination.

- You must differentiate between Vitamin K1 and K2.

- 258,000 US hospital admission annually for hip fractures among people 65 and older. 20% die within 1 year.

Essential Enzymes (Gut Health): Enzymes are considered the "spark of life," needed for virtually all biochemical processes in the body. Human life could not exist without the actions of enzymes, even with sufficient amounts of macronutrients, micronutrients, water, and air. Enzymes are catalysts and the body produces many special enzymes that assist in practically all bodily functions, turning food into energy.

Iodine-150-500mcg daily. (As needed per thyroid test.)

Antioxidants: I believe in a rich supply of antioxidants from your food supply and in addition, from added supplements, for cell protection for the brain and to prevent cell damage from free radicals and oxidative stress. (Healthy people may want to employ a pulse dosage regimen.)

Exercise is a healing and regenerative tool for re-growing damaged brain cells. A protein in the brain called BDNF (brain-derived neurotropic factor) triggers the process of growing back damaged brain cells. With exercise, high levels of BDNF are produced, essentially a growth factor the brain: a brain fertilizer if you will, that helps grow neurons back.

If you are in excellent shape, you may want to consider for optimal absorption and metabolism, employing a pulse strategy, which is 4 days on and 3 days off, with your antioxidant supplements.

Aspirin reduces melatonin levels in the body. Studies show that melatonin should be taken at night and may help slow cancer tumor growth and regulate sleep. Less is more with this supplement. I take 1 mg nightly.

Echinacea: No more than 3 months. Start in flu and cold season. More than 3 months has an adverse effect on your immune system.

Astragalus: Acts as a flu shot. Also may aid telomere length. If you don't want a flu shot, and I don't believe in injecting a virus into my system, take Astragalus. Start in October before cold and flu season, as it takes a while to build up defenses. I also take Echinacea in tandem with Astragalus, but no longer than 3months, as it can have a reverse effect on your immune system if taken for longer periods. 500 mg daily in season.

Like CoQ10 and L-carnitine, magnesium is critical to keeping all of your cells supplied with energy, especially the cells in your heart. In fact, your cells need a steady supply of magnesium to keep the smooth muscles in your blood vessels functioning. Plus, magnesium helps to shuttle potassium and sodium in and out of your cells, which is important for healthy blood pressure. Magnesium helps overall absorption of all supplements. I take 200mg of magnesium glycinate, twice daily. Up to 75% of Americans are magnesium deficient.

Krill oil maybe more absorbable, but doesn't have the high EPA/DHA concentration as a good fish oil.

Omega-3 DHA/EPA facts:

- Lovaza is a pharmaceutical-grade brand that requires a doctor's prescription and is 86% concentrated, whereas most over-the-counter brands are around 60% concentrated fish oil, so there is more bio-available EPA and DHA for your body to absorb with Lovaza. Most insurance policies will cover it, so you only have a co-pay that is still more economical than retail OTC, so a win-win!

- Buy the brand highest in EPA/DHA content. Life Extensions Super Omega-3 is a highly OTC rated brand with high level content.

- Telomeres' longevity is stimulated by at least 2.5gm of purified omega-3 fish oil daily.

- Ideal ratio of omega-3 to omega-6 is 1:1, however, the average American is 16:1 to 25:1 or worse, up to 50:1 if consuming fast foods on a regular basis!

- Omega-3 supplementation can reduce stress-induced production of cortisol by 22%.

- AA/EPA ratio blood test is a superior and more accurate test to measure inflammation than the hsCRP test, as the AA/EPA ratio is an early warning system for increased levels of cellular inflammation, and an elevated level of AA/EPA ratio can precede the development of an elevated hsCPR by several years, if not decades.

ADHD Vitamin deficiencies: B6, B9, magnesium, zinc, omega-3, carnitine.

1,000mg polyphenols daily: Research on the Maqui berry, which has the highest level of delphinidins on the planet, a polyphenol, shows that it stimulates the enzyme of life (RNA, ribonucleic acid). Delphinidins inhibit cellular inflammation and activate the enzyme of life, leading to a slowing of the aging process.

Iron: 1 hour before meals or 2 hours after for maximum absorption and utilization and non-nutrient competition for maximum nutrient sufficiency. Take iron separately at mid-day and do not take in a multi-vitamin. Iron can inhibit absorption of many other vitamins, minerals and nutrients. Blood test for it every 3 months, because it can be toxic and you may need to adjust dosage accordingly. You may also be anemic.

Iron 40-60 Optimal <20-low, > 80-high. (Ferritin)

Fertilizer for mitochondria:

- CoQ10

- PQQ

- R-Lipoic Acid

- L-Carnatine

- Carnosine

- Resveratrol

Type II Collagen: Try it for sore knees, especially in the winter.

Studies show that silymarin (milk thistle) fights oxidative damage and inflammation in the liver and fatty liver disease, so, if you drink alcohol and take statins, it might be wise to take milk thistle. 100mg 2X daily.

GI tract cleanse: Triphala, a potent yet gentle tree-fruit herbal complex that uniquely supports GI (gastrointestinal) tract wellness. Cleanses, tones and revitalizes tissues in entire GI tract, creates better digestion and regular elimination. 2-1,000mg tabs twice daily, morning and night.

Metformin, a drug that has been widely used to treat diabetes for about 60 years, is currently being tested on humans for its anti-aging properties. Metformin has demonstrated its ability to slow the aging process in certain microbes and mammals. To analyze the advantage outside treatment of diabetes, the Food and Drug Administration has green-lighted a clinical trial in the US for what has become known as the Targeting Aging with Metformin (TAME) study.

Vitamins, minerals and other supplements have near zero side effects, reduce risks of nearly all modern chronic diseases, increase energy and vitality, slow the aging process, inhibit wrinkling, promote better skin, hair, nails, and extends life! In my opinion, everyone should be taking vitamins, minerals, and other supplements daily or employ a pulse dosage strategy as listed in this handbook.

A 50/50% chance is the same as a coin flip. Why relegate your optimal health to a coin toss when you can increase your odds to 80/20% in favor of prevention and optimal health, wellness, and longevity? That's a 62.5% increase. I like those odds!

As a general rule, supplements will be better utilized and more effectively absorbed if taken with food. Split dosages, early morning, mid-day or night. Space iron supplements 1 hour before or 2 hours after other supplements. Iron can block receptors of other supplements and affect absorption. Do not take iron and calcium supplements at the same time.

"I believe that you can, by taking some simple and inexpensive measures, lead a longer life and extend your years of well-being. My most important recommendation is that you take vitamins every day in optimum amounts to supplement the vitamins that you receive in your food." – Linus Pauling

CHAPTER 44:
Nootropics/Neutraceuticals

"Whatever is good for the heart is probably good for the brain." – Hippocrates

For keen memory and cognitive health don't forget to feed your brain.

Your brain is just like a muscle that needs to be worked out and supplemented for peak performance. If a muscle atrophies you lose it; if your brain atrophies you get dementia. What you keep you lose, what you gain you keep. Neurogenesis, neurotransmission, and neuroplasticity are all enhanced by supplementation and exercise, which keep the brain sharp, firing, and strong.

Brain food to consider:

- Acetyl-L-Carnitine

- Deprenyl

- Life Extension-Brain shield (Gastrodin)

- Magnesium-Theronate

- Phosphatidyl-Choline-Jarrow-Citicoline-CDP

- Phosphatidylserine-Jarrow PS100

- Piracetam

- PQQ (Pyrroloquinoline Quinone)

- Taurine

- Vinpocetine

As your weight increases your brain atrophies, shrinks, and becomes smaller. Is it any wonder, as obesity and type 2 diabetes, which is an inflammatory disease, have risen, so has Alzheimer's disease?

Here Are some additional recommended supplements for brain health, and their daily dosage:

- Alpha lipoic acid (50-150 mg daily)

- N-acetylcysteine (200-600 mg daily)

- Coenzyme Q10 (50-100 mg daily)

- Omega-3 Essential Fatty Acids (1-2 g daily)

- Resveratrol (25-50 mg daily)

- Turmeric (100-300 mg daily)

- Melatonin (1-5 mg daily at night)

- Vitamin B-complex (800 mcg folic acid, 20 mg of B6, 20 mcg of B12)

- Acetyl-L-carnitine (500 mg daily)

- Blueberry powder (25 mg daily) and vitamin C (10 mg daily)

- Ashwagandha (200 mg daily)

- Phosphatidylserine (400 mg)

- DMAE (20 mg daily)

- CDP-choline (100 mg daily)

- Phosphatidylcholine (75 mg daily)

CHAPTER 45:
Politics, Public Health, Socio-Economics, Big Pharma & Big Agra

---

"Nature to be commanded must first be obeyed."

– Francis Bacon

When one lives in a society where people can no longer depend on institutions to tell them the truth, then the truth must come from the culture or nature.

The abundance of food in the United States, enough calories to meet the needs of every man, woman, and child twice over, has its downside. Our over-efficient food industry must do everything possible to persuade people to eat more: more food, more often, and in larger portions, no matter what it does to waistlines or health and well-being of the American population. Like manufacturing cigarettes or building weapons, food is big business.

Our food manufacturer companies are not food companies, they are chemical companies.

The FDA relies on company-backed science to "prove" that a drug or product is safe and effective. This despite the fact that industry funded research is almost never impartial, thanks to obvious and massive conflicts of interest.

Many people still do not take this into consideration. They believe that "FDA Approved" means that the FDA has performed some sort of independent scientific study. It has NOT.

At best, the FDA carefully reviews the research submitted, but there's plenty of room for cherry-picking, bias and other strategies that can skew the safety profile to an unsuspecting consumer.

It is shocking to learn precisely how food companies lobby officials, co-opt experts, and expand sales by marketing to children, members of minority groups, and people in developing countries. We learn that the food industry plays politics as well as or better than any industry, in part because so much of its activity takes place outside the public view. The food industry influences government nutrition policies and cleverly links its interests to those of nutrition experts to get policy approved and mainstreamed before our very eyes, when it's actually killing millions of Americans every year.

Sodas are astonishing products. Little more than flavored sugar-water, these drinks cost practically nothing to produce or buy, yet have turned their makers, principally Coca-Cola and PepsiCo, into a multibillion-dollar industry with global recognition, distribution, and political power. Billed as "refreshing," "tasty," "crisp," and "the real thing," these sodas also happen to be so well-established to contribute to poor dental hygiene, higher calorie intake, obesity, and type-2 diabetes, that the first line of defense against any of these conditions is to simply stop drinking them. Habitually drinking large volumes of soda not only harms individual health, but also burdens societies with runaway healthcare costs. The soft drink industry works overtime to make drinking soda as common and accepted as drinking water, for adults and children.

If insurance companies and the government would take the time to study the enormous benefits of uncovering the causes of illness and disease, then treating those underlying causes and not the symptoms, instead of treating people with truckloads of expensive prescription drugs, perhaps we would be a healthier society and our healthcare system wouldn't be on the verge of collapse. Prevention is the take-home message; not to treat or manage disease, but to prevent and cure.

Big Pharma defines diseases as a marketplace, a business model. The longer you stay sick the more money they make. They are about money and profits, not health. If it can't be patented, Big Pharma is not interested. Nature has cures and it belongs in healthcare; patents do not. Herbal vitamins and supplements are from nature; therefore, they are not patentable. They have few or no side effects, are not killing people and in fact, are preventive.

Seventy-five percent of every healthcare dollar is going to "preventative" medications for high blood pressure, cholesterol, or diabetes. But we are not getting healthier, we are getting sicker and causing other "diseases" or side effects to then be "treated," resulting in an overmedicated healthcare society and putting our healthcare system, not to mention our good health, at risk.

In 2008 Americans spent $2.3 trillion on this type of "healthcare," 3 times the $714 billion spent in 1990, and more than 8 times the $253 billion spent in 1980. Worldwide, 36 million people die of chronic lifestyle diseases and by 2030 they will cost an estimated $47 trillion, crippling the world's "healthcare" system, and all because of the business model to treat the symptoms and not the cause. That in a nutshell is Big Pharma's and standard medicine's business model for keeping you sick, managing you, keeping you coming back for more, and not curing you.

Sad fact #1: Big Pharma's marketing and lobbying efforts tell us it's our fault if we're overweight or unhealthy, and we should eat less and exercise more, and then brainwashing us to believe it.

Sad fact #2: Most of Big Pharma's marketing and advertising is not even based on science and many of their reports have been falsified or incorrectly interpreted to their advantage, using relative vs. absolute findings.

Combine Big Agra, Big Processed Food Industry, and the Fast Food Industry with the US government subsidies of corn, soy, and wheat, coupled with GMOs permitted by the government and 10,000 GRAS chemicals allowed into our food chain and in production of our food supply, complicity by the FDA, USDA, Public Health and other governmental agencies, and it's no wonder we are sick, tired, fat, and dying. It will take a health revolution, not merely reform, and it starts with your education and awareness and then taking action to take control and command of your health.

Politics, food and medicine playbook: First spin or tilt the science, discredit or attack the messenger, lobby the politicians in Washington D.C., and finally, spend millions of dollars on false or misleading advertising and marketing campaigns. The result: Big Farma (Big Agra) and Big Pharma (Pharmaceuticals) and a sick, tired, fat, and dying American public. Unreasonable corporate growth expectations corrupt nutritional science and public health recommendations.

Spin: Ask yourself, "Is the marketing ahead of the scientific research? Was it a human study or an animal study?"

"Everyone is entitled to their own opinion, but not to their own facts." – Daniel Patrick Moynihan

It is the food manufacturers' responsibility to shareholders and their bottom line that has led to a system where scientific truth has been misplaced by advertising doublespeak.

Processed food companies rely on public health advice to be in agreement with their offerings and anything else would be devastating to that same bottom line. If such advice is short of their message, the industry will resort to measures to protect its place as purveyors of "healthy nutritious food," opposed to the truth that a processed food diet will hasten disease and death.

In the US government, there is a disconnect between public health and agriculture, causing a health and nutrition epidemic of obesity, type 2 diabetes, cardiovascular disease, heart attacks, strokes, cancer, and Alzheimer's disease. Subsidies result in cheap unhealthy food, now exported worldwide, along with their modern diseases. The "American Way" is killing the world to keep the American farmer, Big Agra, Big Pharma and big business profitable globally. It will take a revolution of people, money, and education to stop this, but you can start with yourself and your family today. Buy local, eat organic, vote with your wallet and make smart food choices.

"It's not what we don't know that hurts us, it's what we know, that ain't so." – *Will Rodgers*

We resist change, but fear of the unknown can result in clinging to status quo behaviors, no matter how poor they are.

If enough people repeat an untruth long enough and often enough, it becomes accepted knowledge.

Because vitamins and minerals are found in nature and foods that can't be patented, Big Pharma can't profit from it.

The harsh reality is that the medical pharmaceutical industry doesn't make money out of cures; it makes money out of treatments and it benefits them for you to stay sick as long as possible.

Create healthy profits from healthy foods.

We've had decades of bad nutritional advice: nutritionists, doctors, and the government all invested in a false belief. No amount of evidence to the contrary could convince them they were wrong, as it would question their credibility, as well it should. The largest human experiment in US history – the low-fat, high-carbohydrate FDA food pyramid – had unintended consequences: low-fat, high-carbohydrate diets made us fat, sick, and tired. Cognitive dissonance, confronting long-held contradictory beliefs and cultural habits, must be resolved.

Only 25% of medical schools in the US require students to complete a single course in nutrition. That means at 75% of the medical schools in the US a doctor can receive a medical degree without any knowledge of nutrition, yet that is our #1 killer and healer.

The focus since the early 20th century of a medical education is pharmacology and the circumstances to prescribe drugs as defined by Big Pharma, as they control most of the funding for medical schools and their research.

Medicine is all about science, right? No, it's not. Science is often ignored in favor of rigged studies that support profitable drugs. And that's because our medical system is controlled by the pharmaceutical industry.

The USDA promotes commodity agriculture, not good health. The food pyramid produced people who looked like pyramids after eating the diet and became sick and tired, and eventually died.

If you're a corporation or a lobbyist and you want to "buy" a member of Congress, one common and effective way to do so is by secretly promising them a high-paying job once they leave office.

Since such deals are not made public, legislators can pass laws or create special tax cuts that benefit their future employer with little or no accountability. Politicians do not have to disclose job negotiations while in office, and also do not have to disclose how much they're paid after leaving office.

Research is oftentimes more political than scientific. Follow the money trail and you'll discover bias.

Corn, soy, and wheat are all subsidized by the US government, creating a cheap food source.

Vegetables and fruits are considered specialty foods and are not subsidized. Their price index has increased while corn, soy, and wheat have decreased, making them cheaper food sources that appear in almost all processed junk foods, creating "bad" foods, full of "bad" calories, resulting in an epidemic of obesity, type 2 diabetes, cardiovascular disease, heart attack, stroke, and cancer. Unfortunately, many communities don't have access to fresh produce or can't afford it on a limited budget, and eat the cheaper "bad" foods that government subsidies and the food industry have created.

The cost of fresh fruits and vegetables are 100 to 400 times more expensive per calorie than processed foods, refined grains, sugars, and vegetable oils. Ever wonder where our health would be worldwide if we had a McGreen's, a McBroccoli's, a KaleWay, a Dr. Pickles or even a McPaleo's? Instead of SAD (Standard American Diet) being truly sad, it would be the "Super" American Diet, instead of the Super-Sized American Disaster.

Corporations such as McDonald's, Coco-Cola, PepsiCo, Kraft Foods, General Mills, Subway, KFC and the like who were food giants in the 20th century, will become food dinosaurs in the 21st century if they don't start listening. Vote with your wallet. Their stocks will devalue and so will their advertising budgets, especially when marketing to our children. Childhood obesity is nearly 20% and climbing. Make these corporations think people before profits.

The pharmaceutical industry is the wealthiest and most powerful lobby on Capitol Hill. In 2011 the US Supreme Court shielded all pharmaceutical companies for civil liability lawsuits for injury or death caused by an FDA-licensed vaccine. There is no legal accountability for any corporations or individuals who develop, license, recommend, promote, administer, or mandate vaccines that injure and kill Americans. This is a profound betrayal of public trust by the US government.

There are 3 main products America exports to the rest of the world: weapons, entertainment, and food.

"Maintaining vitality in institutions and in people is brought about by change."
– Henry S. Rowen

CHAPTER 46:
The Healthy Choice Food List

The Food List allows you to lose weight and swap bad, unhealthy foods for good, healthy foods. Change your eating habits. Throw in some exercise and supplementation and bingo, you're ready for your close-up.

The list is a template to start. You will lose weight by cutting carbs, starches, and processed foods, reducing calories by ingesting more water and fiber with increased volumes of vegetables and fruits and eating healthy proteins and fats. However, listen to your body. Some of you may do better or lose more weight on fewer fruits as an example, while others may feel more energy with a small serving of brown or wild rice. It's all about maintenance for the long-term, what you can sustain for a lifetime.

If you do a pantry purge so all you have are healthy choices, you will have no temptations. I was able to lose weight while still eating several pieces of fruit a day and always had protein and fat with every meal. Finding your right balance between the macronutrients of carbohydrates, fats, and proteins is the key.

You have the power of choice and the ability to individualize and personalize your eating strategy to make it work for you. You will be eating a lot of food but consuming fewer calories than normal. You will not be hungry or craving junk food. As a result, you are able to lose weight and maintain a desired weight long-term.

These foods will work wonders for the vast majority of people. You will find the results life-changing. You can modify it to fit your own unique, personalized tastes, in a way that works for you. That's how lifestyle change works: you must enjoy it, see results, and reap the rewards and benefits it provides you.

These foods provide your body with the nutrition it needs and eliminates foods that your body does not require: nutritionally empty carbohydrates and calories.

There are no sugars (simple carbohydrates) and no starches (complex carbohydrates) in the list. The carbohydrates on this list are nutritionally dense and fiber-rich. Sugars are simple carbohydrates and empty calories that should be avoided.

Starchy carbohydrates to avoid include: grains (whole and healthy grains; there are no "healthy" grains), rice, especially white rice, all cereals, flour, corn-starch, breads, pasta (even whole-wheat), muffins, bagels, crackers, corn, potatoes, French fries and potato chips. If you are carbohydrate intolerant, you may have to avoid starchy vegetables like beans, peas, parsnips and carrots to lose weight. Avoid margarine and other hydrogenated oils, as they are trans fats.

Eat a variety of organic mushrooms regularly. Choose from white, cremini, Portobello, oyster, shiitake, maitake or reishi mushrooms.

If you want to eat honey, eat raw honey, unfiltered, unprocessed and unheated. It's full of antioxidants, it's antibacterial and antifungal, and it helps with digestive issues and soothes sore throats and stomachs. If you're sick and want a boost, it's great. I don't recommend it on a daily basis, but when you are sick and want a great taste with health benefits, go for it. Manuka honey is best. 10+ or higher. UMF certified. Other acceptable sweeteners, if you can't live without are: stevia and Luo Han Guo, (Lo-Han), both are plant based.

This is not a complete list of all the nutritional foods available on the planet. As you get healthier, your body craves healthy choices. You can individualize and customize healthy alternatives, as there are some exotic and lesser-known foods available that are both tasty and nutritious.

Meats: (grass-fed)

- Beef

- Buffalo/bison

- New Zealand lamb

Poultry/eggs: (Free-range/Pasture raised/Organic)

- Chicken-breast or dark

- Organic eggs

- Turkey-breast or dark

Fish: (Wild-caught)

- Anchovies

- Herring

- Salmon

- Sardines

- Tuna (ahi, albacore)

Vegetables:

- Asparagus

- Beets

- Broccoli

- Brussels sprouts

- Cabbage

- Garlic

- Green beans

- Kale

- Kimchee

- Mushrooms

- Onions

- Quinoa (okay occasionally)

- Salsa

- Sauerkraut

- Spinach

- Sprouts (Broccoli)

- Sweet peppers

- Sweet potatoes

- Watercress

Fruits: (Organic)

- Apples

- Avocadoes

- Bananas

- Blackberries

- Blueberries

- Cantaloupe

- Kiwi

- Lemons

- Limes

- Raspberries

- Strawberries

- Tomatoes

Nuts/seeds: (Raw)

- Almond butter (organic, no salt)

- Almonds

- Macadamia nuts

- Pistachio nuts-raw (green color=phytonutrients/polyphenols, good fat)

- Pumpkin seeds

- Sunflower seeds

- Walnuts

Legumes/beans:

- Black beans

- Chickpeas (garbanzo beans)

- Peanut butter (organic, no salt)

Oils:

- Avocado oil

- Coconut oil

- Ghee (clarified butter)

- Macademia nut oil

- Olive oil

- Walnut oil

Beverages:

- Green tea (Organic)

- Green Vibrance

- Water

Miscellaneous:

- Dark chocolate (70% cacao, organic, no soy)

- Herbs and spices

- Himalayan pink rock salt (if you want salt)
- PlantFusion (plant-based protein powder)
- Seaweed
- Tempeh

Substitutes/swaps:

- Rice: cauliflower rice (Trader Joe's.)
- Pasta: spaghetti squash.
- Bread sandwiches: Portobello mushrooms.
- Mashed potatoes: mashed cauliflower

All produce, vegetables and fruits should be organic whenever possible.

Fresh is best. Frozen is better than canned.

Carbohydrate restriction is becoming more common as the scientific evidence accumulates.

NO To lose weight you must eliminate or restrict the following:

- No sugar
- No alcohol
- No wheat, oats, barley, or rye. (stay gluten-free)
- No cereals (exception: steel cut, gluten-free oats)
- No bagels
- No margarine
- No jams or jellies

- No dairy

- No soy

- No fruit juices

- No pork

- No starches

- No rice (if you must eat rice, a small portion of brown or wild, not white)

- No potatoes

- No pasta

- No pizza

- No crackers

- No potato chips

- No cookies, cakes, pies, ice-cream, or yogurt.

- No processed foods

- No deli meats (packaged)

- No trans fats/fast foods

- No sodas

- No HFCS (high fructose corn syrup)

This program and eating strategy is not just a weight loss tool; it's a prescription for taking command of your health. Eat smart. Eat for your life.

Dairy:

There are vast differences in dairy products, due to multiple factors. These differences mean that dairy products affect the body in very different ways. Example: raw milk that has not been pasteurized or homogenized, that came from a cow that was organically raised, free-roaming, pastured, grass-fed and not given antibiotics or growth hormone injections, will affect the body much differently than milk or meat coming from a genetically modified cow that has been exposed to antibiotic and growth hormone injections, never allowed to roam in a pasture, is fed chemically laced, growth-enhancing, omega-6-grain based feed and has been pasteurized and homogenized. Raw organic milk and meat from grass-fed animals is the answer. Organic raw, unpasteurized, un-homogenized milk, cheese and dairy are incredibly healthy. Gras-fed, grass-finished animal meat (protein), in moderation, is health-friendly. (If you have changed your body to burning fat from sugar, your body will burn the saturated fat from these animals, so there is not so much concern about consuming saturated fats, but consumption must be kept in moderation for overall mortality risks.)

Homogenized dairy products, whether they are yogurt, milk or cheese, are deadly. It's not the fat that is the problem in dairy; it's the homogenization process, which causes scarring of the arteries, leading to atherosclerosis.

CHAPTER 47:
Exercise

"Take care of your body. It's the only place you have to live." - Jim Rohn

Physical fitness is a major determinant of longevity. If you want to prevent disease, exercise! Lack of fitness is second only to smoking as a predictor of early death.

Exercise helps delay the aging process and reduces the risk of many debilitating diseases including obesity, cardiovascular disease, heart disease, strokes, cancer, diabetes, and even depression. Activity and movement forms a counterbalance to eating by burning calories, strengthening the heart muscle and core, improving mood and ameliorating age-related physical decline. The combination of exercise and a nutrition-rich eating strategy also helps build your immune system, lowers inflammation, and keeps your microbiota healthy.

To preserve muscle mass as you age, you must maintain adequate protein intake and reduce cellular inflammation. These processes are controlled by the diet and by daily exercise with intense and interval training techniques outlined in this handbook.

"Move, walk, no matter how slow you go, you are still lapping everyone on the couch." – Unknown

Enhance your fitness without undermining your health. Good health is simply the absence of disease. We can be fit, but not healthy, so the goal is be fit and healthy at the same time. Exercise should enhance health, wellness, fitness, and longevity, but should not be the driving force. Exercise synergistically improves health in tandem with proper nutrition: 80% nutrition, 20% exercise.

In fitness, you keep what you gain and you lose what you keep. It's like a car, if it sits out in an open field and you don't maintain it, it rusts.

"Eat less and exercise more" is doomed to failure. You cannot out-exercise a poor diet. As we grow older, we naturally desire to grow older still, associating life with health, and health with fitness. The idea for longevity is to determine how little exercise is necessary as opposed to how much, so we are able to maintain health and fitness over a lifetime, combined with a proper diet and supplementation and putting it all together.

"You can't do much about a hurricane, but you can sure build a stronger house."
- Unknow

Exercise helps strengthen the immune system and reduces inflammation.

The most beneficial addiction that you can have in your life is the endorphins from exercise.

Exercise up-regulates your mitochondria and ATP energy at the cellular level, so exercise becomes a great metabolic treatment for disease. ATP energy also comes in nutrient-dense foods, which are an important part of the health equation.

Low intensity, steady-state activities like running or jogging at a steady pace do burn fat but will not give you ultimate health, because you are not building strength through resistance training to build lean muscle mass. Instead, muscles atrophy, reducing your muscle mass and the ability of your muscle cells to drain and restore glycogen, or insulin sensitivity. This becomes insulin resistance and storing insulin as fat.

To exacerbate the condition, if you are eating a high-carb diet of processed foods high in sugar and trans fats and drinks full of sugar, you have a recipe for diet-induced inflammation a double whammy recipe for cardiovascular disease, heart attack, stroke, and cancer, our biggest killers on the planet.

Look at the muscle mass of marathoners, atrophied. Look at the muscle mass of sprinters, defined and healthy, because they also do strength or resistance training. That's the science. You must do resistance training so you don't lose muscle. More calories are burned through your muscles. If you lose muscle, it is replaced by fat and you gain subcutaneous and dangerous visceral fat and your health sags as well as your physique.

Strength training is actually the best way to train the cardiovascular system, as it stimulates all the components of metabolism. The heart and blood vessels support the entire functioning of the cells, so every component of metabolism is supported by the cardiovascular system. This is another reason I like to do strength training first, cardio second.

Aerobic activity, or cardio, is a low intensity form of physical activity that allows the mitochondria (burning of energy) to work at a sub-maximal rate, where only one aspect of the cardiovascular system is utilized, unlike resistance or strength training, which utilizes the complete cardiovascular system.

When you have muscle strength from resistance training, your cardiovascular system doesn't have to work as hard to produce energy. When you cardio training only, your body doesn't have the muscle strength resistance training affords it; hence, you have less cardiovascular conditioning.

If you just run or jog at a steady pace, you will not get maximum oxygen into the cells, muscles, and tissues in the rest of your body. Running does not train fast-twitch muscles like resistance training does.

When you don't exercise with resistance training, your muscles and cells are not depleted of glycogen and your glycogen stores are full. Therefore, you have insulin resistance, the metabolic destiny of those glycogen and insulin stores is to be stored as fat, so it's a downward cascade as you feed your body more processed foods, loaded with sugar, combined with no exercise, especially resistance training, and you simply get fatter and less healthy by the day. That's why runners, joggers, treadmill enthusiasts, and aerobics class addicts may not be in the best shape. To me, most marathoners do not look healthy. Thin, yes; healthy, no.

What you are trying to accomplish is to unplug your drains (insulin resistance), while turning off the faucets (restricted carbs). This is accomplished with HIIT (high intensity interval training), combined with high intensity resistance or strength training, to drain your glycogen stores in your muscles and cells, and not allowing your muscles to atrophy as you age or run yourself to death. You will have greater capacity to store, burn, and restore glycogen, creating insulin sensitivity, not insulin resistance, while at the same time reducing carbs; thereby, turning off the faucets.

The process of high glycogen stores coupled with elevated carbohydrate consumption drives up your LDL small particle size and particle numbers, resulting in higher cardiovascular disease risk for heart attack and stroke. This vicious cycle also amplifies inflammation, which is the root cause of most modern disease.

Low-intensity exercisers like runners, joggers, and treadmillers are more at risk for CVD. They do not fully deplete their muscles and glycogen stores of glucose and insulin through resistance training. Insulin stimulates inflammation, including inflammation of the arterial walls, which is patched with LDL cholesterol, resulting in increased CVD risk. This may explain the premature death of Jim Fixx and other marathoners.

Exercise helps prevent Alzheimer's disease.

An increase in muscular demand simultaneously increases your cardiovascular system intensity to a much greater extent than cardio alone, as they are all tied together as one symphony for total health and fitness.

If your only tool is a hammer, then your whole world becomes a nail and you just bang away at steady state activities, such as running, jogging, or treadmilling. Without high-intensity resistance training, you are limiting yourself to one metabolic enhancement. Why not engage the whole symphony?

You lose about a half a pound of muscle a year if you do nothing to stop the loss. Calories are burned primarily in the muscle cells. Losing muscle means you lose calorie-burning ability and gain fat much more easily. Weight or resistance training will significantly slow that loss or even add muscle if you train to do so. It's never too late to start. Even Ronald Reagan started a weight training program at 82 and he gained muscle. Don't let your muscles atrophy or let your body cannibalize or burn its muscle.

You will burn body fat, reduce diet-induced inflammation, without replacing your fat stores with more fat, while at the same time conditioning your body to burn fat, not sugar, as fuel. How many times have you heard runners say "I have to carb load before the race?" This is dead wrong and will kill you prematurely over the long-run (pun intended). In fact, studies show more athletes now eat more fat because it is a high-octane fuel that your body actually prefers and works more efficiently on, especially over a lifetime.

The average person burns roughly 100 calories per mile, whether you walk or run. There are 3,500 calories in 1 pound of body fat, so it would be necessary to run or walk 35 miles to burn 1 pound of body fat.

Strength training tip: 3 pounds of added muscle burns as many calories as a 1-mile jog, and this is while you are at rest.

Metabolic health is controlled by the muscular system, not the cardiovascular system.

Your heart is a muscle, so if you are conditioning your muscles, you are conditioning your heart, increasing your cardiovascular efficiency and mining all the "gold" your system has to offer on your way to total health and fitness.

Exercise, especially resistance training, helps restore insulin balance. That's why proper high intensity resistance training along with high cardio interval training combined with a well-managed eating strategy produces the best results to lose and manage weight.

Strength or resistance training is an important anti-aging tool in combination with aerobic or cardio training because as we age, we lose muscle mass and strength and that effects our posture, our ability to walk, and our balance. Our muscle mass helps protect us against falls, one of the leading causes of injuries and death in the elderly. Aerobic or cardio training alone is not enough. To age more slowly or more gracefully, you must combine cardio with resistance training. A brisk 30-minute daily walk is still better than being a couch potato, but if you can join a gym and get some resistance training in 1-3 times per week, even better. Adding muscle is a key to burning calories, not static-state exercise like a treadmill or running.

As you age, strength will give you the freedom to continue living your life the way you want to, without physical limitations or loss of independence.

Excessive work on a treadmill can actually cause muscle loss, which in turn decreases your body's ability to burn calories, because muscle burns calories even at rest to keep them alive. You do not want to cannibalize your muscles. Furthermore, when working out on a cardio machine, never pay attention to calories burned or other blinking light information, as it's useless and inaccurate. The only thing you need to input is time, resistance, and speed. With the HIIT technique you are only concerned with time, speed (low to high, up and down) and difficulty or resistance (low to high, up and down); hence the name, high intensity interval training, (HIIT).

The metrics on the machine are useless, because they don't measure or take into account lean body mass, body fat percentage, body mass index, height, weight, or age. They are too generic and not factored in an algorithm formula, which could allow them to be accurate or meaningful. So don't go to the gym and set the treadmill for an hour, thinking you can burn off that extra 350 calories you just ate for dessert. You cannot out exercise away a poor diet. You cannot out exercise your mouth.

Don't live for your workout; workout to live. Find the sweet spot of being happy and staying fit.

I am not a body builder but want to be lean, fit, and agile for life. I don't exercise with free weights because of potential injury. I do high intensity interval circuit training on machines (resistance and strength training). A fit healthy body is the best fashion statement. Fit is fab.

Your exercise goal should be a healthy, strong body, with lean muscles and solid bones, capable of burning fat and building muscle definition. This exercise program is applicable for both men and women, as women need resistance training as well. Women should not concentrate on legs, butt, hips, and cardio, or exercise on the treadmill for hours.

I like to do my cardio after resistance training, because I find that I burn fat more efficiently and get better cardiovascular results. Plus, I'm already warmed up and sweating and releasing energy from my muscles. I'm stronger and able to focus on strength training effort and form, resulting in better overall health.

I believe we were built to be sprinters and not marathoners. To me, marathoners don't look healthy. They may be lean or skinny on the outside, but unhealthy or TOFI on the inside, literally rusting away, many with cardiovascular disease. Many professional athletes are hobbled after their careers by osteoarthritis and joint pain in knees, ankles, and shoulders, as well as tissue and joint issues.

If you are trying to build or rehab from injury, you will need to be on a different schedule. But to maintain a healthy, fit body, you do not have to work hours in the gym or treadmill. I believe in moving daily, at least 30 minutes of walking or aerobic activity, preferably a HIIT format, and resistance training in a circuit format 3 times weekly. On rest days from resistance training, still put in your 30 minutes of cardio, even though it's simply a brisk walk. Just move it, daily.

Lift weight to lose weight. I like resistance training on machines because it allows you to focus on the effort as opposed to the mechanics of the movement. Form is important and the machine does that for you, so you can just concentrate on the effort. On a "circuit" you can work all your muscle groups.

Recent studies show that people with adrenal fatigue may need 3 to 5 days of rest between resistance or strength training days. On rest days you still need to move: either the 30 minute brisk walk or 20 minute HIIT on the 4 machines, 5 minutes each. Interval training releases HGH naturally.

If you run outside, sprint for 30 seconds and walk 30 seconds, repeat for 20-30 minutes. Even better on the beach as you can practice grounding at the same time, but you must do it barefoot at the edge of water and sand, known as hard sand. However, soft sand is a superior workout for a full body workout, but you don't gain all the benefits of grounding, when you touch the water residual with your bare feet. You create more resistance in the soft sand and on hard sand you can create more speed, so simply switch it up and alternate. Variety is the spice of life.

This sample workout is designed more for men than women, but women need a full-body exercise program as well and may benefit from this circuit training routine.

Sample routine:

- **Week 1:** Maximum resistance sets. 1 set each machine. 8 reps - M, W, F.

- **Week 2:** High repetition sets. 60% of max weight. 1 set each machine. 20 reps – M, W, F.

- **Week 3:** Super slow sets. 60% max weight. 1 set each machine. 10 reps out to 10 count, back to 10 count. M, W, F.

- **Week 4:** Cable machine – 3 different positions: high, low, medium position. Max weight, 8-10 reps. (Form important, keep chest out, arms straight.)

- Followed by 20 minutes of cardio on 4 machines, 5 minutes each of HIIT (high intensity interval training.) (1) Treadmill (2) Elliptical (3) Stairmaster (4) Lifecycle.

- Followed by 20-30 minutes of cardio: T, Th, S, Sn. Either HIIT with 4 above machines or 30-minute brisk walk. Break a sweat

Sample Circuit:

- Chest press

- Incline press

- Decline press

- Flys

- Pullups (You want some push and pull alternate movements to work all muscle groups.)

- Dips

- Back machine – 25 reps

- Leg press – 25 reps

- Abs – lying on a bench 25 bent knee leg ups, 25 straight leg ups to horizontal position, 50 swim kick alternating legs. (Crunches or bending at the waist are not the best way to work your abs and can injure your back and spine.)

- Followed by 20 minutes of cardio per above.

I throw in 15 pushups in between first four chest exercises, but I had to build myself back up from stroke damage and paralysis.

My exercise regimen is continuously evolving, but this is what it looks like at the present time.

It is Important to work your large leg muscles as you age. Strong leg muscles help your balance and walking ability. Leg exercises also enhance your upper body and overall health.

Back exercise is important to help prevent back strain and pain; however, strong abs usually contribute to a strong back and freedom from back strain and pain.

This combined workout should take about 1 hour, including 20 minutes of cardio. This is a whole-body workout and is considered high value. You can do it 3 times a week, or just do it once or twice a week, but still do cardio the other 5 or 6 days.

Alternative exercises that I include in my regime from time to time, and which are highly recommend, are yoga, Pilates, and tai chi.

Yoga is excellent for relaxation and stress management: an exercise for the body, mind, spirit, and soul. Pilates will strengthen your core. Tai chi will improve your concentration and balance.

After good exercise, there is nothing better than a great massage to relax your body, muscles, and mind, and reduce stress or anxiety. Cranial Sacral massage and Reiki provide additional relaxation.

An infrared sauna sweats out environmental toxins.

Chiropractic adjustments align your muscular-skeletal core and stimulate blood flow.

Proceed with caution as some chiropractic neck adjustments have been known to cause strokes.

Don't forget the massage. It's a wonderful way to promote blood flow and your overall optimal health – and it feels *so* good!

Studies show that massage therapy relieves pain better than other therapies. Massage therapy also improves anxiety, stress, and health-related quality of life.

All these exercises and disciplines, along with a well-managed nutritional eating strategy, build a solid foundation for optimal health, wellness, and longevity.

Listen to your body. You don't have to spend endless hours on the treadmill or in cardio classes doing steady-state or static-state exercises. Everyone is different and results very, but the key is to combine resistance training with cardio and move daily.

"Build a habit of success . . . the important part is to start." – Unknown

The primary reason for resistance training is to retain and maintain lean muscle mass as you age. Between ages 20 and 40 you lose 40% of your muscle mass and then 1% every year thereafter. You have the ability to build new muscle into your 70's and 80's but you will naturally lose muscle as you age if you do not take steps to maintain it. Without lean muscle mass, you will get sicker more often because aging also weakens your immune system, leaving you more susceptible to infections, illnesses, and inflammation.

"Walking is man's best medicine." – Hippocrates

Daily aerobic exercise is not only good for your heart, but good for your brain as well. Studies suggest that regular walkers have brains that in MRI scans look on average 2 years younger than those who are sedentary. There is a persistent and overstated fear that exercise in later life will lead to strokes and heart attacks. Just the opposite is true.

You should always try to push your body to new weight for maximum strength and lean muscle mass over time because your body gets used to the same routine. Proper form is always more important than more weight or more reps, so if your form is sloppy, either back off the weight or the reps until you can complete your sets with perfect form.

Optimal health is 80% diet, 20% exercise. You CANNOT out-exercise a bad diet. You CANNOT out-exercise your mouth!

For every hour of sitting, do 10 minutes of movement: stand, walk, do the stairs. Move.

Remember to breathe. Inhale through the nose. The hairs are there to filter the air. Exhale through the mouth. Don't hold your breath. As simple as it may seem, breathing and form are of the utmost importance. With weight resistance breathe out when you push up or out. Inhale on the way down or back. With cardio, maintain a steady breathing rhythm or cadence.

Exercising helps change your biochemistry to that of a lean person. If your energy stores are low, you will feel lethargic and less likely to exercise, even though you know you should. If you feed your body nutrient-rich food that your body converts into energy, it's a victory. Your body thrives and you thrive, because you have energy to get off the couch and move.

To preserve muscle mass as you age, you must maintain adequate protein intake and reduce cellular inflammation. This can be accomplished by the diet and by daily exercise with intensity and interval training techniques outlined in this handbook.

Fewer than 25% of people over age 45 engage in strength or resistance training.

You may not achieve perfection, but you will achieve results. Any exercise that makes you sweat is generally a good exercise.

"Diet, exercise and supplementation: you get out exactly what you put in. Give it your all and you'll get even more back." – Unknown

Exercising in the morning reinforces healthful sleeping habits at night, creating increased melatonin production. Morning exercise generally is conducted with more energy, allowing for greater muscle tone, greater cardio expenditure and fat burn, leaving you with more energy for the rest of the day.

Exercise benefits your health in a number of ways, including strengthening your heart muscle and lungs, improving your total cardiovascular system, lowering blood pressure, reducing stress, increasing bone density, building muscle, and decreasing appetite. All this can be obtained through cardio interval training (IT) and high intensity interval training (HIIT) resistance/weight training, calisthenics, isometrics and stretching. As little as simply walking 30 minutes a day can be beneficial.

"Exercise is king and nutrition is queen: together, you have a kingdom." – Jack LaLanne

Exercise helps protect and improve your brain function by:

- Improving and increasing blood flow to your brain

- Increasing production of nerve-protecting agents

- Improving development and survival of neurons through neuroplasticity, neurotransmission, and   neurogenesis

- Reducing damaging brain plaques

- Altering the way damaging proteins reside in the brain, slowing the development of Alzheimer's disease

Regular exercise is important to maintain good health. High intensity resistance training and high intensity interval training (HIIT) and cardio techniques, coupled with a sound nutrition strategy will synergistically catapult you into improved health. Add supplements for insurance. Health is wealth. Prevention is the best cure.

If you don't have time to go to the gym or to take a walk, try this: Mini-Trampolining (AKA - Rebounding) for health.

Jump for joy: How rebounding works:

Many types of exercise are done to target specific muscles or just to increase cardiovascular function. Rebounding is unique, since it uses the forces of acceleration and deceleration and can work on every cell in the body in a unique way.

When you bounce on a rebounder (mini-trampoline), several actions happen:

- An acceleration action as you bounce upward

- A split-second weightless pause at the top

- A deceleration at an increased G-force

- Impact to the rebounder

- Repeat

There are many benefits to rebounding, including NASA's research showing that rebounding can be more than twice as effective as treadmill running.

The action of rebounding makes use of the increased G-force from gravity.

Exercises like this affect each cell in the body as it responds to the acceleration and deceleration. The up and down motion is beneficial for the lymphatic system, since it runs in a vertical direction in the body. The increased G-force helps increase lymphocyte activity. The lymph system transports immune cells throughout the body and supports immune function. For this reason, rebounding is often suggested as a detoxifying and immune-boosting activity.

Rebounding, since it affects each cell in the body, also increases cell energy and mitochondrial function, increasing energy production.

Another of the major benefits of rebounding is its benefit to the skeletal system. Just as astronauts lose bone mass in space as a response to the decreased need for strong bones in a zero gravity environment, weight-bearing exercise increases bone mass. Rebounding is especially effective, since it increases the weight supported by the skeletal system with the increased G-force of jumping.

Benefits of Rebounding:

- Cardiovascular benefit. Rebounding requires the use of several muscle groups, similar to jogging, but has the added benefit of causing much lower levels of shock trauma to the skeletal system than running on hard surfaces. Extended use increases lung capacities and red blood cell counts and lowers blood pressure.

- Strengthens every cell, muscle, organ, tissue, bone, and tendon in the body.

- Lower-impact cardiovascular fitness

- Boosts lymphatic drainage and immune function. May help in preventing and eliminating cancer. Rebounding helps in improved circulation of the lymphatic fluid, which helps to destroy cancerous cells in the body. As the fluids collect waste products, bacteria, and damaged cells, it also collects cancerous cells, if present, in the body and drains them into the lymphatic vessels for excretion

- Increases detoxification and cleansing of the body

- Great for skeletal system and increasing bone mass

- Helps improve digestion

- More than twice as effective as running without the extra stress on the ankles and knees

- Increases endurance on a cellular level by stimulating mitochondrial production (these are responsible for cell energy)

- Improves balance by stimulating the vestibule in the middle ear

- Improves the effects of other exercise. Studies show that exercise such as weight lifting, by adding rebounds on a trampoline, got better results than those obtained by a person who lifted weights or runs or jogs only

- Rebounding helps circulate oxygen throughout the body to increase energy

- Rebounding is a whole-body exercise that improves muscle tone throughout the body

- Some sources claim that the unique motion of rebounding can also help support the thyroid and adrenals

- Weight loss

- Strengthens legs, back, and core

- Injury reduction compared to running

- Natural facelift from G-force stress

- Stress reliever

- Relieves incontinence by strengthening the pelvic floor

- Reduce or rid cellulite

- Reduce and combat varicose veins

- Inside format

- Only 10 minutes daily. More effective than 25-30 minutes of walking or jogging

- Fun and effective form of exercise. Rebounding is fun!

Stroke victims, elderly and fall-prone people could particularly get the benefit of mini-trampolining, as researchers found it improved posture and gait, aided balance and helped to increase joint-position awareness in the ankle. (Think drop foot.) A unit with handle bars for stability is recommended

Compelling evidence suggests exercise is an important component of cancer prevention and care. It slashes your risk of developing cancer, improves your chances of successful recovery, and diminishes your risk of cancer reoccurrence.

The longer you exercise, the more pronounced the benefits. Studies show that both men and women who exercise during their early years have a lower risk of cancer later in life.

Exercise lowers your blood sugar levels and normalizes your insulin sensitivity. Exercise creates an environment less conducive to cancer growth.

Exercise promotes mitochondrial health. Mitochondrial damage and dysfunction can trigger genetic mutations that can contribute to cancer. Optimizing mitochondria health is a key component of cancer prevention.

"Life is like a bicycle. To keep balance, you must keep moving." – Albert Einstein

Exercise is the closest thing to a real-world fountain of youth and slowing of the aging process in both the mind and body. In some cases, it even reverses age-related health issues and stops them in their tracks.

Don't live for your workout; workout to live.

"To keep the body in good health is a duty . . . otherwise we shall not be able to keep our mind strong and clear." – Buddha

CHAPTER 48:
Psychology of Lifestyle Change

"You must take personal responsibility. You cannot change the circumstances, the seasons or the wind, but you can change yourself. That is something you have charge of." – Jim Rohn

"When you're going through something hard and you wonder where God is, remember the teacher is always silent during the test." – Unknown

Every action starts with a first move. Break your barriers. Growth is an outcome achieved through awareness, preparation, education, and action. Your life does not get better by chance. It gets better by change. It takes courage to act and strength to follow through. If it's important to you, you will find a way; if not, you will find an excuse. Complete your circles. Have your best day every day, as you never know about tomorrow. If you never give up, you can't be stopped.

There is no greater feeling in the world than having a vision and making it a reality. No words can describe the feeling of accomplishment!

"There are far, far better things ahead than any we leave behind." – C.S. Lewis

The process of change from what you are to what you would like to become can be either arduous and frustrating or easy and rewarding; the effort required for both paths is the same. Choose the first and you will probably have an endless cycle of yo-yo dieting and up and down weight loss and gain, with no stability. Eat from a nutrient-rich list of foods, cut the sugar and wheat, eat a low-carb, higher-protein, higher-healthy-fats, higher-fiber diet and what was once arduous and frustrating will become easy and rewarding. As new lifestyle habits emerge you will crave healthy choices instead of unhealthy choices. You are reducing your risk of heart attack, stroke and cancer. So change, once thought as only a distant possibility, now becomes an absolute certainty. The choice is yours.

Weakness equals compromise, so deal from a position of strength, not weakness. Reach as far as you can and never give up.

"Your life does not get better by chance, it gets better by change." Jim Rohn

There are 5 stages of change:

- Pre-Contemplation. (All's good. Nothing to worry about)

- Contemplation. (I'm thinking about it, that's why I'm here, but I don't have a plan and I'm confused by all the information.)

- Preparation. (game plan, re-education.)

- Action. (execution, discipline, commitment, confidence, results.)

- Maintenance. (lifestyle, rewards.)

1. Pre-contemplation

People in this stage don't want to make any change to their habits and don't recognize that they have a problem. They may be pessimistic about their ability to make change, or even deny the negative effects of their existing lifestyle habits. They selectively filter information that helps confirm their decision not to exercise or eat better. This stage is many times referred to as the "denial" stage.

Unfortunately, it's difficult to reach or help people in the pre-contemplation stage. It may take an emotional trigger or event of some kind, a wake-up call, that can snap people out of their denial. It's highly likely if you are taking the time to read this book or are at one my seminars, you are not in this stage. You are ready to move forward.

"Change before you have to." – Jack Welch

2. Contemplation

During this stage, you are weighing the costs (i.e., effort, time, finances) and benefits of lifestyle modification. You are contemplating whether it's something that will be worth it or beneficial to you. People can remain in this stage for years without preparing to take action.

Setting very powerful, motivating goals and visualizing your results can be very helpful for someone in the contemplation stage. If you can identify ways that making a change will benefit you, the benefits will begin to outweigh the costs. At this level, you have some knowledge of your disease-promoting lifestyle behaviors and are considering making some beneficial changes. You have not made a final pledge to yourself to take action, but you may be attempting to modify your behavior by eating less fast food, as an example, so you're contemplating behavior change. We tend to seek pleasure and avoid pain, so the more pleasure you can ascribe to making a change, the more likely you are to take action and succeed.

"If you don't like how things are, change it. You're not a tree." – Jim Rohn

3. Preparation

People in the preparation stage have decided to change their negative habits within one month. You may have just set up an appointment with a nutritionist, personal trainer or other fitness professional, purchased a fitness program, started a gym membership or decided to read this book or come to a seminar to get educated. You are now able to say to yourself, "I'm going to do this, I'm ready for it." Congratulations if you're in this category. At this stage you are ready to get started and take action. You're ready to make changes and are developing your plan of action.

4. Action

"Behind every success is someone who made it happen. Take action. Never give up." - Unknown

The action stage is the process of changing your lifestyle, whether you are exercising more consistently or eating healthier. Individuals in this stage are at the greatest risk of relapse, so it's key to leverage any techniques you can to stay motivated. At this level, you have allocated the resources, the time, and energy to reaching your goals. This is a tremendous move forward and you should be proud of yourself for your strong belief, conviction, commitment, and desire, the drive of which will bring you more confidence, especially when you start to see and feel the results and hear it from family, friends, and co-workers. Those will be some of the rewards and pleasures: the compliments and "Slim or Skinny fashions" you are now able to wear, giving you confidence that what you are doing is good and worthwhile for your health. Your body will start craving healthy choices. These feelings and rewards will drive you to achieve success.

Take action to improve your health and cut your risks. Worse than failing is failing to try. Better done, is always better than better said. Turn what you know into what you do. Take action.

"Success is nothing more than a few simple disciplines practiced every day." – Jim Rohn

5. Maintenance

"A healthy attitude is contagious, but don't wait to catch it from others. Be a carrier." – Tom Stoppard

This is the stage of successful, sustained lifestyle modification. If you have been exercising consistently for 6 months to one year and have blended positive eating habits into your lifestyle, then you are in the maintenance stage. It will be difficult to think of how you were before and you will never go back. You are now dedicated to your good health. When you reach this level, you know the benefits of lifestyle change because you have felt and experienced what it finally feels like to live a life of good health for a sustained period of time. At this level you will focus on how you feel and look and your body composition compared to before and never want to return to that state. The maintenance stage is the toughest, but most rewarding.

There are psychologists who believe there is a 6th stage in change, Termination, where problems will no longer present any temptation or threat for relapse or a return to your old habits. I believe when it comes to nutrition and health if you have maintained your healthy lifestyle change for 1-3 years, you will never want to go back to your old eating habits. In fact, your body and brain will crave healthy choices and you will enjoy a lifetime of maintenance.

"The body achieves what the mind believes." – Unknown

The secret of taking action and moving forward is simply getting started. First, you must have the desire or mind set; second, educate yourself; third, take the action; fourth and finally, maintain your newfound good health for a lifetime by combining all stages. However, there is the standard or traditional and conventional way as outlined above. The habits that you practice daily are keys to lifestyle change. You need commitment, consistency and persistence.

"The longest journey begins with a single step." – Lao Tzu

"If you do not change direction you may end up where you are heading." – Lao Tzu

"Mastering others is strength, mastering yourself is true power." – Lao Tzu

"When I let go of what I am, then I become what I might be." – Lao Tzu

Learn how to learn. Pursue the truth. Fulfill your potential to thrive. Take charge, take command, take control of your health. One of the reasons we care about tomorrow is we remember yesterday and this allows us to make plans to create a better future. Belief is a very powerful tool.

"It's the start that stops most people. Yesterday you said tomorrow." – Unknown

The psychology of lifestyle change can be broken down into five standard, traditional, or conventional criteria and stages; however, if you are reading this book or are at a seminar, you have already started to prepare yourself for lifestyle change or new behavior modification techniques, because you have the desire and commitment to move forward as you are starting to educate yourself to take action. Just keep on moving on, until it becomes habit and transformation for a lifetime, a true lifestyle change.

"You must do the things you think you cannot do." – Eleanor Roosevelt

Eating unhealthy foods and not exercising are habits we are trying to change. Understand the problem and then have the discipline to apply the solution.

Practice the 4Ds of success:

- Desire

- Discipline

- Determination

- Dedication

You need desire, discipline, determination, and dedication, not just hope and a prayer or books and videos. You need to educate yourself, but then you need to be motivated to act and maintain a healthy lifestyle strategy. With so much information, confusion is inevitable, but not helplessness. Don't be paralyzed by over-analysis. The key is to take action. Just get started.

"Discipline is the bridge between goals and accomplishment." – Jim Rohn

Viewing food as fuel and as an essential ingredient in good health is a necessary step in making behavioral eating changes. While most people are not connecting the dots with eating habits and health or disease, you must recognize this important factor and that a change is needed now, not later, and how this change will benefit you.

The key to any lifestyle change is consistency and persistence. Repetition increases the probability of success. To live well you must take action.

"He who can believe himself well, will be well." – Ovid

You have been thinking about change and you are ready. That's why you are here, reading this book, but you need the next step.Preparation is education. You must educate yourself and feel confident about a pathway to change. Have a plan and work that plan: that's what this handbook does. The next key step is to take action. Make the commitment. Be determined to make a change. Once you take action and you see results and are rewarded with good health and wellness progress, it will make it easier to take the next and final step, which is the hardest. Maintenance is the lifestyle change and a strategy and habits you will use for life. No more fad diets or bad choices. It's knowing the truth about nutrition and good health and practicing it daily for life. The ultimate goal of good health and wellness is quality of life and longevity. You now have the tools.

By acting on your desire for change, you not only resolve your problems, but you create a happier, healthier self. Developing and then articulating a sense of purpose in life will add about 8 extra years to your life expectancy.

Many otherwise intelligent men and women actively resist becoming aware of the ways in which they are endangering, damaging, and even destroying their lives.

The psychology of change comes from within and you have to be mentally and physically ready. No one can make you do it. You are your own master and your own advocate. Only you know how you feel. Only you know how you want to look. Our fullest accomplishments emerge when we have the opportunity to choose that which will enhance our lives, our sense of self, our friends, our family and our society. You will have a new purpose, I promise.

"Mind over matter. If you don't mind, it won't matter." – Mark Twain

Do the right thing at the right time. Timing is everything. Add value to your life. If you are in a rut, downward spiral, or just getting by day to day, unhappy and not making progress, make a change. If you are not moving forward, then you are moving backward and your health and weight are progressively getting worse, it is only a matter of time before reality sets in and weight gain won't be pretty.

You have to remain committed, determined, disciplined, and purposeful in pursuit of your health and dietary strategy. It won't happen by chance. You must plan and work the plan until it becomes habit, a lifestyle way of eating for the rest of your life. Lifestyle for a lifetime. It's a great tradeoff.

You want to lead a sustainable lifestyle, keep weight off, feel good, be happy and healthy.

Positive reinforcement and rewards come as you feel better, look better, are healthier and happier. You have more self-confidence and you are now comfortable with lifestyle changes. It becomes a way of life. You now crave healthy, nutritious foods, instead of unhealthy, fattening ones.

It takes at least 3 weeks before a new way of doing something becomes a comfortable routine and up to six weeks or more to become habit. Be patient, it will pay off.

"It's not so much what you accomplish in life, it's what you overcome. A second act in life." – Anonymous

"There is nothing you can't do when you tap into your inner strength; you can exceed even your own expectations." - Unknown

"A wise man should consider that health is the greatest of human blessings, and learn how by his own thought to derive benefit from his illnesses." – Hippocrates

It is easier to change behaviors and habits when what you're eating supports your brain and body to work properly and you feel good and see results. It takes about 3 weeks of doing something a new way before it becomes a comfortable routine.

"The grass is always greener on the other side of the fence, because you water it." - Anonymous

The pathways that transform us most are the moments that we are most deeply connected to, the ones we invest ourselves in, the ones we are about to overcome. Connect the dots. Take action and go for it. You'll look back and be glad you did. One moment at a time, one step at a time, one day at a time, building your foundation, your core, your strength, your body, your mind. You can do it. Follow your pathway to lifestyle change.

"Unless you change how you are, you will always have what you've got." – Jim Rohn

Changing habits is undoubtedly the most difficult and most important part of any recovery process.

Every step taken should be filled with pride as to how far you have come in your recovery. The little things build the foundation, over time, to bigger things. More confidence produces more progress and greater results. Overcome resistance and procrastination. Find your inner you, your desires, be your best you. Begin, start and move forward. Never give up. Have no regrets. Your level of success will follow your level of commitment.

"Natural forces within us are the true healers of disease." – Hippocrates

When you are clear on how you want to feel, your decision-making will get to the heart of the matter and help you maintain your health for a lifetime, because many people have never truly felt what good health feels like. Once you attain excellent health you never want to lose it and go back to the way you were.

Tap into the power of your mind's intention, the power of the human spirit, and the will to live. If you focus your mind and envision good health, your subconscious mind will help lead you to take action on what you focus on. Your mind will power you to take action. But you must first have the desire, then educate yourself to take the appropriate action and then the results and rewards of that action will inspire and motivate you for a lifetime. Your body and mind will crave healthy choices. Your behavioral and lifestyle changes will all come together in powerful health solutions.

"Don't settle for less than optimal health. You deserve the feeling." – Unknown

Do the little things right, they add up over time. Do the little things wrong, and they will add up to disease and sickness.

If you have trouble with these lifestyle changes, think of them as "drugs" that you must take on a daily basis to sustain your life.

Health is two choices: life or death. Take charge, command, and control of your health.

With greatness comes criticism. The bigger your dream and the faster you climb the ladder of your dreams you will have people there supporting you and a lot of people who want to bring you down. Understanding that this is part of the process makes it easier to not react or respond to the negative comments of other people, but rather stay focused on your mission, your vision, and your passion. Work with those who want to improve their lives. People who are creating value in the world don't criticize others; it's those that are upset with what they aren't doing who try to bring others down to their level.

The only contract you need to sign is with yourself. Give life a chance, give life structure, meaning, and purpose. Life is worth living. Good health will be your reward. You deserve the best.

There is no substitute for substance. The mind that perceives limitations is the limitation. If you put your mind to it, you can do it.

"Live as if you were to die tomorrow; learn as if you were going to live forever."
– Mahatma Gandhi

Accomplishment deserves recognition. We must have a positive state of mind in order to bring harmony to the body. Realize that your body, lifestyle, spirit, desire, mind, and belief must coordinate together on your health journey.

Imagination and action bring dreams to life, but don't leave your effort behind.

"It is better to light a candle than curse the darkness." – Eleanor Roosevelt

Mindset, commitment, desire, determination, drive, and resilience will be key words in your levels of lifestyle change. Don't let your health to be held hostage by poor lifestyle choices. We must hold ourselves accountable for our actions and push ourselves to be better and achieve our goals. Make lifestyle changes for success.

Add more years to your life and more life to your years. Health is a life-long investment. Your friends should be, too. Surround yourself with like-thinking, positive, happy people.

Are you trying hard, struggling more and getting worse? Don't confuse activity for productivity.

"We resist change, but fear of the unknown can result in clinging to status quo behaviors, no matter how poor they are." - Unknown

The psychology of lifestyle change means:

- Change "shoulds" into "musts."

- Don't wait for a cataclysmic health event to change your life.

- Repeat what works.

- Give back to yourself.

- Walk your talk.

- Compete with yourself to be the best you can be.

- Recognize and move past your limiting beliefs.

- A negative mind will not give you a positive life.

"Success is habit forming and the habit of success, once learned, is nearly impossible to forget." - Anthony Robbins

The key to any lifestyle change is consistency and persistence. Get healthy and get happy. Be your own kind of beautiful. The psychology of weight loss is about taking control of your life. The information in this handbook is here for you to do just that. Education and information is a first step, but then you must use this information and take action to empower and master your environment, your mind and your body. By seeing results, benefits, and rewards, you will believe and once you believe, you will have the confidence to adopt lifestyle changes. Enjoy!

"Without health, life is not life, it is only a state of suffering and languor-an image of death." – Buddha

Results and rewards will be many: renewed confidence, better attitude, and zest for life. You will enjoy a better sex life. You will have turned your health around and improved the quality of your life. You will add years to your life and life to your years. You will recapture your life from the addiction of food. You will no longer live to eat, but eat to live.

"Twenty years from now you will be more disappointed by the things that you didn't do than by the ones you did do." – Mark Twain

Educate and learn. Don't let doubt and the fear of the unknown control your life. Procrastination causes paralysis, leading to deterioration and disease.

Shape your destiny, control your future, learn and grow. Don't grow old with misery and bitterness. Aging is optional. Slow it down. Control it. Getting older is inevitable, but aging prematurely or premature death is not. Decrepitude, deterioration, and impairment are not. Growing older is the opportunity to increase one's value and competence.

Never be defined by your past. It was just a lesson, not a life sentence.

"If my mind can conceive it and my heart can believe it, then I can achieve it." - Muhammad Ali

It's about mindset over matter.

CHAPTER 49:
Stress

"Stress is a killer, music is a healer." – Unknown

Stress is a lot more than a mild annoyance; it's a true life shortener.

Stress is an overlooked health management issue that not only contributes to poor overall health, but studies show that stress can cause a two-fold increase in stroke risk. Those living with chronic stress have a four-times greater risk of stroke. Drinking two or more energy drinks per day doubles stroke risk. Stress is already a well-recognized risk factor for heart attacks. Of course, being a positive person instead of a negative person is always a plus. Stress releases cortisol into the bloodstream and cortisol fuels inflammation and chronic inflammation is a cause of coronary artery disease, setting the stage for heart attacks and strokes.

When our body is stressed two things occur:

1. Your immune system is suppressed, making you more susceptible to disease.

2. It turns your body from the natural alkaline pH state, in which disease, illness and sickness cannot survive, into an acidic state in which diseases like cancer, heart disease and diabetes thrive.

Activity trumps stress. Some of my favorite stress busters are yoga, exercise, walking outdoors or on the beach, music, reading, movies, gardening, cooking, and don't forget sleep. I believe it is better to exercise in the morning in order to sleep better at night. I take 1mg of melatonin nightly as a nightly sleep aid.

Another stress buster is a 30 minute Jacuzzi bath with Epsom salt, which has magnesium and is absorbed through the skin. It's very relaxing and does a body good, especially if you have sore or tired muscles from exercising. I prefer bathing at night before bed. Nearly 60% of the US population is magnesium deficient. Use Epsom salt as directed on the package, usually 1-cup per bath.

Daily walking is good exercise. If you can walk in nature outside in mountains, beach, countryside, or nature trails, all the better. Get out in nature and think healthy, happy thoughts. Breathe.

Favorite music can vary widely from person to person and generation to generation, but I found when I was recovering from my stroke and reading, that Mozart's Concertos 1-5 and Vivaldi's Four Seasons and Concerto music, were not only relaxing, but allowed me to absorb more of what I was experiencing while trying to reclaim my health. Studies have shown that when this music is played to babies in the womb, they are oftentimes more intelligent and quicker learners than their counterparts, so I thought why not, I'm being reborn anyway, with my second chance at life. An orchestra playing at its highest level equals a symphony and that's how you want your health.

Reading is very subjective, but I believe you have to educate yourself to take control of your health and to prepare yourself to take action in lifestyle change. The more I read, the more I learn. I hope this book helps.

Someone said about movies: "If you can make a person laugh, cry, and think in 2 hours, you have a hit."

Gardening is a great hobby: it gets you outdoors, helps you communicate with nature, gives you exercise and hopefully, you have a positive experience, because you are participating with and watching something grow, prosper, and thrive through your efforts.

As I've stated many times in this book, the healthiest people are those who eat at home and know what's going onto their plates, forks and into their mouths, by preparing meals with organic, fresh, whole food ingredients. Besides, cooking is great therapy: very relaxing and creative, an enjoyable stress buster.

Don't forget sleep: 7-9 hours per night. Lack of sleep results in the liver pumping out excess cholesterol and if you're stressed that can lead to stroke or heart attack. If you already have inflammation, oxidized LDL, high blood pressure, endothelial dysfunction, you are a ticking time bomb for stroke, as was I.

Stress is a killer, music is a healer. Soothing music lowers the heart rate, calms the mind and body, and reduces stress, all of which help the body to better fight infection, disease, and illness.

"Worry is to pray what you do not want." - Sharon Lecter

Three of my favorite stress busters and relaxation techniques besides yoga and Tai Chi are Thai massage, Cranial Sacral, and Reiki.

Exercise can be like meditation as you focus and relieve stress.

CHAPTER 50:
CVD-Cardiovascular Event-Stroke, Heart Attack

What is the anatomy of a stroke or heart attack? Let's connect the dots.

It starts in the mouth. You may have periodontal disease or missing teeth. Bacteria and plaque build up, permeate the blood stream, and move to the arteries and heart. The cause is bad diet, too much sugar, excessive red meat and grains. Inflammation starts. Gut bacteria becomes imbalanced. Metabolic syndrome sets in, resulting in insulin resistance, type 2 diabetes, obesity, high blood pressure, high cholesterol, toxicity, plaque, and oxidative stress. Throw in a little alcohol and now we have the perfect storm, a toxic time bomb waiting to explode. Sound familiar? Boom!

Pressure bursts pipes. The arteries are narrowed, plaque is built up, inflammation is rampant, high blood pressure is coursing, an artery ruptures, thrombosis occurs from the plaque and inflammation-filled artery, chronic high blood pressure presses against the endothelial walls of the artery, a pimple-like scab in the fissure or dysfunctional endothelium. Suddenly, it is released into the blood stream and becomes a clot that blocks blood flow and oxygen to the brain, causing a brain attack or stroke, or it goes to the heart, causing a heart attack. A tragic cascade of events. I am a witness.

The real cause of death from heart attacks and strokes is not lipid or cholesterol accumulation, but the rupture of atherosclerotic plaque. Soft, foamy plaque is vulnerable to rupture and cannot be detected by CAT scans or other scanning techniques. The artery can burst without warning due to elevated levels of cellular inflammation and high blood pressure. The ruptured plaque releases cellular debris that rapidly forms a blood clot and stops the flow of oxygen-rich blood needed by the heart and brain to survive. The result is a heart attack, stroke (brain attack) or death.

The good news is 80–90% of CVD is preventable.

For many, the first and only symptom of heart disease is death: 1,786 per day in the US;

1 in every 2 women's deaths is due to cardiovascular disease. If you want to live long and well, CVD is best to avoid, and better yet, to prevent.

The cold facts of hardened arteries and cardiovascular disease:

According to a European study, 77% of our disease burden and 86% of deaths are related to our diets and lifestyle.

According to the CDC, 26 million Americans have been diagnosed with heart disease: that's 11% of the adult population.

8 million Americans have had heart attacks. 735,000 will have a heart attack every year. 600,000 will die. It is the #1 cause of death.

One-third of all deaths over age 35 are due to cardiovascular disease.

After age forty, half of all men and one-third of women will eventually have cardiovascular disease (80% preventable).

25% of all strokes occur in those under age 65, and 10% in those under 45. Strokes are occurring earlier and earlier every year.

In a recent survey conducted in 13 states with 71,000 adults, only 1 in 6 knew the warning signs of a stroke or what action to take.

The adverse health effects of added sugar and of saturated fat from meats and dairy look to be almost stunningly commensurate. However, when saturated fat calories were replaced with unsaturated fat calories from nuts, seeds, avocado, olive oil, fish or seafood, rates of cardiovascular disease declined significantly.

The JAMA study, which took place in July, 2016 found increases in all-cause mortality with increases in both saturated fat and trans fat intake; and decreases in mortality with increases in both polyunsaturated fat intake, and monounsaturated fat intake.

Generally, people with excess belly fat (beer belly) have plaque in their arteries, putting them at risk for heart disease. Fat above the waist (beer belly) and heart disease go hand in hand.

There is s connection between erectile dysfunction and cardiovascular disease. Erectile dysfunction is actually a vascular disease, so instead of Viagra or Cialis, get checked for cardiovascular disease.

The vast majority of strokes are preventable by practicing a healthy lifestyle. Emphasizing reduction in diet-induced inflammation, atherosclerosis and blood pressure will reduce your risk of stroke. Seventy-five percent of heart attack victims have normal cholesterol levels.

With improvements in the quality of medical care, stroke death rates have declined since 1990, but stroke-related disabilities have increased by 40%. Stroke is now the 5th leading cause of death in the US. (down from #3); however, stroke is the #1 debilitating disease worldwide, leaving most stroke survivors dependent, disabled, and confined to institutions. There are 50 million stroke survivors worldwide.

If LDL cholesterol is not oxidized and not damaged, it will not stick to your arterial walls, and thus will not rupture and cause thrombosis, heart attack, or stroke. So, it's not the LDL itself the causes the cardiovascular event, but the condition of the LDL. If you have damaged LDL and high blood pressure, you are a stroke or heart attack waiting to happen, as I was.

Cardiovascular disease, heart attack, and stroke can be reversed and prevented. It takes work, dedication, and commitment, but it can be done. It's in your hands and you must take action or the first symptom may be death. I chose life and so should you.

In the US, if you reach age 65 today, you can expect to live on average to 84.3 for men and 86.6 for women. Life expectancy in the US in 1900 was 47.3. People died young from diseases that are now preventable or curable. The incidence of heart attack and stroke (or CVE) deaths are rising and are the leading cause of death in the US, because we are living longer.

Reversing atherosclerosis, with plant polyphenol concentrates found in pomegranates, green tea extract and grape seed extract are excellent additions to your well-designed nutritional strategy, either from foods (preferable), powders added to your "green drink," or supplements in pill form.

Endothelial dysfunction occurs to our arterial lining, the endothelium, as we age. It endures chronic assault from internal and external factors, generally diet or toxin-related, that results in loss of blood flow to the heart, brain, and kidneys. It is the leading reason why most aging people today are dying or becoming disabled.

Having your blood tested at least every 6 months can help identify the markers. Don't ignore the factors that are silently destroying endothelial integrity and killing or disabling us prematurely. It is critical to keep these markers in safe ranges: elevated glucose and insulin (high blood sugar), elevated triglycerides, high LDL, low HDL, high homocysteine, elevated C-reactive protein, evident oxidative stress, and low testosterone in men.

Your risk of suffering a CVE is greatest in the two-hour period after you eat a meal. That's partly because during that time you can experience dangerous blood sugar spikes that acutely impair blood flow through vital arteries, which can ultimately lead to a heart attack or stroke. That's why you must wisely choose your consumption of carbohydrates like sugars, starches, and wheat.

Clinical data, trials, research, meta-analysis, epidemiological studies and scientific evidence demonstrate that a low-carb, healthy higher fat and higher healthy protein diet is the most efficient diet to lose weight, maintain weight long-term, and reduce cardiovascular disease, heart attack, stroke, and cancer.

Lifestyle intervention moves from the disease model to the wellness model. That"s what this seminar/workshop and handbook are all about.

CHAPTER 51:
Vision

First of all, see your optometry doctor (O.D.) at least once a year for an annual exam.

I lost 50% of the vision in my left eye after my stroke. My vision improved significantly thereafter, and I think it is attributable to my lifestyle choices of diet, nutrition, exercise, and supplementation program. Ridding my body of diet-induced inflammation may be the strongest contributing factor.

There is a strong relationship between the AA/EPA ratios of a pro-inflammatory diet vs. anti-inflammatory diet, by reducing retinal inflammation and combined with a diet rich in omega-3s. For those with an AA/EPA ratio of 1.5 , vision gain is twice as great as those with an AA/EPA ratio of 2.5. Since the average American has an AA/EPA ratio of 20, eating an anti-inflammatory omega-3-rich diet, can result in a significant vision improvement.

Lutein is a very good vision supplement that I take. Please refer to Dr. Shokour's letter in the testimonial section for my results.

Contrary to popular belief, deteriorating vision is primarily a side effect of our modern lifestyle. Aging does not automatically mean you will lose your eyesight. The key is to properly nourish your eyes throughout the years and avoid chronic eye strain. Your diet may be paramount. Chronic vitamin A deficiency can lead to total blindness. Other nutrient insufficiencies significantly contribute to the development of macular degeneration.

Age-related macular degeneration (AMD) is the most common cause of blindness among the elderly, followed by cataracts. There are two forms of macular degeneration: dry and wet. Dry macular degeneration is the milder version that causes few symptoms, but it can degenerate into the wet form, in which blood vessels start growing in the back of your eye, causing your vision to blur.

An indication of wet AMD is loss of vision in the center of your field of vision. A healthy diet can likely prevent AMD in the first place, but supplements have also been shown to help slow down or stop the progression from the dry to the more advanced wet form.

As reported by The New York Times on December 17, 2014, "The federally funded Age-Related Eye Disease Study found that people at high risk for advanced age-related macular degeneration could cut that risk by about 25 percent by taking supplements that include 500 milligrams of vitamin C, 400 IUs of vitamin E, 10 milligrams of lutein, 2 milligrams of zeaxanthin, 80 milligrams of zinc, and 2 milligrams of copper." I take all of these.

In addition, macular degeneration and cataracts are largely driven by free radical damage, and may in many cases be largely preventable by eating foods rich in antioxidants, such as:

Anthocyanins, found in blueberries, bilberries, and black currants

Lutein and zeaxanthin, found in green leafy vegetables and orange and yellow fruits and vegetables. Research shows those who consume the highest levels of lutein and zeaxanthin have a 40 percent lower risk of advanced wet macular degeneration compared to those who eat the least.

High-quality animal-based omega3 fats like those found in krill oil and wild-caught Alaskan salmon.

Bioflavonoids found in tea, cherries, and citrus fruits.

Vitamin D, found to some extent in various foods such as meats, but primarily created in response to direct sun exposure on bare skin. Vitamin D is particularly important for those with genetic risk factors for AMD.

Lutein and zeaxanthin are two key nutrients for eye health, as both of them are found in high concentrations in your macula, the small central part of your retina responsible for detailed central vision. Lutein is also found in your macular pigment, known for helping to protect your central vision, and aid in blue light absorption. Zeaxanthin is found in your retina.

Though there's no recommended daily intake amount for lutein and zeaxanthin, studies have found protective benefits at a dosage of 10 mg of lutein per day, and 2 mg per day of zeaxanthin. Lutein and zeaxanthin are often found together in foods, although zeaxanthin is far scarcer than lutein. They're primarily found in green leafy vegetables, with kale and spinach topping the list of lutein-rich foods. Carrots, squash, and other orange and yellow fruits and vegetables also contain high amounts. In fact, the word lutein comes from the Latin word "luteus," which means "yellow." If you remember this, it may help you pick out vegetables likely to contain higher amounts of these two nutrients.

According to a recent study in the British Journal of Ophthalmology, orange peppers had the highest amount of zeaxanthin of the 33 fruits and vegetables tested. Egg yolk from organically-raised, free-range pastured eggs is another source of both lutein and zeaxanthin that is well absorbed by your body. Interestingly, research shows that adding a couple of eggs to your salad can increase the carotenoid absorption you get from the whole meal as much as nine-fold.

Astaxanthin, the red pigment in salmon and krill, is a powerful antioxidant and promotes eye health.

CHAPTER 52:

Blood Tests & Other Tests That Will Save Your Life/ Diagnostic Evaluations/Results

"Without health life is not life, it is only a state of suffering and languor; an image of death." – Buddha

Getting your blood tested is likely one of the single most important things you can do to figure out what diet, supplements, and lifestyle that are right for you. Everyone is different. Blood doesn't lie. Test, don't guess. Otherwise you're throwing darts blindfolded. If you don't measure it, you can't improve it. Don't be normal. Be optimal.

Regular blood testing detects abnormalities before they lead to serious illness or death. Discovering correctable disease factors or markers not only spares you suffering, disabilities and premature death, but will save you money in the long run. Why have minor disorders go untreated, when you can reverse them before they inflict permanent damage or disability on you? Get your blood tested every 6 months, or at least annually. I get mine tested every 3 months.

Quest Diagnostics or LabCorp in many cities and locations.

Comprehensive blood chemistry panel tests are a valuable tool and resource. Your ability to interpret them will give you quick access to understanding your degree of health or disease and will empower your dialogue with your healthcare team. Blood tests establish your baseline bio-markers to determine progress towards optimal health or decline towards illness and chronic disease. Most blood test are economical and are covered by insurance.

No single test can tell the whole story about your health, but the following are essential and simple blood tests that, interpreted correctly, can save your life. Many doctors do not always order these tests. Remember, the third leading cause of death in the US is iatrogenicity (death caused by physician). You are responsible for your own good health. If your doctor won't order a test, get a different doctor. It will save your life.

These tests will not only save your life, but anyone at risk for cardiovascular disease, and that includes almost everyone over age 50, should not only know about these tests, but know how to read and interpret the results. That way, you can understand your situation and take the necessary action to change, reverse, or prevent the behaviors that are having a negative impact on your health and longevity.

You want your blood test results to progress to optimal levels, not merely clinical levels or lab ranges which are averages for the general population. When it comes to your health, you do not want to be an average American, because an average American is fat, sick, tired, and dying. The sooner you know, the easier it is to reverse the long-term, accumulated damage.

Let's start with cholesterol as the word "cholesterol" has been on our radar and in our lexicon since the 70's. "Good" cholesterol, "bad" cholesterol, "eat it," "don't eat it," "low-fat," fat-free," "statins," who do you listen to?

First off, cholesterol ratios and the "type" of cholesterol are more important than single numbers. For years all we heard was total cholesterol, HDL, and LDL.

The importance of measuring LDL cholesterol through common blood testing has now decreased in value, to the point that the American Heart Association (AHA) no longer recommends using LDL cholesterol as a guide in treating the risk for CVD (cardiovascular disease) or prescribing statin drugs.

LDL particle size and number are also very important to analyzing your cardiovascular disease risk factors. The NMR lipid profile test is now available and is a must-order.

Substitute healthy saturated fats in your diet for the carbs you are losing. These will increase the size of your LDL cholesterol particles and protect you against heart disease. They include raw, organic nuts and seeds, avocadoes, pastured organic eggs, grass-fed meats and virgin coconut oil. (You want the big fluffy kind of LDL particles, not the dense, BB kind, prone to sticking in your arteries and causing a CVE.)

A better predictor is the ratio between your high-density lipoproteins (HDL) and total cholesterol (TC). HDL is an important factor in the fight against heart disease. Your ratio between HDL and total cholesterol (or HDL divided by your total cholesterol, multiplied by 100) should ideally be above 24 percent. Triglycerides: This test is used to identify the risk of developing coronary heart disease or when disorders in fat metabolism are suspected.

Triglycerides are another type of cholesterol formed in your body with excess blood sugar from the metabolism of carbohydrates. They are a significant risk factor in the development of heart disease.

- 150: High

- 100: Normal

- <70: optimal

Triglycerides (TG/HDL) ratio is also a predictor and indicator of developing insulin resistance that results in fatty liver disease, cirrhosis and eventually liver failure, if left untreated. Your triglyceride to HDL ratio (triglycerides divided by HDL, multiplied by 100) should ideally be below 2 percent. (Optimal TG/HDL levels should be kept under 1.0, normal below 2.0.)

TG/HDL:

- >3.5 indicates that you probably have pattern B LDL-P size with a predominance of small LDL particles and a good chance for insulin resistance and cardiovascular disease.

- Triglycerides: 50-100 is the normal range.

- The lower your TG/HDL ratio is (<1.0 is optimal), the greater your protection against heart attack and stroke, because you will have a high percentage of non-atherogenic (good) LDL particles in your blood stream.

- The higher your TG/HDL ratio, the more of the dangerous "bad" LDL small particles you will have.

- Lowering LDL cholesterol is secondary to protecting LDL from oxidation.

Total Cholesterol: (TC)

This test is used to determine the risk of developing coronary heart disease and hyperlipidemias.

- Range: 100 - 199mg/dL

- Optimal Range: 160 - 180 mg/dL

HDL Cholesterol:

This test measures alpha lipoprotein and is used to predict heart disease.

- Range: > 39 mg/dL

- Optimal Range: 50+ mg/dL

LDL Cholesterol:

- This test measures beta lipoproteins and is also used to predict heart disease.

- Range: 0-99mg/dL

- Optimal Range: 80-100 mg/dL (< 80 mg/dL may be ideal)

- Pre-existing/high risk cardiovascular disease: <70 mg/dL

Ratio of Total Cholesterol to HDL Cholesterol:

This test is used to determine the risk of coronary heart disease.

Optimal Range: <3.4

VLDL:

- Range: 2–30 mg/dL

- Optimal: 10–14

- The more triglycerides you have in your blood, the greater chance of developing atherosclerosis

- As triglycerides increase, HDL decreases and VLDL remains elevated.

- VLDL carries fat from the liver to other parts of the body.

- VLDL becomes LDL after it unloads fat

Non-HDL-C:

- <130: Normal

- <100: Optimal

- LDL <100: Optimal

LDL-P number ranges:

- Optimal: <1,000

- Moderate: 1,000–1299

- Borderline: 1,300–1599

- High: 1,600+

- Low-carb diet: Triglycerides decrease, HDL increases, LDL-P size increases.

- Small LDL-P is the most dangerous for CVD.

- The combination of Alpha Lopic Acid, vitamin E, grape seed extract, olive extract, green tea extract, quercetin and CoQ10 work synergistically together to prevent LDL oxidation and artery and endothelial dysfunction. If everyone knew the power of grape seed extract and quercetin in reducing LDL oxidation, increasing HDL levels, strengthening arteries, vessels and capillaries, simultaneously decreasing blood pressure, they'd all be on it, right?

This is a sample NMR Lipid Profile: NMR LipoProfile and results ranges:

Using state of the art technology known as nuclear magnetic resonance (NMR) spectroscopy, the NMR LipoProfile® is an advanced cholesterol test used to identify people at risk for lipid-related coronary heart disease (CHD).

The NMR LipoProfile contains the following tests:

- LDL particle number (LDL-P)

- Small LDL particle number (small LDL-P)

- HDL particle number (HDL-P)

- LDL particle size

- A standard cholesterol test (LDL-C, HDL-C, triglycerides and total cholesterol)

- LP-IR

On the other hand, a higher number of HDL-P is considered to be more protective, since HDL removes LDL by transporting it to the liver. In general, people with higher levels of HDL-P are at a lower risk for CHD.

It is also well known that LDL particle size provides extremely important information on cardiovascular health. Small, dense LDL particles are dangerous since they contribute to plaque formation in the arterial wall. Ideally, one would want their results to show large, buoyant LDL particles.

Small, dense particles are also closely associated with insulin resistance and an increased risk of developing type 2 diabetes. In addition to the particle size, the NMR LipoProfile® provides a laboratory developed index called LP-IR, with a higher number increasing the probability of developing insulin resistance.

Unfortunately, these vitally important markers contained in the NMR LipoProfile® are not included in the typical cholesterol test from your doctor. Standard lipid profiles utilize inferior technology and are limited to the use of cholesterol as a surrogate marker for your extremely important LDL particle number.

Why use outdated technology when the NMR® LipoProfile can more accurately identify if you are really at risk for insulin resistance and CHD?

A 12–14 hour fast is required for this blood test. However, drink plenty of water and take your medications as prescribed.

Additional tests and normal to optimal ranges:

hsCRP Optimal

- <0.55mg/L-men and <1.0-women (< = below or lower than)

- Optimal: below .56

- People with the highest levels of CRP have 5 times the risk of developing cardiovascular disease, heart attack, or stroke.

Hemoglobin A1c:

- Normal: < 5.7

- Optimal: < 5.2

Hematocrit: the ratio of the volume of red blood cells to the total volume of blood. The hematocrit blood test determines the percentage of red blood cells (RBC's) in the blood. Blood is composed mainly of red blood cells and white blood cells suspended in an almost clear fluid called serum. The hematocrit test indicates the percentage of blood by volume that is composed of red blood cells. The definition of normal red-blood cell percentage also varies from one medical practice to another. Generally, a normal range is considered to be: For men, 38.8 to 50 percent. For women, 34.9 to 44.5 percent.

- Healthy range (Men) <50.0 (If over 50.0 consult a Hemotologist MD for a phlebotomy.)

- Optimal (Men) 45.0

Homocysteine: Levels should be below 7.0–8.0 and optimally lower than 6.5: the lower, the better. Research shows that lowering homocysteine to 6.5 or below, reducing oxLDL, reduces the risk of heart attacks, stroke, and heart disease many times better than drugs, without any toxic side effects. All of it can be accomplished through diet and supplementation. Around 80–90% of today's diseases are preventable and controllable through nutrition.

B vitamins are particularly affected and depleted by stress and a lack of B vitamins, especially B1, B6, B9 (Folate) and B12 results in increased homocysteine levels, which leads to increased risk of heart attack and stroke. Homocysteine levels become elevated with a deficiency of B vitamins, B-1, B-6, B-12 and folic acid. Be careful of B-6 toxicity as it can cause tingling of the fingers and toes, but blood test regularly to monitor levels.

Homocysteine oxidizes and damages LDL cholesterol, triglycerides and simultaneously the endothelium, and stimulates the growth of atherosclerotic plaque leading to heart attack and stroke. Homocysteine is second only to cigarette smoking in its oxidative destruction, simultaneously causing damage to the endothelium, oxidizing and damaging LDL, causing it to stick to the homocysteine-damaged endothelium, causing atherosclerosis and leading to plaque rupture and heart attack and stroke. It's critical to realize that it's not simply the level of your LDL cholesterol, but whether it is oxidized or damaged, observable through an oxLDL blood test.

The greater the homocysteine level, the greater the oxidation of both LDL and arterial lining, the greater the inflammation, and the higher the CRP. Homocysteine levels and hsCRP may be more predictive than any other test.

- 7-10umol/L - healthy range.

- 6.5-8.0umol/L - optimal.

(Your thyroid hormones also control your homocysteine levels, so this is another reason to balance your thyroid and your hormones.)

Diabetes is a cardiovascular disease. Diabetes contributes more to the development of cardiovascular disease than any other risk factor besides smoking. If you have diabetes and live long enough, you're sure to develop cardiovascular disease and have a heart attack or stroke. Diabetes in the US is epidemic, having tripled since 1980. Approximately 8% of the population, or 24 million people have type 2 diabetes. That number includes 6 million who are undiagnosed and 57 million with pre-diabetes.

A1C above 6.0 pre, above 6.5 diabetic, 2-hour greater than 200.

- Fasting Insulin, Optimal: 2–3

- High: <5 uIU/mL .

(Supplements I take to keep these in optimal levels: 1000 mcg folic acid daily TMG lowers homocysteine.) However, test for optimal results as you may have to adjust dosage from time to time.)

Vitamins, minerals, antioxidants, and other supplements, including omega-3 fatty acids DHA/EPA, reduce inflammation and oxidation without side effects, and lower levels of homocysteine and hsCRP. In addition, vitamins B-1, B-6 and B-12, along with TMG (Tri-methyl-glycine), reduce homocysteine into safer amino acids and reduce inflammation of LDL and the endothelium, thereby reducing atherosclerosis and plaque rupturing; therefore, reducing the risks of cardiovascular disease, heart attack, and stroke. (I take 4,000mg of Lovaza daily, which is the only prescription omega-3 on the market, nearly pure and above all OTC products. Your insurance should pay. If not, Life Extension omega-3 is probably one of the next best.)

IGF-1 (Insulin-Like Growth Factor I)

- Insulin - Optimal fasting blood glucose <80 mg/dl.

Cortisol:

- Adult/child/morning 5-23 micrograms per deciliter (mcg/dL) or 138-635 nanomoles per liter (nmol/L)

- Afternoon 3-16 mcg/dL or 83-441 nmol/L

Uric acid:

- 3.4-7.0 mg/dL normal range

Vitamin D, 25-Hydroxy: Vitamin D is essential for life. So much so that our bodies can manufacture this critical nutrient in the skin upon sun exposure. However, most people do not get enough sun exposure to maintain optimal levels of vitamin D in their bodies; risks of skin cancer and sun damage dissuade many people from spending much time in the sun. Sun exposure is not the only way to increase your vitamin D levels. Supplemental vitamin D also efficiently boosts blood levels of vitamin D, which are typically measured as 25-hydroxyvitamin D. This is fortunate, because research over many years has firmly established vitamin D as a key mediator of health throughout the body. Vitamin D was thought to primarily support calcium homeostasis, but it is now known that vitamin D has many other crucial functions, including helping balance the immune system, suppressing abnormal cell growth and supporting brain health.

Vitamin D deficiency has been associated with a host of diseases ranging from cancer and cardiovascular disease to osteoporosis and cognitive impairment. Maintaining a blood level of 25-hydroxyvitamin D is of paramount importance to optimal health.

Vitamin D. Around 42% of US adults are vitamin D deficient and are subject to many health issues, including immune system disorders. There are 30,000 genes in your body and vitamin D influences about 3,000 of them.

- Normal range: 40–60 ng/mL

- Optimal: 60–80 ng/mL

- Fighting cancer: 80ng/mL or above

Thyroid: TSH: (thyroid stimulating hormone)

- Optimal: 1.0-2.0 mIU/L

T4 (Free): Thyroxine

- Range: 0.82–1.77 ng/dL

- Optimal upper ranges: 1.4–1.5 ng/dL

T4 (Total): Thyroxine

- Optimal: 8.5–10.5 mcg/dL (Men)

- 9.0–11.0 mcg/dL (Women <60)

- 8.5–10.7 mcg/dL (Women >60)

T3 (Free) Tri-Iodothyronine: Bioavailable

- Optimal: 3.4–4.2 pg/mL

T3 (Total): Tri-Iodothyronine

- Normal range: 71–180 ng/dL

Testosterone: I believe in maintaining the 500–750 range and, depending on age, up to 1,000. A Life Extension study claimed that men who maintained a range between 500 and 750 stopped having CVEs. My testostoerone, when first measured post-stroke, was less than 100, so not only do I recommend HRT, I recommend a range between 550 and 750, but no higher than 1,000. Optimal is 700–900.

PSA: (Prostate-Specific Antigen)

- Normal: <4.0 ng/mL

- Optimal: 1.0–2.5 ng/mL

Lp-PLA2/PLAC:

- Optimal: <200ng/Ml

ApoB

- Normal range: <100

- Optimal: <80

Lp(A):

- Healthy Zone: <30 mg/dL (standard blood test) <10 mg/dL

OGTT (oral glucose tolerance test for insulin resistance)- 2 hour

- Optimal range: <6.0 - <7.8 mmol//L

Glucometer: blood sugar levels tester. Ketone meter: levels of ketones or fat.

LP-IR Score

- <45

AA/EPA (cellular inflammation/SIP: silent inflammation profile)

omega-6 versus omega-3 score. Arachidonic acid is toxic fat created by an inflammation-induced diet. SAD. (Standard American Diet.)

Reduce the AA/EPA omega score ratio in your blood, you reverse toxic fats in the blood and brain. Rich in omega-3s: salmon, herring, sardines, mackerel, anchovies, and tuna.

- AA/EPA ratio under 3.0.

- Optimal: 1.5, no less than 1.0. (omega Score: AA/EPA ratio blood test is a superior and more accurate test to measure inflammation than the hsCRP test, as the AA/EPA ratio is an early warning system for increased levels of cellular inflammation, as an elevated level of AA/EPA ratio can precede the development of an elevated hsCPR by several years, if not decades.

- Low: 1.5–3 (future state of wellness: excellent)

- Moderate: 3–6

- Elevated: 7–15

- High: >15 (future state of wellness: poor)

- The ideal ratio of omega-6 to omega-3 is 1:1 to 3:1, however, most Americans consume a very unhealthy ratio of 20:1 to 50:1. The average ratio in Asia is 3:1.

- Minimum - 2,500 mg daily. (However, I take 4,000mg of prescription Lovaza daily.)

Mixing saturated fats with trans fats is a recipe for disaster. The metabolic effect saturated fats have on your body is dependent entirely on what else you consume with it. Saturated fat: if carbs are low, insulin is low, saturated fat is handled more efficiently and you're burning the saturated fat as fuel and your body makes and stores less fat.

ApoE: A DNA test is a gene test or your blueprint that requires a certain environment. Epigenetics is gene expression, so you are no longer just stuck with your genes, you can express them with the right nutrition for a different outcome. (You only have to take this test once.)

- Optimal: 3:3

ApoE genotype testing: best type of eating regimen for your body type.

IL-6 interlukin-6 test-inflammation:

- Range: 0–14 pg/mL

Coenzyme Q10 (CoQ10): This test is used to check the blood level of CoQ10 and will enable more precise dosing for anyone seeking to achieve and maintain high levels of this critical antioxidant. Coenzyme Q10 is produced by the human body and is necessary for the basic functioning of all cells. It is known to be highly concentrated in heart muscle cells due to the high energy requirements of this cell type.

- Ranges: 0.37–2.20 µg/mL

- Optimal: 3–7 µg/mL; At least 3 µg/mL for general health, at least 4µg/mL for cardiovascular issues and up to 7 µg/mL for maximal anti-aging and neurodegenerative protection.

- Healthy Zone: 1.0–1.8 ug/mL

hsCRP-Reactive Protein (CRP) (cardiac) (high sensitivity)

This test is used to assess risk of cardiovascular and peripheral vascular disease.

- Healthy zone: <0.8 mg/dL

DHEA: Dehydroepiandrosterone sulfate:

This test is used to diagnose female infertility, amenorrhea, or hirsutism and to aid in the evaluation of excess androgen/adrenocortical disease, including congenital adrenal hyperplasia and adrenal tumors.

- Optimal levels: 350–500 mg/dL-Men and 275–400 mg/dL-Women

- <200–100 mg/dL (supplement 25mg daily dose.)

Fibrinogen:

- Healthy Zone: 180–350 mg/dL

Optimal Blood Pressure: (BP):

- Normal: 120/80

- Better: 115/75

- Optimal: 110/70

Fasting insulin level: Any meal or snack high in carbohydrates like fructose and refined grains generates a rapid rise in blood glucose and then insulin to compensate for the rise in blood sugar. The insulin released from eating too many carbs promotes fat accumulation and makes it more difficult for your body to shed excess weight. Excess fat, particularly around your belly, is one of the major contributors to heart disease.

Fasting blood sugar level: Studies have shown that people with a fasting blood sugar level of 100-125 mg/dl had a nearly 300 percent increase higher risk of having coronary heart disease than people with a level below 80 mg/dl.

Insulin:

- Optimal insulin level: <10.0 uIU/mL

Fasting Insulin:

- Normal range: 5–10

- Optimal: <8

Ketones

- Normal range: 1.5–3.0

Iron (Ferritin):

- The healthy range of serum Ferritin is between 20 and 80 ng/ml. Below 20, is iron deficient, and above 80 is an iron surplus. Ideal iron range is 40–60 ng/mL.

- Optimal: 40-60 ng/mL

- Deficient: <20-low ng/mL

- Surplus: > 80-high ng/mL

Iron can be a very potent cause of oxidative stress, so if you have excess iron levels you can damage your blood vessels and increase your risk of heart disease. You should monitor your ferritin levels and make sure they are not much above 80 ng/ml. The simplest way to lower them if they are elevated is to donate your blood. If that is not possible, you can have a therapeutic phlebotomy and that will effectively eliminate the excess iron from your body. Do not take a multi-vitamin that includes iron. You want to take iron separately, so you can adjust dosages. Iron blocks the pathway to several micronutrients and should be taken an hour before or two hours after other vitamins and minerals so they are all absorbed biochemically to their maximum efficiency.

Test for all vitamin and mineral deficiencies

Test for toxic and heavy metals panel:

- Mercury

- Arsenic

- Lead

- Cadmium

- Chromium

- Cooper

- Zinc

Oxidative Stress Analysis 2.0 Blood Test. (antioxidant reserve)

BMI does not differentiate between fat or muscle, that's why I like the body fat percentage measurement best. Optimal body fat percentage in men 12% or less; women 20% or less. Optimal waist line: men 35" or less; women 30" or less.

People with vitamin D deficiency have higher risk for insulin resistance, type 2 diabetes and metabolic syndrome.

Facts about high blood pressure (hypertension):

- One in three US adults has high blood pressure

- Nearly a third of people with hypertension don't know they have the condition or symptoms

- Over 40 percent are not being treated

(*Source: Journal of the American Medical Association (JAMA), 2003*)

Approximately 1 in 11, or 8.8% of Americans suffer from kidney stone disease each year and many don't even know they have it. Annually, nearly 3.3 million Americans seek out medical care for kidney stone removal and pain relief at a cost of about $5.3 billion per year.

Nearly 12 percent of men and 5 percent of women in the United States will feel a kidney stone during their life—and it's not pleasant. Although they're often described as "the worst pain I've ever experienced," kidney stones rarely cause long-term damage. Kidney stones can occur at any age, but men are more likely to develop stones between the ages of 40 and 70, while women are more likely to develop a kidney stone in their 50s. Often kidney stones are a recurring problem; having had one kidney stone puts you at increased risk for a second.

Kidney stones can form anywhere along the urinary tract, including the kidneys, bladder, ureter, or urethra. A kidney stone starts as a microscopic crystal. Over time, the crystal enlarges or multiple crystals can aggregate to form a single large kidney stone. Pain develops when the stone breaks away and becomes lodged in the urinary tract, either partially or totally blocking the passage of urine. Blood in the urine is a good indication that you have a breakaway stone.

If you have kidney stones you may have calcium buildup in your arteries, a precursor to atherosclerosis or hardening of the arteries. Kidney stones may lead to high blood pressure or hypertension. Obesity, type 2 diabetes, high blood pressure, and atherosclerosis can all be early markers for heart attack and stroke. A kidney stone is often times discovered during scanning and testing for other diseases. Something so benign as a kidney stone can seem a non-life threatening inconvenience and pain, but could be a precursor of coming serious health events. This is another reason to test and don't guess. Blood doesn't lie.

Common kidney stone therapies: ureteroscopy and laser lithotripsy.

Kidney stones are totally unrelated to gallstones, which form in the gallbladder.

(Sample blood tests suggestions from Life Extension:)

Male Blood Test Sample Report: The male panel is a comprehensive blood test that addresses cardiovascular health, hormone status, and general health.

- Chemistry Panel (metabolic panel with lipids): The cornerstone of any complete physical, the chemistry panel provides an array of markers to help assess cardiovascular risk, metabolic function, electrolyte status, minerals important for bone health, plus liver and kidney function.

- Complete Blood Count (CBC): The CBC test evaluates three types of cells that circulate in the blood (red blood cells, white blood cells, and platelets). These markers can help to provide information regarding the immune system, possibility of an infection, blood disorder, nutritional deficiencies, your body's ability to clot, and more.

- Free and Total Testosterone: Known as the feel-good hormone, testosterone helps maintain a man's bone density, fat distribution, muscle strength, sex drive, mood, energy, sperm production, and more.

- Dehydroepiandrosterone sulfate (DHEA-S): Produced primarily by the adrenal glands, DHEA is the most abundant steroid hormone in the human body. DHEA plays a fundamental role in hormone balance, as well as supporting one's immune function, energy, mood, and maintaining muscle and bone mass. Since orally administered DHEA is mostly converted to DHEA-S, coupled with the fact that DHEA-S levels are more stable in the blood than DHEA, measurement of DHEA-S is preferable to DHEA.

- Prostate-Specific Antigen (PSA): PSA is produced exclusively by cells of the prostate gland. Used in conjunction with a digital rectal examination, PSA is a useful screening test for benign prostate hyperplasia (BPH) and prostate cancer development.

- Estradiol (E2): The primary female sex hormone, estradiol is a form of estrogen that is also present in males. In men, high levels of estradiol are associated with excessive abdominal fat, enlargement of the prostate, and increased cardiovascular risk. Conversely, levels that are too low are associated with osteoporosis.

- Homocysteine: A risk factor for cardiovascular disease, high homocysteine levels can directly damage the delicate endothelial cells that line the inside of arteries, resulting in vascular inflammation, arterial plaque rupture, and blood clot formation.

- C-reactive protein (High sensitivity): CRP measures general levels of inflammation in your body, but cannot show where the inflammation is located or what is causing it. Uncontrolled, systemic inflammation places you at risk for many degenerative diseases like heart disease and stroke.

- TSH (thyroid stimulating hormone): TSH is produced by the pituitary gland, and stimulates your thyroid to produce thyroid hormones T3 and T4. TSH can be used to screen for thyroid disease and other thyroid imbalances,

- Vitamin D, 25-Hydroxy: Known as the sunshine vitamin, vitamin D is important to every cell and tissue throughout the body. Offering benefits from proper immune function and bone density to heart health and mood disorders, vitamin D is critical for optimal health.

HDL/Cholesterol ratio: HDL percentage is a very potent heart disease risk factor. Just divide your HDL level by your total cholesterol. That percentage should ideally be above 24 percent.

Triglyceride/HDL ratios: You can also do the same thing with your triglycerides and HDL ratio. That percentage should be below 2.

Fasting insulin level: Any meal or snack high in carbohydrates like fructose and refined grains generates a rapid rise in blood glucose and then insulin to compensate for the rise in blood sugar. The insulin released from eating too many carbs promotes fat accumulation and makes it more difficult for your body to shed excess weight. Excess fat, particularly around your belly, is one of the major contributors to heart disease.

Fasting blood sugar level: Studies have shown that people with a fasting blood sugar level of 100-125 mg/dl had a nearly 300 percent increased higher risk of having coronary heart disease than people with a level below 79 mg/dl.

An 8 to 12 hour fast is required for most blood tests. However, drink plenty of water and take your medications as prescribed.

If you are supplementing with any hormones, it is important to take them approximately 2 hours prior to having your blood drawn. Ejaculation within 72 hours preceding the blood draw may elevate the PSA in some men.

Female Blood Test Sample Report: The Life Extension female panel is a comprehensive blood test that addresses cardiovascular health, hormone status, and general health.

- Chemistry Panel (metabolic panel with lipids): The cornerstone of any complete physical, the chemistry panel provides an array of markers to help assess cardiovascular risk, metabolic function, electrolyte status, minerals important for bone health, plus liver and kidney function.

- Complete Blood Count (CBC): The CBC test evaluates three types of cells that circulate in the blood (red blood cells, white blood cells, and platelets). These markers can help to provide information regarding the immune system, possibility of an infection, blood disorder, nutritional deficiencies, your body's ability to clot, and more.

- Free and Total Testosterone: Known as the feel-good hormone, testosterone helps maintain a woman's libido, bone and muscle mass, cardiovascular health, mood, and sense of well-being. Testosterone in conjunction with estrogen is crucial in minimizing hot flashes, sleep disturbances, night sweats, and vaginal dryness.

- Dehydroepiandrosterone sulfate (DHEA-S): Produced primarily by the adrenal glands, DHEA is the most abundant steroid hormone in the human body. DHEA plays a fundamental role in hormone balance, as well as supporting one's immune function, energy, mood, and maintenance of muscle and bone mass. Since orally administered DHEA is mostly converted to DHEA-S, coupled with the fact that DHEA-S levels are more stable in the blood than DHEA, measurement of DHEA-S is preferable to DHEA.

- Progesterone: Instrumental in balancing the powerful effects of estrogen, an imbalance between progesterone and estrogen is linked to weight gain, insomnia, anxiety, depression, migraines, cancer, uterine fibroids, ovarian cysts, and osteoporosis.

- Estradiol (E2): The primary female sex hormone, estradiol is a form of estrogen responsible for menstrual cycle regulation, skin elasticity, bone strength, and bladder and vaginal health.

- Homocysteine: A risk factor for cardiovascular disease, high homocysteine levels can directly damage the delicate endothelial cells that line the inside of arteries, resulting in vascular inflammation, arterial plaque rupture, and blood clot formation.

- C-reactive protein (high sensitivity): CRP measures general levels of inflammation in your body, but cannot show where the inflammation is located or what is causing it. Uncontrolled, systemic inflammation places you at risk for many degenerative diseases like heart disease and stroke.

- TSH (Thyroid stimulating hormone): TSH is produced by the pituitary gland, and stimulates your thyroid to produce thyroid hormones T3 and T4. TSH can be used to screen for thyroid disease and other thyroid imbalances. Healthy Zone: 0.1–2.8

T4 (Free): Thyroxine

- Healthy Range: 0.82-1.77 ng/dL

- Optimal upper ranges: 1.4-1.5 ng/dL

T3 (Total): Tri-Iodothyronine

- Normal range: 71-180 ng/dL

Vitamin D, 25-Hydroxy: Known as the sunshine vitamin, vitamin D is important to every cell and tissue throughout the body. From proper immune function and bone density to heart health and mood disorders, vitamin D is critical for optimal health.

Hemoglobin A1C (HbA1C): HbA1C shows the average level of blood sugar (glucose) over the previous 3 months. HbA1C is a useful indicator of how well blood glucose is being controlled, and is also used to monitor the effects of diet, exercise, and drug therapy in diabetic patients. Healthy Zone: <6% of total HGB.

An 8 to 12 hour fast is required for this blood test. However, drink plenty of water and take your medications as prescribed.

If you are supplementing with any hormones, it is important to take them approximately 2 hours prior to having your blood drawn. Any type of contraceptives that contain hormones will invalidate hormone results.

Comprehensive Thyroid Panel Test: Your thyroid gland sits in the lower portion of your neck and acts as the metabolic throttle for every cell in your body. When your thyroid doesn't function efficiently, it can affect every cell in your body. An estimated 27 million Americans have thyroid disease, and about 13 million of them are undiagnosed. Since symptoms can often be vague (fatigue, depression, and weight gain), many people are not tested for thyroid dysfunction.

- Thyroid-Stimulating Hormone (TSH)

- Total Thyroxine (T4)

- Free Thyroxine (T4)

- Free Tri-iodothyronine (T3)

There is a connection between AFib (atrial fibrillation) or Aflutter and thyroid function: Your thyroid gland is located over your voice box in your throat. It controls your metabolic rate, which means it is responsible for how fast or slow all of the processes in your body occur. If your thyroid is healthy, the processes occur at an optimal rate. Studies have shown that thyroid function has an impact on the frequency with which atrial fibrillation occurs. This is important information if you have a diagnosis of either AFib or thyroid disease. (Hypothyroidism is the most common.)

Additional Test Ranges

- Apolipoprotein A-1 (ApoA):

This test is used to evaluate survival rate or risk factors for patients with myocardial infarction and peripheral vascular diseases. APO A-1 deficiency states include Tangier disease, HDL deficiency, and hypoalpha-lipoprotein anemia. Apolipoprotein levels may be a better indicator of atherogenic risks than high-density lipoprotein (HDL), low-density lipoprotein (LDL), and very-low-density lipoprotein (VLDL) measures.

Reference Ranges:

- Men 110–180 mg/dL

- Women 110–205 mg/dL

BUN (Blood Urea Nitrogen):

This test is used to measure liver function and to indirectly assess renal function and glomerular filtration rate.

- Range: 6–20 mg/dL

BUN/Creatinine Ratio:

This test is used to diagnose impaired renal function. With creatinine, BUN is used to monitor patients on dialysis.

- Range: 8:1–20:1

Sodium: This routine test is used to evaluate and monitor fluid and electrolyte balance and therapy.

- Range: 135–144 mmol/L

Potassium: This routine test is used to evaluate and monitor electrolyte balance and is especially important for cardiac patients.

- Range: 3.5–5.2 mmol/L

Chloride: This test by itself does not provide adequate information. However, as part of a multiphasic testing for electrolytes, it can give an indication of acid-base balance and hydration status.

- Range: 97–108 mmol/L

Carbon Dioxide: This test is used to assist in the evaluation of pH and electrolyte status.

- Range: 19–28 mmol/L

Calcium: This test is used to evaluate parathyroid function and calcium metabolism

Range:

- 18–59 years old: 8.7–10.2 mg/dL

- \> 59 years old: 8.6–10.2 mg/dL

- Optimal Range: 9–10 mg/dL

Phosphorus: This test is used to measure serum phosphorus levels. An imbalance could indicate the possibility of any number of conditions.

- Range for people between 12 and 60 years old: 2.5–4.5 mg/dL

Protein/Albumin/Globulin: This test is used to assist in the diagnosis of many diseases that affect blood proteins as a whole or one single fraction of protein.

Range:

- Total Protein: 6.0–8.5 g/dL

- Albumin: 3.5–5.5 g/dL

- Globulin: 1.5–4.5 g/dL

Albumin/Globulin Ratio: This test is used to evaluate renal disease and other chronic diseases.

Range: 1.1:1–2.5:1

Bilirubin: This test is used to evaluate liver function.

- Healthy range: 0.2-1.2 mg/dL

- Total Bilirubin: 0.0–1.2 mg/dL

Alkaline Phosphatase: This test is used to detect and monitor liver or bone disease.

- Range: 25–150 IU/L

CBC (Complete Blood Count) with Platelets and Differential: This is a series of tests of the peripheral blood that provides a variety of information about the blood components.

White Blood Cell Count:

- Range: 4.0–10.5 x10E3/uL

Red Blood Cell Count:

Ranges:

- Men: 4.14–5.8 x10E6/uL

- Women: 3.77–5.28 x10E6/uL

Hemoglobin:

Ranges:

- Men: 12.6–17.7 g/dL

- Women: 11.1–15.9 g/dL

Platelet Count:

- Range: 140–415 x10E3/uL

Estradiol: This test is used to assess hypothalamic and pituitary functions, menopausal status, and sexual maturity. In males it is helpful in the assessment of gynecomastia or feminization syndromes.

- Men: 7.6–42.6 pg/mL

- Women: (Varies by menstrual cycle and menopausal status.)

Estrogens Total: Estrogen measurements are used to evaluate sexual maturity and menstrual and fertility problems in females. This test is also used in the evaluation of males with gynecomastia or feminization syndromes. In pregnant women, it is used to indicate fetal-placental health. In patients with estrogen-producing tumors, it can be used as a tumor marker.

Ranges:

- Men: 40–115 pg/mL

- Optimal: 40–77 pg/mL

- Women:

- Optimal: 75–200 pg/mL (with HRT)

Glucose (Serum) (Fasting): This test is used to detect diabetes mellitus. It is used to evaluate carbohydrate metabolism disorders including alcoholism. It is also used to evaluate acidosis, ketoacidosis, dehydration, coma, hypoglycemia, insulinoma, and neuroglycopenia.

(These tests require a fasting blood level, meaning that a 12-hour fast is required before the collection of a blood sample.)

Reference Ranges:

- Normal: 65–99 mg/dL

- Pre-Diabetic: 100–125 mg/dL

- Diabetic: > 125 mg/dL

- Optimal Range: 70–85 mg/dL

Glucose (2 hours postprandial): Normally, your blood glucose levels increase slightly after you eat. This increase causes your pancreas to release insulin so that your blood glucose levels do not get too high. Blood glucose levels that remain high over time can damage your eyes, kidneys, nerves, and blood vessels. This test measures blood glucose exactly 2 hours after eating.

Ranges:

- Normal: 65–139 mg/dL

- Pre-Diabetic: 140–199 mg/dL

- Diabetic: > 200 mg/dL

- Optimal Range: 110–125 mg/dL or < 40 mg/dL increase over baseline

Heavy Metals Profile: This test is used to monitor exposure to arsenic, lead, and mercury.

Optimal Range: As low as possible

Insulin Fasting: This test is used for insulin measurement in patients with fasting hypoglycemia or hyperglycemia. High fasting insulin is a sign of insulin resistance and the start of type 2 diabetes or syndrome X.

- Range: 2.6–24.9 µIU/mL

- Optimal Range: < 5 µIU/mL

Interleukin-6 (IL-6): This test is used to identify elevated levels of interleukin-6. Elevated IL-6 serum or plasma levels may occur in sepsis, autoimmune diseases, lymphomas, AIDS, alcoholic liver disease, tumor development, Alzheimer's disease, and in concert with infections or transplant rejection. Elevated levels of IL-6 may be associated with an increased risk of heart attack or stroke.

- IL-6: 0–14 pg/mL

Insulin-Like Growth Factor I (IGF-1): A test for insulin-like growth factor-1 (IGF-1) may be used to help identify growth hormone (GH) deficiency; it is not diagnostic of a GH deficiency but may be ordered along with GH stimulation tests to offer additional information. As follow-up to abnormal results on other hormone tests. Evaluate pituitary function.

Lipoprotein (a): Lp(a): This test is used to measure excess small dense lipoprotein. Elevated lipoprotein (a) is a strong indicator of premature coronary disease and atherosclerotic vascular disease and is associated with increased risk of cardiac death.

- Ranges: 0–30 mg/dL

- Desirable: <20mg/dL

- Borderline High Risk: 20–30 mg/dL

- High Risk: 31–50 mg/dL

- Very High Risk: >50 mg/dL

Magnesium (serum): This test is used to evaluate magnesium levels. Decreased levels of magnesium have been associated with cardiac arrhythmias, hypocalcemia, hypokalemia, long-term hyperalimentation, intravenous therapy, diabetes mellitus (especially during treatment of ketoacidosis), alcoholism and other types of malnutrition, malabsorption, hyperparathyroidism, dialysis, pregnancy, and hyperaldosteronism. Magnesium deficiency produces neuromuscular disorders causing weakness, tremors, tetany, and convulsions. Renal loss of magnesium occurs with cis-platinum therapy. Increased magnesium levels relate mostly to individuals in renal failure or with Addison's disease. Marked increases may be found in individuals who take magnesium salts (e.g., antacids, which contain magnesium) or magnesium-containing cathartics and in pregnant woman with severe preeclampsia or eclampsia who are receiving magnesium sulfate as an anticonvulsant. High magnesium levels are manifested in decreased reflexes, somnolence, and heart block.

- Range: 1.6–2.6 mg/dL

Pregnenolone: This test is used to determine ovarian failure, hirsutism, adrenal carcinoma, and Cushing's syndrome.

Ranges:

- Men: 10–200 ng/dL

- Women: 10–230 ng/dL

Optimal Range:

- Men: 125–175 ng/dL; max 200 ng/dL

- Women: 130–180 ng/dL; max 230 ng/dL

Selenium: This test is used to monitor selenium deficiency and occupational exposure. Because selenium is a very important supplement for the extension of life, optimal levels are in the upper half of the normal range.

Ranges:

- Environmental Exposure: 79–326 μg/L

- Normal Range: 46–143μg/L

(*Reference source: LifeExtension.com*)

Additional Blood Test Results:

- ALT (alanine aminotransferase)

Healthy range: 8 to 37 IU/L

This test looks at levels of the liver enzyme ALT. When all's well with your liver, your score on this test should be within range. Anything higher may indicate liver damage.

- Albumin

Healthy range: 3.9 to 5.0 g/dL

A protein made by the liver, albumin levels can be an indicator of liver or kidney problems.

- A/G ratio (albumin/globulin ratio) or total protein test

Healthy ratio: a bit over 1, favoring albumin

There are two types of protein your blood — albumin (see above) and globulin. The A/G ratio test compares levels of these proteins with one another. Elevated protein levels could indicate a health condition in need of attention.

- Alkaline phosphatase

Healthy range: 44 to 147 IU/L

This enzyme is involved in both liver and bone, so elevations may indicate problems with the liver or bone-related disease.

- AST (aspartate aminotransferase)

Healthy range: 10 to 34 IU/L

This enzyme is found in heart and liver tissue, so elevations suggest problems may be occurring in one or both of those areas.

- Bilirubin

Healthy range: 0.1 to 1.9 mg/dL

This provides information about liver and kidney functions, problems in bile ducts, and anemia.

- BUN (blood urea nitrogen)

Healthy range: 10 to 20 mg/dL

This is another measure of kidney and liver functions. High values may indicate a problem with kidney function. A number of medications and a diet high in protein can also raise BUN levels.

- BUN/creatinine ratio

Healthy ratio of BUN to creatinine: 10:1 to 20:1 (Men and older individuals may be a bit higher.) This test shows if kidneys are eliminating waste properly. High levels of creatinine, a by-product of muscle contractions, are excreted through the kidneys and suggest reduced kidney function.

- Calcium

Healthy range: 9.0 to 10.5 mg/dL (the elderly typically score a bit lower)

Too much calcium in the bloodstream could indicate kidney problems; overly active thyroid or parathyroid glands; certain types of cancer, including lymphoma; problems with the pancreas; or a deficiency of vitamin D.

- Chloride

Healthy range: 98 to 106 mEq/L

This mineral is often measured as part of an electrolyte panel. A high-salt diet and/or certain medications are often responsible for elevations in chloride. Excess chloride may indicate an overly acidic environment in the body. It also could be a red flag for dehydration, multiple myeloma, kidney disorders, or adrenal gland dysfunction.

- Creatinine

Healthy range: 0.5 to 1.1 mg/dL for women; 0.6 to 1.2 mg/dL for men (The elderly may be slightly lower.)

The kidneys process this waste product, so elevations could indicate a problem with kidney function.

- Fasting glucose (blood sugar)

Healthy range: 70 to 99 mg/dL for the average adult (the elderly tend to score higher even when they are healthy)

Blood sugar levels can be affected by food or beverages you have ingested recently, your current stress levels, medications you may be taking, and the time of day. The fasting blood sugar test is done after at least 6 hours without food or drink other than water.

- Phosphorus

Healthy range: 2.4 to 4.1 mg/dL

Phosphorus plays an important role in bone health and is related to calcium levels. Too much phosphorus could indicate a problem with kidneys or the parathyroid gland. Alcohol abuse, long-term antacid use, excessive intake of diuretics or vitamin D, and malnutrition can also elevate phosphorus levels.

- Potassium

Healthy range: 3.7 to 5.2 mEq/L

This mineral is essential for relaying nerve impulses, maintaining proper muscle functions, and regulating heartbeat. Diuretics, drugs that are often taken for high blood pressure, can cause low levels of potassium.

- Sodium

Healthy range: 135 to 145 mEq/L

Another member of the electrolyte family, the mineral sodium helps your body balance water levels and helps with nerve impulses and muscle contractions. Irregularities in sodium levels may indicate dehydration; disorders of the adrenal glands; excessive intake of salt, corticosteroids, or pain-relieving medications; or problems with the liver or kidneys.

Lipid Panel Results (Lipid Profile)

The lipid panel is a collection of tests measuring different types of cholesterol and triglycerides (fats) in your bloodstream.

Total cholesterol

General rules (best to worst):

- Healthy: Below 200 mg/dL (below 5.18 mmol/L)

- Borderline high: 200 to 239 mg/dL (5.2 to 6.2 mmol/L)

- High: Above 240 mg/dL (above 6.2 mmol/L)

- Optimal: 180-200 for prevention of all-cause mortality

This test measures combined levels of both LDL (bad) and HDL (good) cholesterol. The test may be done simply to record an individual's cholesterol levels or for comparison purposes (e.g., to determine if cholesterol-lowering medications or nutrients are working).

- Triglycerides

Healthy range: 40 to 160 mg/dL

These fats are found in the bloodstream and may contribute to heart disease and other health problems.

- HDL (good) cholesterol

- Best   Above 60 mg/dL

- Good 50 to 60 mg/dL

- Poor   Below 40 mg/dL for men; below 50 mg/dL for women

Also known as "good" cholesterol, HDL (high-density lipoprotein) protects against heart disease. Low scores are risk factors for heart disease.

- The lower your TG/HDL ratio is <1.0 is optimal, the greater your protection against heart attack and stroke, because you will have a high percentage of nonathergenic (good) LDL particles in your blood stream.

- The higher your TG/HDL ratio, the more of the dangerous "bad" LDL small particles you will have.

- TG/HDL is less than 2.0 your LDL is predominantly large and fluffy, the good "bad" cholesterol. If your ratio is greater than 4.0, you have a lot of small, dense LDL particles, the bad "bad" LDL cholesterol that accelerate the development of atherosclerotic plaques.

- Those with the highest TG/HDL ratios, over 7.0, have a 16 times greater risk of a heart attack than those in the lower ratios. That's a huge increase in the most common cause of death in the US. Again, 80% preventable by eliminating diet-induced inflammation.

- Elevated TG/HDL is also a marker for metabolic syndrome, developing insulin resistance, obesity, Type 2 Diabetes, as well as, accelerated cardiovascular disease.

- Lowering insulin levels lowers both inflammation and "bad" cholesterol levels.

High-dose omega-3s-EPA/DHA reduces all types of inflammation.

- TC/HDL < 4.

- LDL/HDL< 3.

(The higher the LDL, the greater risk of CVD; the higher the HDL, the lower the risk.)

Visceral fat is measured by your TG/HDL ratio and your fasting insulin levels.

Oxidized LDL (oxLDL):

- Low risk: < 60 U/L

- Moderate risk: 60–69

- High risk: >70 or higher

Three additional life-saving preventative tests:

1. cIMT (Carotid Intima Media Thickness and FMD-flow mediated dilation):

2. CT Coronary Calcium Score:

- <10 is ideal.

- 0-optimal.

- Over 400 serious

CT Coronary Calcium score:

- <50 for women - Normal

- <60 for men - Normal

Coronary artery calcium is a good indicator of how stiff the vessels are becoming: higher calcium suggests more atherosclerosis, and therefore the greater the risk of a cardiovascular event, heart attack, or stroke.

3. Aortic Aneurysm:

- Abdominal ultrasound or CT scan

5 common must do cardiology tests:

- Electrocardiogram (EKG): is a test that checks for problems with the electrical activity of your heart. An EKG shows the heart's electrical activity as line tracings on paper. The spikes and dips in the tracings are called waves. The heart is a muscular pump made up of four chambers.

- Echocardiogram (ECG): uses sound waves to produce images of the heart.

- Nuclear Exercise Stress Test (Treadmill): is a diagnostic test used to evaluate blood flow to the heart.

- Holter Monitoring: A Holter monitor is a small, wearable device that keeps track of your heart rhythm, usually worn for 24-48 hours.

- BNP: is a substance secreted from the ventricles or lower chambers of the heart in response to changes in pressure that occur when heart failure develops and worsens. The level of BNP in the blood increases when heart failure symptoms worsen, and decreases when the heart failure condition is stable. BNP is a naturally occurring signaling hormone in the blood, and is produced by human heart muscle.

A colonoscopy and endoscopy done simultaneously, throat to anus in one visit, about every 5 years after age 40 will save lives, regardless of what governments say.

One last test you may want to consider:

Mitochondria (ATP) are the secret to longevity as they provide energy and repair to our cells, which equates to longevity. Most diseases are rooted in mitochondrial dysfunction and inflammation. The GKIC (glucose ketone index calculator) test looks at your glucose to ketone ratio. Ketones must be measured by blood, not urine, and your glucose must be entered in mmol, not in milligrams per deciliter (mg/dL).

When you have a glucose ratio of 1.0 or below, you know your mitochondria are in the optimal healthy range.

Getting down to a 1.0 may be difficult. You may need to fast in order to get that low. You don't have to remain in that ultra-low zone for long periods of time, unless, you have cancer, then you'll want to maintain that level as much as possible.

"What you do today can improve all your tomorrows." – Ralph Marston

CHAPTER 53:
Statistical Reference Guide

Know the statistics. Don't be one!

Heart disease remains the most common form of death in the United States, taking the lives of more than 614,000 people annually. Cancer takes the lives of nearly 592,000 Americans annually, placing that class of disease as the second leading cause of death in the United States. Medical errors have now risen to no. 3 on the list of most common causes of death. Behind accidental deaths, stroke comes in as the no. 4 killer with 133,100 fatalities annually, while Alzheimer's disease rounds out the top 5, taking the lives of more than 93,500 Americans each year, the CDC reports.

According to the National Cancer Institute in 2016, an estimated 1,685,210 new cases of cancer will be diagnosed in the United States and 595,690 people, or 35%, will die from the disease.

National expenditures for cancer care in the United States totaled nearly $125 billion in 2010 and could reach $156 billion in 2020.

Cancer is among the leading causes of death worldwide. In 2012, there were 14 million new cases and 8.2 million cancer-related deaths worldwide. The number of new cancer cases will rise to 22 million within the next two decades.

Obama Care - Affordable Care Act:

- Newly insured 16.4 million

- Still uninsured 28.6 million

Iron causes type 2 diabetes. Many multi vitamins and supplements contain iron. Read the labels. Cooking in iron skillets can cause an increase in iron levels. Excessive red meat increases iron levels as well. The best and most altruistic way to rid your body of built up iron or hematocrit is through donating your blood. If you can't donate for any reason, you should have a medicinal phlebotomy. Ideal iron level is 60-80; 100 or over is high; 300 is toxic. Do not take a multi-vitamin supplement with iron in it. Take an iron supplement separately, only after testing your levels.

The US is 3rd in world population, (4.45% of the world's population), behind China (1.4 billion) and India (1.3 billion). The US experiences a birth every 8 seconds and a death every 12 seconds.

The most common chronic diseases cost the US economy more than $1 trillion annually and that figure threatens to be more than $6 trillion by mid-century. 80–90% of these diseases are preventable.

The US is the most medicated country in the world. We live on 1/4 of the food we eat and our doctors live on the other 3/4. We have the greatest emergency room acute care and diagnosis in the developed world, but rank near the bottom for chronic illness and treatment. We spend more per capita on medical care than any other nation on the planet and we get less in return. The US healthcare system, especially, Medicare and Medicaid, is nearly bankrupt.

The focus of a medical education since the early 20th century has been pharmacology and the circumstances in which to prescribe drugs as defined by Big Pharma, as they control most of the funding for medical schools and their research. There is no money in healing through food because you can't patent the food. So instead they treat the symptom, not the cause. Our healthcare system is on the verge of collapse under the weight of a lifetime of prescription drugs. Meanwhile, 80–90% of all modern illnesses are preventable through proper nutrition. To live longer, our #1 tool should be diet and nutrition, not the prescription pad.

75% of all deaths from coronary artery disease are from atherosclerosis or hardening of the arteries. It affects half of all Americans and claims 500,000 lives annually. It is progressive and accumulates throughout life. Studies show that 1 in 6 teenagers already have damaged arteries.

Studies show that 7 out of every 10 deaths in the US are due to preventable chronic diseases such as heart attacks, stroke, cancer, obesity, and diabetes and 80% of those deaths are preventable with proper nutrition, diet, exercise, and supplementation.

Only 7% of people who suffer a heart attack outside of a hospital can be saved. One-third of heart attack victims die without ever experiencing any symptoms. Don't wait to have the first heart attack or stroke to transform your life, as I did, or it could be too late.

- Average age for a stroke in the US is 68 for men, 72 for women.

- Heart attack average age is 65 for men, with risk steadily increasing after age 45. For women, the average age is 70.

- Under age 50, women's heart attacks are twice as likely as men's to be fatal.

- Cancer average age men - 66, women - 70.

It's clear from these statistics that the average age of men and women in the US with an incidence of heart attack, stroke, or cancer is the late 60s. This means possibly dying nearly 10 years early, when the average life expectancy in the US is 79 as of 2012.

We spend more than double any other nation on healthcare, yet the World Health Organization ranks us 37th in results, worse than Costa Rica. The US is the sickest civilized nation on earth.

Obesity started rising in America in 1971 when the USDA recommended a low-fat, high-carbohydrate diet. Today, 66% of American adults are obese; 24 million, or 8%, are diabetic; it is projected that by 2025 we will have 50 million diabetics.

In 1977 the FDA food recommendations started changing, adding vegetable oils and omega-6s, and going low-fat, high-carb, which was probably the worst health experiment in history, killing millions of people. In 1992 genetically modified crops (GMOs) were green-lighted by the FDA/USDA.

Our hunter-gatherer ancestors consumed omega-6 and omega-3 fats at a ratio of 1:1. The modern American SAD diet gives us an omega-6 to omega-3 fats ratio of 16:1, up to as high as 40:1 if you eat fast foods.

The inflammatory toxins added to our food supply after 1977, and even more so after 1992, won't make you sick in a month, but over time the toxic ingredients cause your body tissues to become inflamed, and that creates the environment for degenerative diseases to take root and grow. That's why people are so shocked when they get a cancer diagnosis or suffer a heart attack or stroke, or are told they have type 2 diabetes, or gain weight they can't lose, or suddenly develop crippling joint pains or chronic digestive problems. These diseases do not come out of the blue. Medical researchers tell us they take 10, 15, 20, even 30 and 40 years to develop and always under conditions of chronic body inflammation.

Cancer treatment is a $150 billion a year industry. Chemotherapy, radiation, and post-cancer drugs create a firestorm of inflammation that can cause new cancers and many other diseases.

In a major full-life study with lab animals fed a 33% GMO diet (to approximate average human consumption), cancer occurred in human years as early as age 10, and exploded between ages 40 and 50. Their premature death rate was 6 times higher than normal for females, and 5 times higher for males.

Over 80,000 chemicals are registered in the US, with 1,000 new chemicals introduced every year. Many of these industrialized chemicals act as obesogens: disrupting your endocrine system, causing hormonal issues, weight gain, and toxic overload.

According to the Working Group on Primary Prevention of Breast Cancer, 232 chemicals were found in newborns' placentas and in breast milk.

Stress or anxiety plagues 80% of Americans. Stress contributes to many degenerative diseases, including cardiovascular disease, heart attack, stroke, and cancer. B vitamins are particularly affected and depleted by stress, especially B1, B6, B9 (folate) and B12, resulting in increased homocysteine levels, which increases risk of heart attack and stroke.

More than 15 million Americans suffer from cardiovascular disease, the #1 killer of both men and women in the US, and some 525,000 Americans per year suffer their first heart attack. More than 100 million Americans have high cholesterol. Approximately 50% of Americans have at least one of the three major risks for cardiovascular disease: high cholesterol, high blood pressure, or a smoking habit. Every year, 600,000 Americans die from heart disease; that's 1 in every 4 deaths.

- 75 million Americans have metabolic syndrome.

- Nearly 90% of people diagnosed or living with type 2 diabetes are overweight or obese.

- 35% or 78.6 million adults, 9.3% or 29.1 million have type 2 diabetes.

- 8.1 million adults are undiagnosed.

Two-thirds of all Americans have insulin resistance, which leads to type 2 diabetes, and the number keeps growing. One-third of US adults are affected by high blood pressure, which is a risk factor for stroke and heart disease. Thirty million Americans have diabetes, which is a nutritional disease. Another 86 million are pre-diabetic. By 2020 it is estimated that 50% of all Americans will have one of the two conditions, putting over 150 million people at risk for cardiovascular disease.

The average American eats 200 pounds of meat and drinks 45 gallons of soda per year, equivalent to ingesting 150 to 170 pounds of sugar per year. The beverage industry produced 15 billion gallons of soft drinks in 2014, twice as much as 1974. That's 1.6 12-ounce cans per day for every man, woman and child. Boys aged 12-19 who consume sodas drink an average of more than two 12-ounce sodas per day, or 868 cans per year.

Many US babies are born into junk food taste and addiction. Childhood obesity has increased to over 18% of US children, quadrupling since the 1980s.

Your body only has two ways of handling toxic overload: the toxins wreak havoc in your body and cause thyroid issues, neurological damage, or cancer, or, preferably, you have enough nutrients, vitamins, and minerals in your system to fight for natural detoxification to absorb or chelate them and then eliminate or excrete these toxic contaminants.

This is another reason to supplement specifically antioxidants: vitamins A, C, E, alpha-lapoic acid, magnesium, selenium and zinc. Zinc is also an immune strengthener, which promotes tissue healing and is necessary for the functioning of many detoxifying enzymes that protect cells from pollutants and toxins. I also supplement with chlorella and chlorophyll for mercury and heavy metals detox.

In the 1950s commercial farmers discovered that feeding antibiotics to livestock, cattle, hogs, and chickens would make them grow faster and get fatter, increasing their bottom line, but these tactics came at the expense of human health. Today, 80% of antibiotics are used for veterinary purposes and not treating human diseases. America's obesity and diabetes epidemics, as well as other chronic modern diseases, started shortly thereafter.

Chances are if your neck size is over 16 ½" for a man and 16" for a woman you will snore. Good health recommends keeping neck size under those numbers. Your waist should be half your height.

Over 78 million Americans are obese and the number is growing at epidemic rates. Half of all adults, 117 million people, live with one or more chronic conditions and diseases, most of which are diet-induced and can be prevented, reversed, and cured by the food or nutrition we eat and consume. Nearly two-thirds, or 67% of Americans are overweight.

Around 10% of our life expectancy is due to genetics, 90% due to lifestyle. The human body is engineered to live to 90-100 years of age or older, free of diseases; however, the life expectancy in the US is only 78 years. Why are we leaving all those additional enjoyable years on the table?

There are 320 million people in the US; 4.02 billion prescriptions written annually equals 12.5 prescriptions per capita at a cost of $320 billion. That's $1,000 per person.

The body uses 20 amino acids from protein. The body manufacturers 11 of its own, called non-essential amino acids. The other 9 must come from foods and are called essential amino acids. Complete proteins contain all the essential amino acids and are found in all animal products such as meats, poultry, fish, dairy, and eggs.

Dairy products are the only animal-based products that contain a significant amount of carbohydrates. Most carbohydrates come from plant-based foods, fruits, vegetables, grains, and legumes.

Every day, 2,600 Americans die of some sort of cardiovascular disease – that's 1 death every 34 seconds. It is a myth that strokes only occur in older people. 25% of strokes occur in people under 65 and 10% under 45, and the numbers are rising. Strokes affect 800,000 people annually.

One-third of people who experience a TIA (transient ischemic attack) or "mini-stroke" go on to have a major stroke within a year. A stroke is like a heart attack in the brain, often referred to as a brain attack.

The biggest mistake people make when experiencing a stroke is denial, indecision, and waiting too long to get help. Time is your best ally against a stroke. Time is brain-saving and affects long-term disability or life itself. Timely hospital treatment can stop, reduce, or even reverse stroke damage.

I didn't get to the hospital for nearly 15 hours after my stroke and I paid the price, not knowing the consequences of stroke and its devastating aftermath. There is a 21st Century "magic bullet" which provides a 2-3 hour window for a clot buster, tPA, but I missed that window. Luckily, I was able to fight through the damage and paralysis and recover, but it was a lot of hard work.

In 2015, 5.3 million people will be diagnosed with Alzheimer's disease. The number is expected to grow each year as the US population ages and the number of people above age 65 continues to rise. By age 85, half of all people will have some form of Alzheimer's. If a person has diabetes they are twice as likely to develop Alzheimer's.

The global cost of dementia is now above $600 billion per year and will soar even further. The WHO predicts that by 2050 the number of people living beyond their 80th birthday will quadruple to 395 million people, and 1 in 6 will be living with dementia. An Alzheimer's forecast: 19 million Americans will be age 85 by 2050 and more than half will have some form of dementia or Alzheimer's.

- The brain is 60% fat.

- The human body is 2/3 water.

- Optimal body fat%: men 12% or less; women 20% or less.

- Optimal waist line: men 35" or less; women 30" or less.

The cost of fresh fruits and vegetables are 100-400 times higher per calorie than processed foods, refined grains, sugars, and vegetable oils.

Half of all Americans eat one or more sandwiches per day. Any way you slice it, sandwiches are your waistline's worst nightmare.

Is it a coincidence that we spend $175 billion per year on processed foods and nearly as much on prescription drugs, $160 billion per year?

- 10%, or 33 million Americans, do not have healthcare insurance.

- 40%, or 130 million people, have no dental insurance.

- 35%, or 111 million people, do not see a dentist annually.

According to the American Association of Cancer Research, 50% of the 585,720 cancer deaths in the US in 2014 were preventable. More action is urgently needed to help educate people about maintaining a healthy weight and developing and implementing preventative lifestyle strategies and eating habits.

More than 1 million Americans and 10 million worldwide are expected to be diagnosed with cancer this year, and 90–95% of these cases can be linked to environmental or lifestyle choices. Of those, 35% are a result of diet, and 70% of colorectal cancers are blamed on diet. That's nearly 500,000 cancer cases in the US and 5 million worldwide that may be preventable through diet.

Disabled life expectancy is now rising faster than total life expectancy, meaning the number of years you can expect to live in good health is decreasing. Studies show that if we can slow the aging process, we can delay the onset and progression of many fatal and disabling diseases simultaneously. We need to treat the cause, not the symptom. The underlying cause of fatal and disabling diseases is aging itself. The increase in healthy years of life from an investment of slowing aging and preventing diseases would generate enormous economic benefits.

GMOs are found in over 80% of all packaged foods in the US. GMOs deplete the nutrients in plants and crops and in turn, do the same thing to the animals and humans who consume them.

GMO seeds were created in the laboratory to grow plants that would resist diseases and pests, and thus produce bigger, more profitable crop yields. To that end, lab scientists altered the plant DNA to tolerate much larger doses of poisonous herbicides and pesticides.

It worked. Crop losses to diseases and pests were greatly decreased while yields were greatly increased. But this also increased the residues of inflammatory carcinogenic toxins in all foods with GMO ingredients. Processed foods with GMOs also contain inflammatory sugars, omega-6 vegetable fats, and chemical flavor enhancers, a surefire disease-causing combination. Consider that most foods containing GMOs also contain inflammatory sugars, omega-6 vegetable oils, and chemical additives. This is a health disaster.

Cardiovascular disease is a gradual disease, starting in childhood as early as age 5.

The average American consumes 5 pounds of additives or artificial ingredients per year. Add sugar, and the average American consumes 135 pounds per year. Remember, we only need 1 teaspoon of sugar in our system at one time to survive.

- 70% of all diseases in the US are diet-related.

- 95% of dieters gain back lost weight and more within 5 years.

- 40% of Americans consume a diet containing only 60% of proper nutritional value.

- 40% of all cancers in the US are diet-related.

The bottom line is we either get our essential nutrients, vitamins, and minerals from our food or from supplements, or we don't get them at all. The Food Industry Complex is perpetuating a culture of junk food that is literally making people sick. You can buy a hamburger for less than an apple.

Sick soil equals sick plants, sick animals and sick people. North American agricultural soil is 85% mineral depleted. We are being starved of essential minerals from our food, no matter how much of it we eat. Vitamin and mineral deficiency results in disease and disorder. Vitamins control the body's appropriation of minerals, but in the absence of minerals, vitamins do not perform their function. Lacking vitamins, the system can make some use of minerals, but without minerals from our food, vitamins are useless.

Farmers are paid on maximum yield, not maximum nutritional value. If it's not in the soil, it's not in our food. That is why it is highly recommended eating organic, grass-fed, and wild-caught and supplementing with vitamins and minerals.

Adding to the mineral deficiency in traditional agricultural soil, our air and atmosphere has more CO_2 carbon emissions than past generations. Higher carbon content in the air lowers plants' ability to extract an already-depleted soil mineral reserve out of the ground. The air further saps plants' ability to produce minerals and proteins necessary for good health. The plants instead produce higher sugar, starch, and carbohydrate content, a double whammy. This reduction in nutritional value of plants has a profound impact on human health. If the plants are sick, the animals are sick, and we are sick.

Studies show that 68% of Americans are magnesium deficient.

Today, 70% of the American diet comes from processed foods and represents 90% of food expenditure. In 1970 Americans spent $6 billion on fast food, in 2000 $110 billion, and in 2011 $168 billion. The average American eats 3 fast food burgers and 4 orders of fries a week, trading our health for convenience. Those who eat at home are the healthiest. You know what's going into the ingredients on your plate.

A 2010 report concluded that consumption of sugary drinks, sodas, and fruit juices, leads to 133,000 deaths from diabetes, 45,000 deaths from heart disease, and 6,450 deaths from cancer, worldwide.

According to the USDA, more than 96%, or 304 million Americans, are nutrient-deficient from the food supply based on the RDAs of vitamins and minerals needed to maintain minimum basic health levels. Bear in mind that the government's RDAs are minimums. Since the average American is sick, tired, and dying, you don't want to be an average American. You want to be the best you can be and that's OPTIMAL.

- 162.5 million Americans are affected either by heart disease, cancer, diabetes, or osteoporosis.

- 40 million Americans are living with osteoporosis, due to low bone mass.

- Diabetes affects 29 million Americans, the 7th leading cause of US deaths.

- 75% of heart attack victims have normal cholesterol levels.

One million Americans and more than 10 million people worldwide will be diagnosed with cancer this year and as many as 950,000 Americans and 9.5 million people worldwide could prevent this horrifying disease with a few simple dietary and lifestyle changes.

- 1.7 million new cancer cases in America each year.

- 40.8% chance of developing cancer in your lifetime.

- 13.5 million Americans are living with cancer.

- 20–25% from tobacco

- 30–35% from diet

- 15–20% from infections

- 830,000 total deaths, almost a third of which are preventable

- 25% all-cause mortality deaths

- 50% are preventable

Annual US deaths:

- 2.5 million

- 1.3 million heart disease, stroke, and cancer

- Heart disease - 611,000. (1,675 per day, 70 per hour, more than 1 per minute)

- Cancer - 585,000. (1,600 per day, 67 per hour, more than 1 per minute)

- Stroke - 130,000. (356 per day, 15 per hour, 1 every 4 minutes)

- 1,675 people die every day from heart disease; 1 in 4 deaths

- That's 3,562 per day, 148 per hour, 2.5 per minute from heart disease, stroke, and cancer

- Up to 80% preventable

You are what you eat and science is proving the validity of this powerful statement. You have true power over your own health through nutrition and a well-formulated eating strategy. But, equally as important, you are what you do with what you eat, whether you burn it as energy or store it as fat, so the proper nutritional eating strategy is of utmost importance.

In a 2009 study, researchers showed that those who took multivitamin supplements had younger DNA, which equated to living 9.8 years longer.

70 million US adults, or 1 out of every 3 adults, are affected by high blood pressure (hypertension), known as the silent killer, causing a 62% increase in deaths from 2000–2013. Another 1 in 3 US adults have pre-hypertension. High blood pressure is one of the leading causes of heart attacks and strokes. High blood pressure costs the US healthcare system $100 billion annually in healthcare services, medications and missed work days and is nearly 100% preventable and reversible through proper nutrition and exercise.

A damaged heart or brain usually means a damaged life. Stroke generally results in lifelong disability, loss of independence and quality of life, or permanent confinement to a nursing home (or cemetery).

- Smokers double their risk of stroke.

- Atrial fibrillation (or Afib) increases stroke risk 5-fold.

- High blood pressure or hypertension is the leading risk factor for stroke.

- 90% of stroke survivors experience some degree of paralysis.

An individual stroke prevention program includes annual, if not quarterly blood testing, regular monitoring of blood pressure, blood sugar, and blood fats. The blood tests must include stroke risk factors such as elevated levels of homocysteine, hsCRP, fibrinogen, oxLDL, and hormone imbalances.

Over 100,000 people die annually from FDA-approved drugs. Many are removed from the market every year. The leading cause of cancer deaths is medically induced, most notably, from chemotherapy and radiation. Studies show that 97% of all cancer patients treated with chemotherapy die within 5 years. Chemotherapy is derived from mustard gas, which was used to kill people in world wars, is a known carcinogen. It damages other vital organs in the body, causes other new cancers, and kills healthy cells. Why is the standard of care in America to give a known carcinogen to treat cancer? If it's a cure, why do 97% of people die from the treatment?

The food industry spends $1.8 billion per year marketing junk food to children.

ADHD children (2011 stats):

- 6.4 million diagnosed, ages 4–17. Avg. age - 7.

- Symptoms first appear age 3–6.

- 6.1% of US children are being treated for ADHD.

- 42% increase in last 8 years.

- 89% - affected by artificial colors.

- 71% - affected by artificial flavors.

- 71% - affected by preservatives.

- 59% - affected by MSG.

- HFCS in sodas is linked to ADHA in children.

- Gluten is a significant trigger in neurodevelopment disorders.

All found in processed foods and cereals.

Possible solutions for ADHD can be obtained thorough diet and supplementation with an anti-inflammatory nutritional diet: low in carbohydrates, but rich in healthy fats, antioxidants, phytonutrient-dense vegetables, and clean, healthy protein. Maintaining microbiome/gut health balance with probiotic and essential enzyme supplements is also important.

When was the last time you went to a doctor and he asked you what you were eating? How many times have you gone to the doctor for a cold or flu and he wrote a prescription for an antibiotic? Antibiotics kill bacteria, not viruses. Colds and flu are viral, not bacterial.

According to the *Journal of Biomedical Education* in 2015, most US medical schools (86/121, 71%) fail to provide the recommended minimum 25 hours of nutrition education. Most doctors rationalize: "If food be thy medicine, why wasn't I taught it in medical school?"

The jury has deliberated and the votes are in, if you ask me.

CHAPTER 54:
Colds & Flu

I'm not a big fan of flu shots and have never had one. Multiple studies show they provide very little, if any, protection against flu. Why introduce a virus into your body? Another government and Big Pharma misinformation program. Many flu shots are made from egg protein, dog kidney cells, Army worm (caterpillar) cells, mercury, aluminum, and other toxins and carcinogens. Do you really want this in your body? Most people don't die of the flu anyway; they die from bacterial pneumonia and a flu shot does not protect against pneumonia, let alone flu.

Research shows that during the 2012–2013 flu seasons, the flu vaccine's effectiveness was found to be just 56% across all age groups reviewed by the CDC – essentially the statistical equivalent of a coin toss. In seniors aged 65 and over, the US flu vaccines were even worse, only 9% effective.

The gold standard for independent scientific evaluation and analysis, The Cochrane Database Review, has issued five reports between 2006 and 2010, all of which obliterate the myth that flu vaccinations are "the most effective flu prevention method" available. According to the Cochrane report, with average environmental conditions, when a flu vaccine, at least marginally, matches the circulating flu virus, 100 people needed to be treated and vaccinated to avoid only 1 onset case of influenza symptoms. Unfortunately, in addition to the fact they may not be nearly as effective as advertised, flu vaccines can, and do, cause harm.

Your best bet is to increase your immune system's chances of successfully fighting off infections. Sugar inhibits healthy immune system function, leaving you vulnerable to colds and flu. Get plenty of sleep. Eat right, exercise, take a good multivitamin, at least 2,000 mg of vitamin C daily in divided doses from a whole food source, like Garden of Life brand.

Vitamin C has both antiviral and antibacterial activity as it boosts the immune system. N-acetylcysteine (NAC), which is a precursor to glutathione, is the body's preeminent antioxidant. Take 600 mg of NAC during the fall and winter. Other proven immune-enhancing supplements include zinc (30–60 mg per day, as high as 200 mg daily), vitamin D, and probiotics. D3 (cholecalciferol) is best. Test your blood for vitamin D levels and keep in the optimal range of 50–80 ng/mL; 5,000–10,000 IUs daily.

Although probiotics are best known for their effects on gastrointestinal health, these beneficial bacteria are also a boon for the immune system, as 80% of your immune system is in your digestive tract. If you get sick, temporarily increase your intake of vitamins D (50,000 IU per day for three days) and C (500 mg every two to three hours), and find a clinic that offers intravenous (IV) vitamin C, which will get into your blood stream the fastest and with most effective bioavailability.

I also add Astragalus-500 mg daily and Echinacea-400 mg daily, for 6–8 weeks in the heart of cold and flu season, but for no more than 3 months, as it can then have a reverse effect on your immune system. I take Astragalus year-round as studies have shown it supports telomere length.

Only about 20% of all influenza-like illnesses that occur every year are actually associated with influenza viruses, because many types of respiratory illnesses with flu-like symptoms can be mistaken for influenza. The other 80% of cases of suspected influenza sent to the CDC lab for analysis test negative for type A or type B influenza.

CHAPTER 55:
Epigenetics

O ur DNA is not our destiny. Your life choices are. Gene expression (epigenetics) is controlled through nutrition, which consists of what we put in our mouths, and which we control completely. Maximize your expression of ideal health. Turn off disease-promoting genes. What we eat becomes us. Make your diet speak to your genes.

Cells can change based on the environment they live in and that environment is influenced by the nutrition you do or do not feed to that environment. You are stuck with your genes or DNA, but you are not stuck with the environment in which they express themselves. Most of our health is determined by how we live our lives.

Genes play a major role in how you respond to diet and exercise. You may not lose much weight from vigorous exercise, but your genes may be programmed to be responsive to the stimulus of a carbohydrate-restrictive diet. That's why many people get frustrated and depressed because they are exercising like crazy and not dropping weight, while staying on a low-fat/high-carb diet that has been promoted since the 70s.

You have to not only change your diet, but change your way of thinking, because in most cases, it's exactly the opposite of what you have been told for decades. But it is wrong? Just look at the statistics since the 70s: increases of obesity, type 2 diabetes, heart attacks, strokes, and cancer to epidemic levels.

You cannot exercise yourself out of a bad diet. The 80/20 rule applies: 80% diet, 20% exercise. They not only complement one another, they become synergistic.

The combination of a low-carb diet with resistance training will result in better maintenance of muscle mass, strength, and body composition during weight loss.

Diet, environment, and lifestyle all affect your ability to express and influence your genes. Turn on the good, turn off the bad.

Genetics are the hardware of your computer, (body). Epigenetics are the software. Software drives the hardware. It's the brains. By eating the correct nutrition, taking the right supplements, doing the proper exercise and practicing a healthy lifestyle you will express to your genes the exact message to take control of your health and live a longer, healthier life!

"Genes load the gun, but environment pulls the trigger." – Scott Kahan, MD

CHAPTER 56:
Iatrogenics

Studies show that 251,454 annual deaths in the US in 2015 were due to medical errors and prescription drugs, as reported by the *British Medical Journal*. This ranks as the third leading cause of death behind heart attacks and cancer. Prevention is the best cure and that starts with nutrition, exercise and supplementation.

Today's healthcare is disease management.

If your doctor is unhealthy and overweight, how can he or she give good health advice?

Zero people die per year taking vitamins, minerals, and supplements. Fewer than five die annually from iron overdose or toxicity, but if those people were getting their blood tested regularly, as we recommend in this handbook, then those would drop to zero as well.

But many doctors will warn you to be careful about taking vitamins and supplements that kill no one, yet are quick to write a prescription that could kills many people. Make sense? Yes, dollars and cents.

Vitamins, minerals, antioxidants, and other supplements are not only safe, but have few, if any, side effects, are inexpensive and provide multiple health benefits. Combined with a well-designed nutritional diet and exercise, vitamins are truly the safest and healthiest substances you can ingest to reduce your risk of nearly all chronic diseases and premature death.

Modern medicine focuses on getting a specific diagnosis and prescribing specialized treatment. If someone suffers from anxiety, modern medicine focuses on making drugs for the brain. If someone has arthritis, modern medicine focuses on making drugs for the joints. This shift in medical thought since Hippocrates' day has caused a serious problem. Modern medicine is blind to the hidden epidemic behind the exploding disease statistics. It has almost completely stopped looking holistically at the entire body.

Prescription drugs kill far more people than illegal drugs. While most major causes of preventable deaths are declining, those from prescription drug use are increasing, as revealed by an analysis by the *Los Angeles Times* of recently released data from the US Centers for Disease Control and Prevention (CDC). Their analysis of 2009 death statistics showed:

For the first time ever in the US, more people were killed by drugs than motor vehicle accidents.

Drug fatalities more than doubled among teens and young adults between 2000 and 2008, and more than tripled among people aged 50 to 69.

These drug-induced fatalities are not being driven by illegal street drugs. The most commonly abused were prescription drugs like Oxycontin, Vicodin, Xanax, and Soma, which now cause more deaths than heroin and cocaine combined.

In a June 2010 report in the Journal of General Internal Medicine, study authors said records that spanned from 1976 to 2006, the most recent years available, showed that, of 62 million death certificates, almost a quarter-million deaths were coded as having occurred in a hospital setting due to medication errors.

An estimated 450,000 preventable medication-related adverse events occur in the US every year.

The costs to society of adverse drug reactions are more than $136 billion annually, greater than the total cost of cardiovascular or diabetic care.

Adverse drug reactions cause injuries or death in one out of five hospital patients, 20%.

The reason there are so many adverse drug events in the US is that so many drugs are used and prescribed and many patients receive multiple prescriptions at varying strengths, some of which may counteract each other or cause more severe reactions when combined.

There was a 36% increase in hospital admissions and a 28% increase in emergency room visits among children age five and younger who had accidentally ingested prescription medication. Emergency room visits for ingestion of prescription opioid painkillers, such as Oxycodone, increased 100 percent.

In 2009, there were nearly 4.6 million drug-related visits to US emergency rooms nationwide, with more than half due to adverse reactions to prescription medications, most of which were being taken exactly as prescribed by the doctor.

Doctors' illegible handwriting kills more than 7,000 people annually and injures more than 1.5 million.

The "war on drugs" has focused nearly exclusively on the illegal trafficking of drugs like cocaine, heroin, and marijuana, while the most powerful drug dealers of all, the pharmaceutical companies, are now allowed to grow their businesses with the US government's seal of approval.

Prescription drugs can be just as addictive as illegal drugs. In fact, in many cases there's no difference between a street drug and a prescription drug. Example, hydrocodone, a prescription opiate, is synthetic heroin. It's indistinguishable from any other heroin as far as your brain and body are concerned, so, if you're addicted to hydrocodone, you are in fact, just simply a good-old-fashioned heroin addict.

So, is this the fault of the doctor, or Big Pharma, or the US government? The US government allows Big Pharma to produce drugs that injure and kill people, while doctors prescribe them because that's what they were taught in a medical school that is funded by Big Pharma, or informed by a Big Pharma salesman at a convention, but did the doctors actually take the time to read the scientific literature? Probably not.

At the end of the day, you are your own master and your own advocate and you must take command of your own health.

There are 225,000 deaths per year from iatrogenic causes, and that constitutes the third leading cause of death in the US, following heart disease and cancer. Additional deaths by doctor, hospitals, and medications include the following:

- 12,000 unnecessary surgery

- 7,000 medication errors in hospitals

- 20,000 other errors in hospitals

- 80,000 infections in hospitals

- 106,000 non-error, negative effects of drugs

- 59 deaths due to Aspirin poisoning

- 147 deaths associated with acetaminophen-containing products

Drugs, surgery, and hospitals are rarely the answer to chronic health problems.

CHAPTER 57:
Grounding/Earthing

Grounding/Earthing is defined as placing one's bare feet on the ground, whether it be dirt, grass, sand or concrete, especially when humid or wet. The Earth is a natural source of electrons and subtle electrical fields, which are essential for proper functioning of immune systems, circulation, synchronization of biorhythms, and other physiological processes. It may be the most effective, essential, least expensive, and easiest antioxidant to attain.

The benefits include better sleep and reduced pain. They can be obtained from walking barefoot outside or sitting, working, or sleeping indoors connected to a conductive system that transfers the earth's electrons from the ground into the body.

Modern science has thoroughly documented the connection between inflammation and all chronic diseases, including the diseases of aging and the aging process. It is important to understand that inflammation is a condition that can be reduced or prevented by grounding your body to the Earth.

Studies show when you practice grounding, there's a transfer of free electrons from the Earth into your body. These free electrons are probably the most potent antioxidants known to man. These antioxidants are responsible for clinical observations from grounding studies showing beneficial changes in heart rate and blood pressure, decreased skin resistance, decreased levels of inflammation, increased immune function, faster tissue repair, and relief from muscle pain. Researchers have also discovered that grounding actually thins your blood, making your hematocrit less viscous.

This can have a profound impact on cardiovascular disease. Virtually every aspect of cardiovascular disease has been correlated with elevated blood viscosity. Studies show when you ground to the Earth, your zeta potential quickly rises, which means your red blood cells have more charge on their surface, which forces them apart from each other. This action causes your blood to thin and flow more easily and not stick or cause clotting that leads to heart attacks and strokes. Your blood pressure will also drop.

The ideal location for walking barefoot is on the beach, close to where the water and sand meet, known as "the hard sand," as sea water is a great conductor. Your body also contains mostly water, so it creates a good connection.

I practice HIIT on the beach by walking, then running, then walking, then running in 30 seconds to 1 minute intervals for approximately one hour to get the full benefits of grounding and HIIT, combined. In addition, you get the sunshine for vitamin D3 and the fresh air. You will sleep like a baby.

With a grounding unit (see Tools) make sure there is a built-in resistor.

An advisory: if you are on a blood thinner, especially Warifin/Coumadin, thyroid hormone or diabetes meds, have your blood tested as you may need to reduce or eliminate dosages.

Grounding is the battery for all planetary life.

CHAPTER 58:
MRI Technique

Relaxation, breathing rhythm, and visualization are the keys to enduring MRIs successfully, especially if you are claustrophobic.

If enduring multiple MRIs is motivation enough to not have a stroke, I don't know what is. An MRI is probably one of the most uncomfortable tests on the planet, yet one of the most sophisticated to reveal a health problem. If you are claustrophobic, an MRI is almost unbearable, unless they hit you in the head with a rubber mallet or otherwise sedate you.

I've taken several and developed a technique that will help you survive this test effortlessly. First, relax your arms to your sides or even lightly clasped on your waist, lightly close your eyes, not tightly, before you ever go into the MRI tube. You do not want to look at the inside of the tube. Start your breathing relaxed and controlled, in through your nose and out through your mouth, a nice, relaxed rhythm.

Relaxation, breathing rhythm, and visualization are the keys. Start thinking pleasant thoughts about huge open spaces, blue sky, sunshine, mountains, beach, beauty, sex, smiles, laughter, anything pleasant, other than space and time.

The more you think about the small space you are confined in and the prolonged or elapsed period of time you are confined, the more anxiety you will build up, so if you close your eyes from the beginning, you will never picture in your mind a claustrophobic, confined space. Just relax in a meditative, almost sleep-like state or trance, with visions of open spaces and pleasant thoughts in your mind and no concern for elapsed time. Simply take a nap and you will sail through this test effortlessly. Time will fly by and there will be no need for the rubber mallet.

Tools

Weight scale (Digital)

Blood pressure monitor/cuff

Blood glucose meter/monitor-tester

Blood Ketone Meter

Light relief

Spinner

Ab-roller wheel

Twister

Weight vest

George foreman grill

Coffee grinder-eggs-calcium. (Non-soy feed.)

WaterPik-Superflosser

Electric toothbrush

Steel, cast iron or ceramic skillets and cookware

Steamer

Toaster oven

Thermal belt

Grounding unit

Set up an Amazon account

Join Life Extensions

Vitamin Shoppe

Whole Foods

Trader Joe's

Sprouts Famers Market

Conclusion

"Just when the caterpillar thought the world was over, it became a butterfly." – Old Japanese Proverb

It's never too early or too late to start putting life into your years and years into your life. Prevent, don't treat. Take control of your health! Wellness keeps illness away.

To access quality of life and longevity, it requires a shift in thinking, knowledge, and taking action for new ways to age. Time is our only non-renewable resource.

Time costs nothing but is priceless. Work with it, not against it. Put time on your side. Don't count the time. Make time count.

Take preventative measures to slow aging, prevent disease and extend healthy longevity, to remain healthy and alive, so we may benefit from breakthrough scientific and biomedical advances. If you are dead, there is no advancing.

The simple take-home message is: Cut the sugar, wheat and starches, and eat real, whole foods, as many green and colorful vegetables as you want. Control your hormones, especially insulin and leptin. Don't worry about counting calories, carbs, fat, or protein as long as you only eat good food choices, not processed or manufactured foods. Exercise, take a good multi-vitamin, a probiotic, omega-3, CoQ10, and an antioxidant like R-Lipoic Acid, Astaxanthin or Glutithione. Brush and floss your teeth morning and night. And test, don't guess, and you will be well on your way.

Being informed is your first line of defense in prevention of disease. It's never too late to start. Make the rest of your life the best of your life!

We truly are what we eat. I hope this helps you on your journey to a healthy, longer, more vibrant life!

No one gets out of life alive, so you might as well live as long as you can. Birthdays are actually good for you. The more you have the longer you live!

Eliminate unnecessary pain, suffering, and death.

Don't wait for something small to get big. Prevention is the best medicine.

Life is short, don't make it shorter! Eat real, live, whole foods. Processed foods are dead and they will kill you prematurely!

Are you sick and tired of being sick and tired? Your diet is the very foundation of your health. The goal is to look and feel great for life. My health for the last few years has been my job and my life. I saved my own life and now I want to help others save theirs. That's my new purpose in life and I hope my experiences, suggestions, and tools will help you achieve your health goals and live a longer, more vibrant life.

Many Americans today are overweight, overwhelmed, and depressed. Remember the old adage: "Know thyself." One diet does not fit all. The nutritional food lists and educational information in this book will help you lose and maintain your weight, improve your health long-term and live a longer, healthier, more more energetic life. We live by our choices. We truly are what we eat!

Don't wait for something small to get big. Prevention is the best medicine. I had a choice between life and death. I chose life. I'm now training for life. I take it seriously, as should you. Don't wait for a near-death experience, life threatening or a life changing event. Prevention is the best cure. Your good health is a responsibility: your responsibility. The human body is constantly rejuvenating itself with new cells, rewiring, neuroplasticity, neurogenesis, angiogenesis, new blood vessels, pathways and circulation, so it's a continuum. Put in the work, see the results and never give up.

Don't start your day with the broken pieces of yesterday; every new day that we wake up is the first day of the rest of our lives. Take action. Start today.

I hear people say all the time: "I don't have time to be healthy." Do you have time to be dead? You can rest when you are dead.

Become your own "Diet Doctor" and you will actually be practicing medicine with the power of practical nutrition. The more educated you are the better decisions you will make about your health. "Let food be thy medicine and medicine be thy food." – Hippocrates

Eliminate all artificial ingredients, preservatives, additives, flavors and colors, along with sugar, wheat, and artificial sugars such as sucralose. Eat whole, live foods, organic vegetables and fruits. Avoid foods with a barcode or ingredients you can't pronounce or recognize. Eat wild-caught fish, such as Alaskan sockeye salmon, organic, pasture-raised chicken and eggs, grass-fed beef, bison, or lamb. Take vitamins and supplements. Exercise regularly. Maintain good oral and gut health. This will take you a long way toward having more years in your life and more life in your years – a pretty simple lifestyle change and recipe for healthy success.

A massive amount of data, research and studies conclude that lifestyle, diet, nutrition, supplementation, and exercise, these five simple behaviors, can reduce risk of heart attack, stroke and many cancers by a percentage greater than the effect of any drug on the planet. The body has a remarkable ability to respond to healthy habits, so it's never too late to develop them. The body will heal itself with proper nutrition.

The combined benefit of these five elements acting in concert will be greater than its parts. Synergy is generated by combining the individual components. One element by itself is an improvement but does not a recovery make. When you mix the components, your body and mind attain true health homeostasis, a body-mind symphony. You will feel better than ever.

Homeostasis means life in balance and internal stability. Lifestyle and nutrition are the key components. Don't be trapped by dogma, living with the results of other people's thinking and opinions. Don't let their noise drown out your own thoughts, goals, and ambitions. Have the courage to follow your inner voice, your heart, and intuition, and most of all, take action!

How many times have you thought about starting a diet, exercising, or stopping smoking without doing anything about it or lapsing back into bad lifestyle habits and choices? The psychology of change is not an easy one. What motivates you? If you don't have your health, you have nothing and prevention is the best cure.

Don't wait for a cataclysmic event or think you will get a second chance if you survive. Life is not a dress rehearsal. There are no guarantees of a second chance or life extension. Most preventative diseases are progressive, so stop or eliminate the progression before it's too late. Life is short and there are no mulligans so do it right the first time. The sooner you start the longer you will live. Birthdays are actually good for you – the more you have, the longer you will live!

"Nothing tastes as good as fit and strong feels." – *Anthony Robbins*

For many health crisis survivors, their cancer diagnosis or heart attack or stroke was a bittersweet opportunity to make lifestyle changes that ultimately saved their lives. The same habits that make for health, wellness, and longevity before an illness apply after, so why not prevent as opposed to waiting for that second chance that may not come, because your first symptom could be death. There are no guarantees in life. All you can do is maximize your chances and reduce your risks. If you practice healthy lifestyle choices and habits, you are less likely to experience life-threatening illnesses such as heart attack, stroke, or cancer, and you can maximize your outcome no matter what.

Getting healthy and helping others do the same will become your new purpose in life. We need a health revolution in this country, not just reform. Habit change, healthy lifestyle design, optimal health and wellness all start with an attitude.

"I have never let my schooling interfere with my education." – Mark Twain

Just as being in top physical shape is the best way to prevent disease or injury, being in top mental shape makes it less likely that you will engage in self-destructive behaviors and make the necessary lifestyle changes. Good nutrition, vitamins, and supplements give you clarity and peace of mind from stress, disease, and illness.

"Those who don't know history are destined to repeat it." – Edmund Burke (1729-1797), British Statesman and Philosopher

Food is information and you need the right information to program your mind and body to perform at their best. People are destroyed by lack of knowledge. Knowledge is power.

Wellness means more than mastering the facts about healthy eating. You have to turn those facts into action to promote and protect your health. Transform your relationship with food that is truly nourishing, nutritional and empowering. Degenerative diseases occur when the body's own healing capabilities are overwhelmed by a person's bad habits and lifestyle choices, including poor nutrition. Feed the body properly and it will heal itself. Let food be thy medicine and medicine be thy food.

You may not be able to turn back the clock as time marches on, but you can certainly slow down the aging process and have the best health of your life. In today's world, you must eat as if your life depends on it, because it does. Aging gracefully is what health, wellness, and longevity are all about.

Increase your food literacy. Not only do you need to know where your food comes from and who made it; you also need to know what you are eating and what was eaten by what you are eating ate. You are what you eat; you get out what you put in. "The grass is always greener on the other side of the fence," because we water it.

Make your diet work for you by identifying foods whose biochemistry make you strong and healthy and which ones make you ill and weak. Your goal is to promote health, not disease.

"Everybody dies, but not everybody lives." – Drake

Forget low-fat diets. They have been spreading incorrect information for decades now. Look around. We are fatter, sicker, and more addicted to sugar and carbs than any time in history. Sadly, we're passing these poor eating habits on to our children. This may be the first generation that lives shorter lives than their parents.

Don't live in the past, but learn from the past. Live in the present and plan for the future. We want to live longer, disease free, disability free. How do we do that? Decrease and reduce inflammation, which is the leading cause of all modern chronic diseases.

Utilize all three food categories (carbohydrates, fats, and proteins) for a healthy nutritional balance. Focus on foods that do not cause inflammation and are easily assimilated, metabolized, and excreted from your body. Choose natural whole foods that are not processed. You won't know what healthy feels like until you get there and then you won't want to let that feeling go. Your body will start craving healthy foods instead of the old crappy junk. Eating style=Lifestyle. Eat well and fall in love with yourself all over again.

Some simple rules to live by: Have gratitude and be thankful, contribute, have purpose, spirit and soul, reduce your stress, eat a healthy diet, move or exercise, and drink plenty of water.

Never stop achieving. Always reach for better, to be the best you can possibly be at any age. Live up to your full potential. Capture the belief that you can do it. Look into the mirror and envision the thinner, fitter, shapelier, healthier, new you.

Don't count calories; count chemicals and work from the inside out.

Develop a partnership with your genes through expression created by nutrition. Provide the right fuel. You're stuck with your genes, but you're not stuck with the environment in which they express themselves. You control your genetic environment by the food you ingest. What you put in your mouth controls your genetic destiny.

Age reversal happens internally. Slow the aging process by building a strong immune system. Rid the body of diet-induced inflammation and environmental toxins. Strengthen muscles and restructure arteries and veins, making them more flexible by reducing plaque and atherosclerosis. At the same time lower blood pressure, reduce weight and insulin resistance.

"I believe that health is more than merely the absence of disease, it is a total state of physical, mental, emotional, spiritual and social well-being." – Dr. Frank Lipman

People will come and go in life, but the person in the mirror will be there forever, so take good care of yourself.

Embrace the power of cellular nutrition and gene expression or epigenetics. Fetal programming, what your mother ate and ingested before pregnancy and during, plays a significant role by transmitting and amplifying adverse epigenetic markers that affect metabolism from one generation to the next, meaning that your increased weight gain and weight maintenance and metabolic health may be a multi-generational struggle. Epigenetics is genetic expression, not genetic destiny, so you're not stuck with weaknesses in your DNA. Genetic expression is modified through proper nutrition.

Food is more than calories. It is also vitamins, minerals, nutrition, fuel, energy, and life. Biochemically we are each as unique as our fingerprints.

Our instinct to survive is a powerful motivator; I know from experience. But why wait for a near-death experience or a life changing event to motivate you? It seems that's what it takes for people to change their habits, but by then it is too late for many, because the first symptoms are often fatal. Many of us believe we're bulletproof, when we're actually advancing our degenerative diseases every day.

Mindful awareness is a way of life. The only person who has control of what goes in your mouth is you. You are the one-person consumer protection agency over your food intake.

Successful aging entails avoiding chronic modern diseases that rob us of our quality of life and debilitate or kill us prematurely. A diet-induced inflammation-reducing eating strategy should be your target goal.

You will become intoxicated with the process of discovery. When you eat processed foods you are giving permission to the food industry to use your body as a science experiment and a toxic waste dump.

"The best way to predict your future is to create it." – Abraham Lincoln

Watch yourself deliver dramatic and permanent results, a profound transformation. Where you are now is a step in the journey forward. Every day above ground is a good day. Keep waking up on the right side of the dirt and be happy, thankful, and grateful.

Practice resilience. If you have a bad day, bounce back the next day, next meal, or next workout. I don't believe in cheat days. For me it's a committed eating strategy and a lifestyle program.

The essential macronutrients that we can't live without, are defined as protein, fat, and carbohydrates; however, you must tweak your thinking to protein, fat and vegetables, (fruits, seeds and nuts) as your three major dietary sources, as there is no daily requirement for carbs and carbs are the only macronutrient we can live without,

Low-carb living is synonymous with high-octane living. When it comes to your health and lifestyle, be in the "want" business, not the "need" business. Look at pleasure and happiness as essential nutrients in your life. You have to eat, so you may as well eat smart. Oh, and I found I like the sound of smart people talking.

A simple goal is to create a healthier version of yourself. However, if you mobilize a mass action, you can change the world, one person at a time; a nutritional revolution, healing the world. Health is wealth.

NO Food either supports health or it doesn't. If it doesn't, it should be considered a junk food and not fit for consumption; as in, poison. Pretty simple: label it pro-health or poison with a big red X label across the package so kids and uninformed adults will only eat at their own peril.

What made McDonald's and Coca-Cola food giants in the 20th century will make them dinosaurs in the 21st century if they don't change. Their sales are already declining, their stock prices reversing, and insiders are positioning themselves to sell. People are getting smart and voting with their wallets.

People are tired of being sick. People are hungry for a change. People want to eat real food, not Frankenfoods or scientifically engineered foods. GMOs fool with Mother Nature and you don't want fool with Mother Nature.

People want to eat foods that put them in a position of strength to defend, to grow and to heal. If instead of McDonald's we had McGreen's or McBroccoli's, wouldn't it be neat to have babies born with a silver sprout in their mouths. Baby McSpouts. Isn't there something wrong when you can go into a fast food restaurant with $5 and buy five hamburgers or only one salad for the same price?

We don't hunger for information, as we live in the information age; we hunger for correctly applied information.

Adapting a philosophy of self-experimentation can make a tremendous difference in your life. Choosing to experiment with diet, nutrition, supplementation, and exercise can help you discover a health and fitness strategy that works for you. That's what I have done since my stroke, modifying and fine-tuning to where I am today. If you follow the nutrient-rich food choices in this manual and cut out sugar, wheat, processed foods, fast foods, trans fats, and high fructose corn syrup, you will not only lose weight, but you will be healthier, happier, and live longer. As in most things in life, your mileage may vary.

Eating less and exercising more is not a good health strategy and won't work long term. That's the old calories in/calories out mentality. It is true if you have a calorie deficit, by the laws of thermodynamics, you will lose weight. But that cannot be sustained for long. What we want is a total eating or lifestyle plan and strategy that can be sustained and practiced for a lifetime. Remember, it is quality of calories, not quantity, that matters. A bad diet cannot be corrected with exercise. You cannot eat anything you want and exercise it into a desirable body style.

Timing and frequency of eating, by eating throughout the day, creates thermogenesis or calorie burning to keep your furnace revved up and your energy abundant, while keeping blood sugar and insulin low, at a slow steady burn, with a faster, hotter metabolism.

Exercise is important, along with a low-carb, moderate healthy protein and higher healthy fat. Low-carb diets only work with moderate protein and higher fat.

You have to work at living. Your health should be your job. So help yourself by taking control of your health and pass it on. It's contagious.

Empowered people will be the future revolution of healthcare. It's not an informed choice unless you have all the information.

"People often say that motivation doesn't last. Well, neither does bathing, that's why we recommend it daily." – Zig Ziglar

Details make the difference in your results. The little things, day by day, brick by brick will advance your health further than you ever thought possible. It took you years to sabotage your health in a day by day assault, now reverse that to a day by day return of taking control of your health. Pay attention to detail. The little things will add up to big things. Keep growing, learning, and evolving to be the best you that you can be.

A prevention strategy is health assurance, not health insurance. Life is short; don't make it shorter.

"It's not over 'til it's over." – Yogi Berra

Knowledge is power. Knowledge with action is super power. Knowledge is the best medicine.

It's a sign of wisdom, not weakness, to seek more knowledge through your active participation as a patient with your doctor. This handbook is intended to provoke thought and inform. Always get a second or third opinion and take charge, command, and control of your health.

My hope is this handbook will dramatically improve your health and may even save your life.

Medicine and science can be very slow, but you cannot afford to be left behind. Today, to survive and have any chance of being truly healthy, you must be informed about pollution, detoxing, genetic profiling, EMF dangers, inflammatory foods, GMOs, food labels, the gut microbiome, inflammatory markers, glucose metabolism, blood tests, vitamins, minerals, supplementation, nutrition, exercise, lifestyle, and so much more.

Becoming health literate is the only way to radically transform your health and become optimally healthy.

Becoming health literate is a matter of life and death.

YOURS!

Becoming health literate means you have the tools and the knowledge to take control of your health.

It's up to you, so start today.

This is my story, now it's time to write yours. Oh, what a beautiful life . . . life is worth living!

"True joy comes when you inspire, encourage, and guide someone else on a path that benefits him or her." – Zig Ziglar

Appendix -1-
Corporate Health & Wellness Management Strategy

"Maintaining vitality in institutions and in people is brought about by change." – Henry S. Rowen

Healthcare is a monumental issue with employers and too much is at stake to be reactive. It's time for companies to be proactive and educate employees about long-term personal health and wellness and to institute and offer programs that help more than just standard health insurance. An ounce of prevention is worth a pound of cure.

Advantages include the following:

- Show employees you care.

- Cut health insurance costs, control costs of poor health.

- Increase bottom line.

- Follow a good business strategy.

- Cultivate a healthy work environment and workforce.

- To create a culture of health takes education and passionate, persistent, persuasive leadership.

- Improve health, happiness, attitude, and productivity.

- Employee behavior improvement through knowledge.

- Research consistently shows that costs to employers from health-related lost productivity dwarfs those of health insurance costs.

Employees who exercise regularly are 15% more efficient than those who do not. That means a fit employee only needs to work 42.5 hours per week to do the same amount of work as an average employee does in 50. Combine a sound nutrition program and eating strategy with exercise and a healthy, fit, happy employee becomes a productive employee and boosts the company's bottom line.

Unhealthy employees with bad eating habits are more prone to illnesses, take more sick days, are lethargic, unmotivated, and prone to mistakes that are costly and dangerous. This negatively affects the bottom line through increased healthcare costs, absenteeism, workers' compensation, short and long-term disability claims, lost productivity, turnover, and damage to the healthcare system with a cumulative effect on the entire economy.

Being overweight and obese are the two most contributing factors to unhealthy employees. They cause most modern debilitating diseases, including heart disease, stroke, cancers, diabetes and asthma. Thirty-five percent of American adults are obese, creating medical costs of over $150 billion annually. Obese, unhealthy employees file twice as many workers' comp and illness claims, 7 times higher medical claims and 13 times more missed work days due to illness and injury.

By adopting healthy lifestyle choices, improving eating and drinking habits, and adding exercise and stress management, 75–80% of healthcare costs and diseases are preventable.

Most people have never been taught to live healthy or felt the benefits and rewards of optimal health, wellness, and longevity. Most people are dependent on the healthcare system, where symptoms are treated rather than the causes, and they are never taught simple solutions to their afflictions. People need progress-based results. Companies have a responsibility and an investment in employee wellness for profitability, lower risks, and ultimately saving lives in the community and leading by example. Healthy employees are a good business strategy. It's a health movement that makes dollars and sense.

Most people blame everything except what they are eating for the causes of their poor health, physical miseries, and premature aging. Why they are suffering is always a mystery to them. The average person does not know how horribly unclean and unsafe the inside of their bodies are, with internal poisons and clogging toxic wastes, literally rusting from the inside out. Some people even look thin on the outside, but are fat on the inside (TOFI) with visceral fat damaging their organs.

A comprehensive, strategically designed investment in employees' social, mental, and physical health pays off. Johnson & Johnson management estimates that wellness programs have cumulatively saved the company $250 million on healthcare costs over the past decade; from 2002 to 2008, the return was $2.71 for every dollar spent.

Wellness programs have often been viewed as a nice extra, not a strategic imperative. Newer evidence tells a different story. With tax incentives and grants available under recent federal healthcare legislation, US companies can use wellness programs to chip away at their enormous healthcare costs, which are only rising with an aging workforce.

A 2010 study by Harvard economists concludes that medical costs fall by about $3.27 for every dollar spent on wellness programs and absenteeism costs fall by about $2.72 for every dollar spent. Not a bad investment for increasing employee productivity, retention, health, and long-term happiness.

Japan requires employers, not employees, to bear healthcare costs through substantial corporate tax penalties if more than 25% of employees have metabolic syndrome, knowing that a future tsunami of health problems, obesity, and Alzheimer's is in their future. Japan is planning ahead. The US is not.

Appendix -2-
Measurement Conversions

Blood work/Lab tests

gm: grams

g/dL: grams per deciliter

mcg: micrograms

mg/dL: milligrams per decimeter

ng: nanograms

pg: pictograms

L: liter

dL: deciliter (1/10 of a liter = 100ml)

fl: fraction of one-millionth of a liter

mEq/L milliequivalents per liter

ml: milliliter (1/1000 of a liter)

mmol/L: millimoles per liter

U: unit

mcmol/L: millimoles per liter

mcU: microunit

IU: international unit

IU/ml: international units per milliliter

mIU/L: milli-international units per liter

mlU/ml: milli-international units per milliliter

u/ML: units per milliliter

Mm: millimeter

cmm: cells per cubic millimeter

mmHg: millimeters of mercury

mm3: cubic millimeters

mEq: milliequivalents

micron: micrometer

mM: millimoles

ng/ml: nanograms per milliliterPG/ml: one-trillionth of a gram (pictogram)

There is a difference in measurements of dry versus wet ingredients. On wet measuring instruments, generally fractions of cups, you will see a space between the top line and the lip of the cup, so you avoid spillage and don't make a mess. Spoons or fractions thereof are meant to be leveled off at the top, therefore, there is a slight difference between dry and liquid measurements and will be denoted accordingly. Variances can range from 13–26%. Measuring spoons are generally tablespoons (tbsp) and teaspoons (tsp) versus grams (gm), milligrams (mg) or micrograms (mcg) measurement conversions. Cups or fractions thereof are generally both wet and dry. (Volume versus weight are factors, as are powder versus liquid, so these are approximations.)

This is what I go by:

Abbreviations:

gm: grams

mg: milligrams

mcg: micrograms

tbsp: tablespoon

tsp: teaspoon

pt: pint

qt: quart

gal: gallon

gr: grain

lb: pound

oz: ounce   fl oz: fluid ounce

Wet and dry conversions:

5 gm = 1 tsp

3 tsp = 1 tbsp

15 gm = 1 tbsp

1 gm = 1,000 mg

1 mg = 1,000 mcg

2 pints = 1 qt

4 qts = 1 gal (128 oz)

2 qt = ½ gal (64 oz)

1- cup/glass = 8 oz

1qt = .964 liters

1 liter = 33.814 fl oz

1gr (grain) = 14.342 gm

2 tbsp = 1 oz

1/16 tsp = a dash

1/8 tsp = a pinch/ 6 drops

16 tbsp = 1 cup

1/4 tsp = 15 drops

1/2 tsp = 30 drops

1 cup = 1/2 pint

2 cups = 1 pint = 16 fl oz

4 cups = 2 pints = 32 fl oz

8 cups = ½ gallon = 64 fl oz

16 cups = 1 gallon = 128 fl oz

2 tbsp = 1 oz

16 oz = 1 lb

1/4 tsp = 1000 mg (dry)

1/2 tsp = 2000 mg (dry)

15 Almonds = 1 portion size

7 gm protein = 1 oz of cooked meat (chicken breast, turkey breast, beef.)

Appendix -3-
Tips & Tricks

We are creatures of habit, but switch things up. Make your brain think, from simple things like switching sides of the bed you sleep on, to putting your contact lenses in a different order: left eye first, then switch to right eye first. Challenge your brain to perform and think differently. Challenges both mental and physical will make your brain react in a positive manner of growth and stimulation. "You lose what you keep and you keep what you gain." Your brain is like a muscle and you must keep it exercised or, like muscle without exercise, it shrinks and atrophies. Try to learn or do something new every day, even if it's a new vocabulary word.

Zoom-Zoom. Make your own whitening toothpaste:

- 1 tbsp baking soda

- 1 tsp hydrogen peroxide 3%

While you're at it sanitize your toothbrush-soak in hydrogen peroxide or apple cider vinegar overnight to remove bacteria from your toothbrush, once per week, at least once per month.

I don't provide a bunch of recipes in this book. Instead I give you a list to replace "bad" food choices with "good" food choices in your own recipes, and the information to formulate a well-managed eating strategy. With that said, here are some tips and tricks I learned along the way:

When you're hungry many people eat carbs or processed food snacks and gain weight and experience poor health as a result. Oftentimes when you think you're hungry, it's simply that you're actually thirsty, so try drinking a big glass of filtered or alkaline water with fresh lemon squeeze, if you can tolerate and are not allergic to citrus.

If that doesn't do the trick, instead of carbohydrates, try a fat or protein. Fat has 9 calories per gram so it is more satiating than 4 calories per gram from a carb. If that doesn't work and if you're hungry at night, one of my favorite late night or before bed snacks is a piece of turkey breast (adds tryptophan for sleep) and some raw spinach leaves or kale. Add some olive oil and lemon juice to the leaves and you're all set with protein, fat and healthy carbs. Alternatively, have a half avocado with the turkey.

Options: grilled eggplant or scooped-out cucumbers, cut length-wise in place of the bun.

When I grill a grass-fed burger, instead of using a bun (fattening carbs), I grill or sauté two Portobello mushrooms in place of the bun, add lettuce, tomato, onion, mustard, just like at the burger shop, but no wheat or carbs. Very healthy, delicious and filling at the same time. Other bun replacements can be grilled eggplant or cucumbers.

In place of spaghetti or pasta, I steam spaghetti squash, drizzle it with olive oil or ghee butter, add garlic powder and pepper and make a little alla checca sauce. Add shrimp, chicken breast or grass-fed beef, turkey or chicken meatballs and voila, you're in Italy without the carbs and weight gain. It tastes good and is good for you.

Steam a dozen eggs for about 6 minutes after the water boils. They look like hard-boiled eggs, but are healthier because they are steamed rather than boiled and you have a ready breakfast or healthy snack at your fingertips in your fridge. Don't scramble eggs, as that oxidizes the cholesterol and we don't want to oxidize anything in our bodies, as we are trying to rid oxidative stress and inflammation.

Soft poached eggs are a good substitute too, but can't be stored like the ones in the shell. I soft boil eggs. Eggs are one of the true super foods on the planet, especially the yoke.

I grill chicken or turkey in advance, cut it into strips, and store it in containers in the refrigerator, so I have several pre-cooked, ready-to-eat meals. All I have to do is arrange them in a bowl or plate and I'm all set for quick meals during the day or on the run. I use powdered garlic, coarse ground pepper and blackened spice seasonings. Delicious.

I like to have a kale salad in the fridge too. I take a big glass mixing bowl, fill it with organic kale, add 2-tbsp of olive oil, 2-tbsp of lemon juice and a ¼ tsp of Himalayan pink rock salt. Toss and you have several ready-made salads and snacks.

I always have nuts like raw almonds, walnuts, pistachios, pumpkin seeds, sunflower seeds; and veggies like broccoli, carrots, tomatoes, sweet red, yellow and orange peppers, celery, raw beets, sweet potatoes and mushrooms, that I dip in hummus, tapenade, Tahiti or pesto for great healthy snacks. Try frozen seedless grapes and frozen dark cherries. Pull them out of the freezer and pop 'em into your mouth.

Buy green avocadoes when they go on sale at your local grocer or buy in bulk at Trader Joe's or Smart & Final and refrigerate them, as they will not ripen in the fridge. Take them out a night or two before use and place in a paper bag or a container and they will ripen for use overnight. If they turn brown, pitch them out, as they have oxidized and are not healthy. Avocadoes are a healthy fat and should be introduced into your diet daily. I eat them in the morning to jumpstart my fat as fuel, which gives me energy all day long.

Organic raw cacao beans can be ground in a coffee grinder and added to your green drink. The nutrients are too numerable to mention. Buy them at Whole Foods or online at Amazon.

When cooking, instead of using non-stick spray oils like olive oil, coconut oil, walnut oil or ghee, use a splash of water. Foods won't stick and no added calories. Or use a combination of a smaller amount of oil with more water. It's a great combo for steaming or sautéing your veggies.

Don't overheat oils when cooking. If it smokes, it's too hot and you've ruined the oil. It's now unhealthy to ingest the oil and has become a trans fat. I use a little water and cover the pan or skillet with a lid and steam/cook veggies on a medium/low heat. That way it's more like a sauté.

If you must eat a high glycemic carb, pair it with a low glycemic carb so you have balance or homeostasis. In addition, if you eat a lot of sugar, say a piece of cake at a birthday party, when you arrive home, eat some sauerkraut, kimchee or fermented sea vegetables to sop up that sugar and restore your gut microbiome to a net positive gut bacteria position. Little tricks like this will help you maintain your health.

Myers Cocktail for migraines and asthma:

CoQ10, magnesium, calcium, vitamin Bs and vitamin C.

Do the little things right, they'll add up to big things.

Drink water before you're thirsty.

Any exercise that makes you sweat is generally a good exercise.

Lemon water upon rising in mornings is invigorating (if you're not allergic to citrus), as is apple cider vinegar (ACV) at night, before dinner. ACV helps balance your gut flora and can make you less hungry, so you don't overeat at night. If you ever get the hiccups and can't get rid of them, take a 1-oz shot of ACV and away they go almost instantaneously, like magic.

Start your day by making your bed. This helps to clear and declutter your sleeping space and your mind. It also gets you taking action and building positive momentum toward getting results for a new day.

If you weigh yourself once a week, weigh yourself first thing Wednesday morning before eating or drinking anything. You will weigh the least on Wednesdays.

After you drink green tea, cut the leaves out of the pouch or bag, dry them, grind them up in a coffee grinder and add them to your green drink. If they were good once, wouldn't they be good again?

Hydrogen peroxide (H_2O_2) is useful in cold and flu season. One capful in each ear will lessen the length of colds and flu. Tilt head to one side, pour in one capful, wait about 5-10 minutes, drain, wipe clean, and do the same in the other ear. This seems to be effective about 80% of the time if done when symptoms first appear, but not as effective later. The key to preventing colds and flu is to keep your immune system strong and healthy. Colds are a virus, not a bacteria and should not be treated with antibiotics. Antibiotics won't work and will foul up your gut microbiome balance and damage your immune system. Take antibiotics only when absolutely necessary.

Skin tags under your arms usually means you are insulin resistant and have type 2 diabetes.

I brush my face and body skin daily in the shower. This not only helps rid the outer layer of dead skin cells and debris, improves circulation and your skin's ability to breathe, but keeps your lymphatic system flowing, giving your skin a nice tight, vibrant glow. Guys, don't be reluctant to moisturize your face daily. I then spritz it with a water spray to lock in the moisture. Try it, you'll like it and so will your skin, and you'll look younger than your years.

Rules of the road:

- Wear your seatbelt

- Use your turn signal

- Slow down

- Don't drive and text

- Don't smoke

- Eat organic

- Learn to read labels

- Exercise (Get at least 30 minutes of exercise each day.)

- Test your blood (blood does not lie.)

- Supplement

- Stop multi-tasking

- Prioritize what's important

- Recycle

- Be present with the task at hand

- Do less, be more

- Find a few minutes for quiet each day

- Fill your mind with energizing uplifting content

- Don't be judgmental

- Be inspired by the success of others and extend compassion to those who need it

- Be thankful and grateful for what you have and not be negative or want what you don't have

- Be positive

- Replace anger and hostility with empathy, compassion and understanding.

- Smile! Smiles are FREE and have the power to bring so much joy to the world.

- The best things in life are free: smiles, hugs, friends, family, love, laughter and great memories

- Life is short so spend it with those who make you laugh and make you feel loved

- Live a longer, healthier, happier life

"The secret to living well and longer is: eat half, walk double, laugh triple and love without measure." - Tibetan Proverb

Appendix -4-
Preventive Doctor Tools (head to toe)

- Chiropractor (alignment)

- Optometrist D.O. (eyes)

- Dentist D.D.S. (oral health)

- Dermatologist (skin)

- Endocrinologist (thyroid health)

- Functional medicine specialist (M.D. or D.O.)

- Neurologist (brain/nervous system)

- Cardiologist (heart)

- Endocrinologist (thyroid, pituitary, adrenal, endocrine, your master switches)

- Urologists (men)

- Gynecologist (women)

- Nutritionist (diet, most doctors know very little re: nutrition or supplementation.

- Internal medicine specialist-Internist (captain of the ship-integrative/alternative M.D.)

- Podiatrist (feet)

You want head to toe specialists. Your body is a symphony, not a rock and roll band. If one instrument is out of tune, the symphony will not hit on all notes. If your body is out of tune, you will not perform at your best. Don't settle. Test, don't guess. If you don't measure it, you can't improve it.

Be an ageless wonder . . . all you need are the right tools.

"When a man has his health he has a thousand dreams, when he is sick, he has but one." - Unknown

Appendix - 5 -
Doctor Testimonials

RANCHO LOS AMIGOS
NATIONAL REHABILITATION CENTER

**Los Angeles County
Board of Supervisors**

Hilda L. Solis
First District

Mark Ridley-Thomas
Second District

Sheila Kuehl
Third District

Don Knabe
Fourth District

Michael D. Antonovich
Fifth District

Jorge Orozco
Chief Executive Officer

Ben Ovando
Chief Operations Officer

Mindy Aisen, MD
Chief Medical Officer

Aries Limbaga, RN
Chief Nursing Officer

7601 E.Imperial Highway
Downey, CA 90242

Tel: (562) 401-7111

*To ensure access to high-
quality, patient-centered,
cost-effective health care to
Los Angeles County
residents through direct
services at DHS facilities
and through collaboration
with community and
university partners.*

September 29, 2015

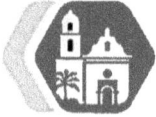

To Whom It May Concern:

As one of his inpatient rehabilitation physical therapists, I met Steve Dimon very early in his physical and mental recovery. Steve's physical transformation has been remarkable. Following an ambitious diet and exercise regime, he has been successful toward his weight loss and recovery goals. What I remember most about Steve was the moment he rejected the notion of being a victim to a very severe stroke and seized control of his recovery and became a stroke victor. His transformation continued, and he began asking questions regarding prevention, nutrition and exercise. He attended every stroke specific education session and began to seek out opportunities to practice activities that presented challenges for him, including walking. He embraced the notions of "hard-work payoff" and activity-based neuroplasticity. He also recognized the roles that repetition, practice and challenge have in the recovery of the body and brain after a stroke. I vividly remember Steve in our self directed practice gym for hours at a time practicing what he learned during formal therapy sessions. I always knew that more was better but Steve really brought that fact to life. I now find myself sharing his story to many of my current patients. His story is a testament to the power of the human spirit and the will to **live** and not just be alive.

Covey J. Lazouras PT, DPT, NCS, ATP
Physical Therapy Supervisor
Neurological Rehabilitation Service
Rancho Los Amigos National Rehabilitation Center
562-401-6239

Keck School of Medicine

University of Southern California
Department of Neurology
Nerses Sanossian, M.D.
Associate Professor, Clinical Scholar

September 17, 2015

Re: Steve Dimon

To Whom It May Concern:

Steve Dimon is under my care at the RTH Comprehensive Stroke Clinic of USC. He suffered a major stroke, which most often leads to significant, profound and prolonged disability. He was paralyzed on the entire left side of his body and had to relearn to walk again, and gain the use of his arms, hands and legs. In my experience this type of recovery from such a devastating stroke is rare and is a reflection of neurological restoration and not luck. In general response to physical, occupation and speech therapy is extremely dependent on the amount of effort put into it by the stroke survivor.

Mr. Dimon is an example of what can be achieved when someone with a devastating neurological disability from stroke commits himself to his neurological recovery and restoration program. Recovery from stroke is a full-time job and Mr. Dimon put more hours into that process than anyone else I have met, and the results are remarkable!

Sincerely,
Nerses Sanossian, M.D.
Associate Professor of Neurology (Clinical Scholar)
Director, Roxanna Todd Hodges Comprehensive Stroke Clinic
Director, Vascular Neurology Training Program

1540 Alcazar St., Suite 209
Los Angeles, California 90089
Tel. (323) 442-0049
Fax. (323) 442-7689

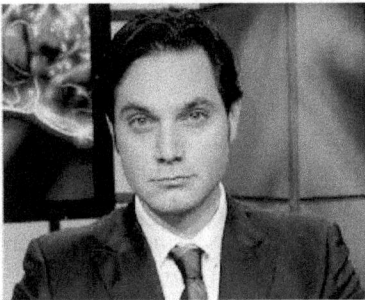

Dr. Nerses Sanossian is Assistant Professor of Neurology and Associate Director of the Neurocritical Care/Stroke Section at the University of Southern California. His research interests are in prehospital stroke therapies, vascular cognitive impairment, lipids/lipoproteins and stroke prevention in underserved populations. He was born in Beirut, Lebanon and grew up in Southern California. He is a graduate of UC San Diego, and obtained his medical degree from the Albert Einstein College of Medicine in the Bronx. He completed residency in Neurology at Albert Einstein in the Bronx, and returned to Los Angeles for fellowship in Vascular Neurology at the UCLA Stroke Center. His research in lipids and stroke has been funded by the American Heart Association and the Zumberge foundation. Dr. Sanossian serves as an investigator in clinical trials of stroke care and has published over 100 papers and abstracts. He serves as a spokesperson and grant reviewer for the American Heart Association, and as director of fellowship training in Vascular Neurology at USC. Dr. Sanossian was recently awarded the Keck School of Medicine excellence in teaching award.

October 19, 2015

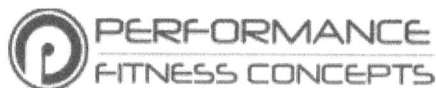

To Whom It May Concern:

Steve Dimon came to me as a patient in 2012. He was still suffering from aftershock from his stroke. He was determined to reverse his metabolic syndrome and stroke effects through nutrition, exercise and supplementation. It didn't take me long to recognize that this person was not just beyond lucky to survive his stroke, but was dedicated to an exhaustive research and study program in which he applied relevant research to not only his lifestyle, but to an everyday life that is exemplary of a person who goes beyond what I call the norm.

Steve is an example that should be followed by anyone trying to recover from illness and disease. Steve has successfully rescued a life that is worth living! I believe that a person can prevent and reverse illness and disease through nutrition and Steve is a living example of that process.

Dr. Philip Goglia, PhD, Author of *Turn Up The Heat*

2800 28th St., Suite 130
Santa Monica, CA 90405
310.392.4080
e: philip@pfcnutrition.com

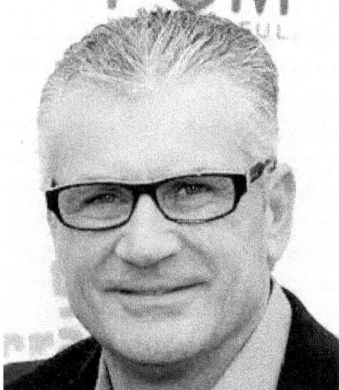

Dr. Philip Goglia is the founder of Performance Fitness Concepts, one of the most elite performance nutrition and rejuvenative health and wellness clinics in the United States. He has been a certified nutritionist for over 30 years and has been recognized as the recipient for the 2009 and 2010, 2011, 2012 and 2013 Best of Santa Monica Award in the Dietician category by the US Commerce Association. Most recently he was awarded the 2013 "Deborah Constance Children's Inspiration" award for his commitment to health and wellness mentoring at the inner city charitable foundation "A Place Called Home."

Dr. Goglia holds a PhD in Nutritional Science, and is a graduate of Duke University, The American College of Sports Medicine and the National Academy of Sports Medicine. Additionally, he serves as the official nutritionist for Gold's Gym International, exclusive nutritional consultant for the Amgen/UBS Masters Cycling Team, Lux, Team Helen's and Velo Club LaGrange. He is a board member for Visions and 449 Recovery Centers, a spokesperson for TriFit Athletic Center, Glaceau Corporation, makers of Vitaminwater and Smartwater, Nozins, Bonk Breaker nutritional bars, and Sharkies nutritional energy chews. Bestselling author: 'Turn Up the Heat – Unlock the Fat Burning Power of Your Metabolism.'

Harrington Media, Inc.

October 7, 2015

To Whom It May Concern:

I met Steve Dimon less than two years after he suffered a massive stroke in the course of writing a book about successful survivors of stroke. Steve was in remarkable shape when we first met, and remains so, because of the continuous effort he puts into his recovery. Steve decided very early on, while in a rehabilitation center, that his life after stroke was "all on him."

He has worked at gaining and maintaining his health, employing to the fullest extent, both traditional and alternative medical practices. He went from paralysis to a state of exceptional health and wellness by going far beyond the work expected in rehab.

Although Steve thinks his recovery was not miraculous, it is very rare. Steve's life after stroke is a stellar example of the astonishing healing power of our bodies, stretching the idea of neuroplasticity to its furthest borders. Steve is now an advocate for a healthy lifestyle, willing to use his own story as a teaching tool.

Few of us are capable of doing what Steve has been able to accomplish, but we can learn from his example and sample his hard-earned knowledge.

Maureen Harrington
President
Harrington Media, Inc.

925 North Sweetzer Avenue
Suite Number Three
West Hollywood, CA 90069

323 654 4413 (office)
310 567 8288 (cell)

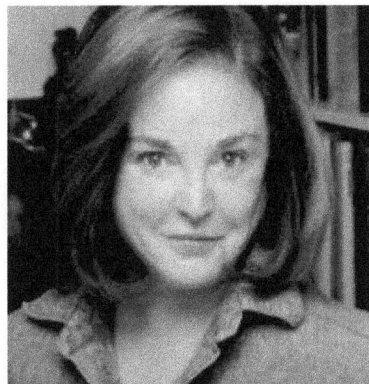

October 12, 2015

To Whom It May Concern:

I would start by saying that Steve Dimon is an extraordinary guy. That means that he is a guy just like all of us who decided to step into the "extra" of who he really is. We all have this "extra" and we know it. The question we have to ask ourselves is "Are we willing to be all that we came here to be and to express our gifts and talents and be that "extraordinary" person who we really are?" Steve's journey to wholeness began when he answered that question with a resounding "YES".

When Steve came to me, he was in shock. How could this happen to him? His life force was low. His vitality diminished. I began by giving him a constitutional remedy to stimulate that life force and he changed fairly quickly from being a victim to deciding to be a hero. With the help of Feldenkrais, he eventually began to run and the rest is history. When I asked Steve if he thought he could run he said "No" and I said "Run". He ran a short distance that day and he ran a football field within 2 weeks only to move on to a boot camp. He had made a decision to be his true self and he has lived that life ever since.

When Steve initially came to me, he asked if I thought he could heal completely and I said "Yes". He asked me how he would know when he was healed and I told him that would be when he knew this was all a blessing. Indeed, today we realize this was a blessing and the new blessing is the inspiration that Steve is on the planet. It has been my honor to work with such an extraordinary individual.

Deborah McMahon
Homeopath and Guild Certified Feldenkrais Practitioner
12812 Stanwood Dr.
Los Angeles, CA 90066
310.306.5479
e: hugdoctor@gmail.com

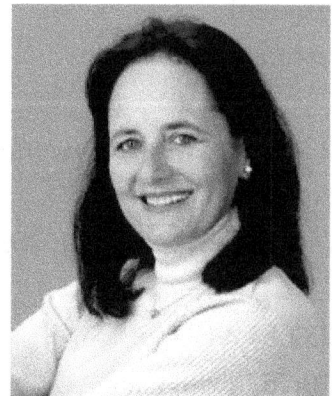

October 22, 2015

To Whom It May Concern:

Steve Dimon is a patient of mine that I have been seeing for 10 years, since 2005.

Steve came to me after his stroke in 2012, complaining of lost vision in his left eye suffered from his stroke, as he had been tested in the hospital during his stroke rehab and it was determined that he had lost 50% of the vision in his left eye from collateral stroke damage.

We changed his contact prescription accordingly into a mono-vision format.

Steve returned to me a year later for a re-exam and check-up and to my surprise his eyes had improved to the point where he had regained 40% of what he had lost from the stroke. We just thought it was probably a healing of the damage done. However, on his next year's exam, his eyes had improved again, now we became curious about this pattern of improvement, but we gave it another year.

In February of 2015, Steve came in for his annual exam and after examining his eyes, I was amazed at the results! Steve's myopia had improved 2 full diopters, improved his corneal hydration, an increase in BEST corrected vision and resolved chronic Blepharitis and MGD, massive improvements, literally off the charts! This is not only very unusual to observe in a man in his 60's to improve his vision, as it's more common for vision to deteriorate and become more problematic with age, but in Steve's case as a stroke survivor with collateral damage, to improve his vision this dramatically is not only rare, but I can only attribute this to his determination, dedication and discipline, with his self-designed-diet-nutritional program, exercise regime and supplementation program.

Steve's positive progression has been a wonderment to observe and his self-designed programs to recovery are a true testament to not only what hard work, determination, dedication and discipline can accomplish, but that nutrition, exercise and supplementation can reverse and prevent disease and Steve is living proof!

Dr. Bita Shokouh, O.D.

Beverly Hills Optometry
210 South Robertson Blvd.
Beverly Hills, CA 90211
310.623.4848
e: bitash@yahoo.com

Dr. Shokouh graduated from University Of California, Los Angeles (UCLA) with distinction, Summa Cum Laude, and completed her doctorate degree at Southern California School of Optometry. She returned back to UCLA where she is currently associate physician at the Jules Stein Eye Institute. She is currently involved in several studies at UCLA on Age-Related Macular degeneration and Diabetic Retinopathy. Dr. Shokouh's achievements include but not limited to being the Chairman of Education and the past President of California Optometric Society.

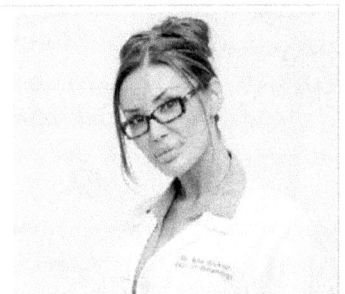

MICHAEL A. BUSH, M.D.
MARK G. BAMBERGER, M.D.
ASHKAN L. NARAGHI, M.D.

INTERNAL MEDICINE
ENDOCRINOLOGY & DIABETES CARE
PULMONARY & CRITICAL CARE MEDICINE

8920 WILSHIRE BOULEVARD, SUITE 635
BEVERLY HILLS, CALIFORNIA 90211
PHONE (310) 652-3870
FAX (310) 652-4317

November 20, 2015

Re: Steve Dimon Testimonial

To whom it may concern,

Steve Dimon has been under my care since March of 2015. Prior to our initial visit, I thoroughly reviewed Mr. Dimon's medical records and must say that I was shocked when he walked through the door, Steve has turned back the clock! Immediately after his stroke, very few expected Steve to ever walk again, talk properly, or even be able to eat again. Despite this and after nearly two months in the hospital, Steve made a complete recovery and is now a model of good health. With his robust physique, many often doubt that he is actually 67 years old. He has an immaculate biophysical profile and is a model patient. As a physician, to me Steve demonstrates that anything is possible and that people control their own destinies. Moreover, he demonstrates the importance of bio feedback in the treatment of most metabolic disorders.

Sincerely,

_____
Ashkan Naraghi, M.D.

8920 MEDICAL ASSOCIATES, INC.
A MEDICAL CORPORATION

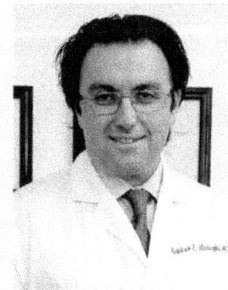

To whom it may concern,

I have known Steve Dimon as a neighbor and then, over the past three years, as someone that I know on a completely different level. I have come to know Steve as a survivor, someone I admire for his amazing perseverance and his ability to focus all of his energy into shaping his amazing recovery from an ischemic stroke.

As a Gerontologist, I work with occupational therapists, physical therapists, nutritionists and medical practitioners, such as physicians and nurses. All of this is aimed at understanding aging processes, including the physical, mental and social components of healthy aging. Steve Dimon's experience as a stroke survivor is unique and complex. He has battled back from a debilitating event that might have been, at best, a partial disability, to eliminate all apparent physical symptoms of what he experienced just three years ago. Upon seeing what seems to be a miraculous recovery, one must ask, "How is this possible?" To find the root cause of this recovery, one must look at his dynamic approach to physical and occupational therapy and his diet and exercise regimen. In the last three years, he has been a man on a mission – possessed with the idea of demonstrating that one does not have to give in to the notion that, after suffering a major stroke, one must accept the unalterable prospects of disability and a life of emotional scars. He was determined not to accommodations and adaptations of mental and physical functioning limitations, that many professionals said were inevitable, but to overcome them.

Steve's recovery of his mental and physical functioning, while not unheard of, is truly remarkable in the sense that, by adopting a rigorous diet and exercise plan, he has completely turned his life around and become a model of fitness and mental acumen. He has written a book that recounts his experiences as a stroke survivor and his resolve to surpass his previous levels of mental and physical functioning.

I respect his overcoming all obstacles and his boldly asserting that he is a concrete example of how hard work and determination can help all of us overcome, seemingly, impossible odds.

George Shannon MSG, PhD
Assistant Professor
USC Davis School of Gerontology
3715 McClintock Ave. # 231
Los Angeles, CA 90089

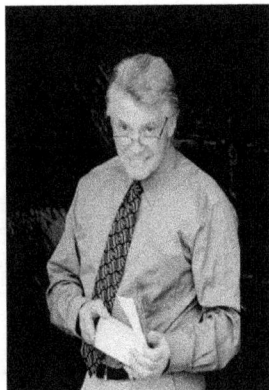

University of Southern California
Andrus Gerontology Center, Los Angeles, California 90089-0191 • Tel: 213 740 5156 • Fax: 213 740 0792 • www.usc.edu/gero

Dr. George Shannon has a Master's and a PhD from the Leonard Davis School of Gerontology at the University of Southern California (USC). He is an active member of Phi Kappa Phi, the All-University National Honor Society and Sigma Phi Omega, the National Gerontology Academic Honor Society. In 2006, he completed a postdoctoral fellowship at the VA Greater Los Angeles Center of Excellence leading the Quality of Life (QoL) section of the Minimum Data Set Evaluation Project as part of a multidisciplinary team of investigators from the VA, the RAND Corporation, the University of California at Los Angeles (UCLA), and Harvard University. Dr. Shannon currently (2010) teaches classes in Program Evaluation, Social Policy and Aging, Economics and Aging, and Society and Adult Development at the Leonard Davis School of Gerontology at the University of Southern California.

Glossary

AA/EPA: omega score. arachidonic acid (omega-6) vs. eicosapentaenoic acid (omega-3). The higher the AA/EPA ratio, the greater the likelihood you will develop a chronic disease in the future. The lower the ratio, the less likely. Detects inflammation at the cellular level. 4:1 or less for optimal cardiovascular health.

Acidic: pH versus alkaline. The body is generally alkaline - 7.2–7.3 pH range. Sugar is acidic. Cancer feeds on acid and sugar.

Acute: health conditions are sharp, severe, and sudden in onset. Chronic condition by contrast is a long-developing health syndrome that may last a life time.

ADD: Attention Deficit Disorder.

ADHD: Attention Deficit Hyperactivity Disorder.

Adrenal Gland: the adrenal glands are endocrine glands that produce a variety of hormones that are vital to life. We have two of them and they are located just above kidneys in the middle of the lower back area. They are not symmetrical. The right adrenal gland is triangular. The left is half-moon shaped. They are 2.5 inches long and 1 inch wide and yellowish in color. The adrenal glands are important to controlling stress and kidney function.

Aerobic: relating to or denoting physical exercise that is intended to improve the efficiency of the body's cardiovascular system in absorbing and transporting oxygen. Physical fitness.

AGE: Advanced Glycation End Products. Advanced glycation end products (AGEs) are proteins or lipids that become glycated as a result of exposure to sugars. Damage from AGEs have been associated with aging and in the development or deterioration to many degenerative diseases, such as diabetes, atherosclerosis, cardiovascular disease, chronic renal failure, and Alzheimer's disease.

A-FIB, (AF): Atrial Fibrillation. An irregular (arrhythmia), often rapid heart rate that cause poor blood flow or clots leading to heart attack or stroke. Quivering heart.

A-Flutter, (AFL): Atrial flutter is a rapid but organized rhythm (tachycardia) in the top chamber of the heart (either from the right or left atrium). It's a type of abnormal heart rate, or arrhythmia. It occurs when the upper chambers of your heart beat too fast. When the chambers in the top of your heart (atria) beat faster than the bottom ones (ventricles), it complicates your heart rhythm. Can accompany A-FIB.

ALA: alpha-linolenic acid. Plant source omega-3, as opposed to EPA/DHA.

ALA: Alpha Lopic Acid, a powerful antioxidant. R-Lipoic is the best supplement to consume.

Alkaline: a pH value greater than 7.0. Ideal is 7.30–7.45.

Alternative medicine or alternative doctor: any of a range of medical therapies that are not regarded as orthodox by the medical profession, such as herbalism, homeopathy, chiropractic, naturopathy, Ayurveda or acupuncture. Complementary medicine is different from alternative medicine. Whereas complementary medicine is used together with conventional medicine, alternative medicine is used in place of conventional medicine.

All-cause mortality: all deaths that occur in a population, regardless of the cause. Also a measurement in clinical trials and used as an indicator of safety or hazard of an intervention, treatment or drug.

Allergen: a substance that causes an allergic reaction. A type of antigen that produces an abnormally vigorous immune response in which the immune system fights off a perceived threat that would otherwise be harmless to the body. Such reactions are called allergies.

Allopathic: drugs and surgery versus diet and lifestyle or naturopathic therapies.

Alzheimer's disease: Alzheimer's is a type of dementia that causes problems with memory, thinking and behavior. Symptoms usually develop slowly and get worse over time, becoming severe enough to interfere with daily tasks. Alzheimer's is the most common form of dementia, a general term for memory loss and other intellectual abilities. Alzheimer's disease accounts for 60 to 80 percent of all dementia cases. Alzheimer's disease is now being referred to as type 3 diabetes.

AMA: American Medical Association.

AMD: Age-related Macular Degeneration.

Amylopectin A: modern wheat is high in amylopectin A, a carbohydrate that is converted to glucose faster than just about any other carbohydrate.

Anaerobic: anaerobic exercise is an intense physical exercise. It is used by athletes in non-endurance sports to promote strength, speed, and power and by body builders to build muscle mass. Muscle energy systems trained using anaerobic exercise develop differently compared to aerobic exercise, leading to greater performance in short duration, high intensity activities, which last from mere seconds to up to about 2 minutes. Any activity lasting longer than about two minutes has a large aerobic metabolic component.

Anecdotal: Not necessarily true or reliable. Based on personal experiences rather than scientific facts or research. It is, however, within the scope of scientific method for claims regarding particular instances, for example the use of case studies in medicine.

Angiogenesis: literally means creation of new blood vessels. The word "angio" means blood vessels while "genesis" means creation. The physiological process through which new blood vessels form from pre-existing vessels.

Antibiotic: a drug used to treat bacterial infections. Antibiotics have no effect on viral infections. An antibiotic medicine (such as penicillin or its derivatives) that inhibits the growth of or destroys microorganisms, (bacteria). Kills both good a bad gut microbiome, as opposed to a probiotic, which feeds good gut bacteria.

Antioxidants: A substance that reduces damage due to oxygen, such as that caused by free radicals. A supplement that inhibits oxidation, such as vitamin C or E that removes potentially damaging oxidizing agents in a living organism.

Antioxidants may possibly reduce the risks of cancer. Antioxidants clearly slow the progression of age-related macular degeneration.

Anti-inflammatory: a medication used to reduce inflammation. Chronic inflammation is the root cause of many serious illnesses - including heart disease, many cancers, and Alzheimer's disease. Inflammation can occur on the surface of the body as local redness, heat, swelling, or pain. It is the cornerstone of the body's healing response, bringing more nourishment and more immune activity to a site of injury or infection. But when inflammation persists or serves no purpose, it damages the body and causes illness. Stress, lack of exercise, genetic predisposition, and exposure to toxins like secondhand tobacco smoke and other pollutants can all contribute to chronic inflammation, but dietary choices play a major role as well.

Apoptosis: The death of cells that occurs as a normal and programmed sequence of events that leads to the elimination of cells without releasing harmful substances into the body. Apoptosis plays a crucial role in developing and maintaining the health of the body by eliminating and excreting old cells, unnecessary cells, and unhealthy cells. The human body replaces nearly one million cells per second. When apoptosis does not work correctly, cells that should be eliminated may persist and become immortal, leading to diseases such as cancer and leukemia.

Artificial sweeteners: a sugar substitute is a food additive that provides a sweet taste like that of sugar while containing significantly less food energy and are noncaloric. Some sugar substitutes are natural and some are synthetic or man-made. Those that are not natural are in general called artificial sweeteners. Sucralose (Splenda), aspartame (Nutrasweet) and Equal are some of the more common artificial sweeteners and are found in sodas, "sugar free" or "fat-free" products and processed foods. Should be avoided at all costs.

Astaxanthin: an antioxidant nutrient found in some foods. As a supplement, heralded as one of the most powerful antioxidants ever discovered.

Atherosclerosis: Atherosclerosis is a general term for the narrowing, thickening, and hardening of the arteries, a condition in which plaque builds up inside the arteries. Plaque is made of cholesterol, fatty substances, cellular waste products, calcium and fibrin (a clotting material in the blood). Part of the metabolic syndrome and coupled with high blood pressure (hypertension), can lead to heart attacks and strokes. Starts at 10 years of age andprogrsses from teens into 20's and 30's.

ATP: Adenosine Triphosphate is a source of energy for physiological reactions in every cell and muscle. It stores and supplies the cell with energy needed for sustaining life. Energy is the currency of life.

Autoimmune disease: The body's immune system protects you from disease and infection. But if you have an autoimmune disease, your immune system attacks healthy cells in your body by mistake. Autoimmune diseases can affect many parts of the body. There are more than 80 types of autoimmune diseases. First symptoms are fatigue, muscle aches, and a low fever. A classic sign of an autoimmune disease is inflammation, which causes redness, heat, pain, and swelling.

Autophagy: (both neuronal and systemic) the process by which cells clean themselves up and recycle all the unnecessary and dysfunctional junk that's been accumulating within.

Bacteria: Bacteria are microscopic living organisms, usually one-celled, that can be found everywhere. They can be dangerous, such as when they cause infection, or beneficial, as in the process of fermentation such as in wine.

Big Agra: Big Agra equals big agricultural corporations. Resulting in Big Food and phony FDA nutritional science leaving a world sick, fat, and dying.

Big Food: Big Food companies are manufacturers of processed and junk foods that are unhealthy contributing to many chronic diseases including metabolic syndrome, obesity, diabetes, heart disease, strokes, cancer, and Alzheimer's. Junk and processed food consumption is a much more serious problem today than Big Tobacco ever was.

Big Pharma: pharmaceutical companies collectively as a sector of industry.

The term Big Pharma is used to refer collectively to the global pharmaceutical industry. The term has come to connote a demonized form of the pharmaceutical industry. Conspiracy theorists use the term Big Pharma as shorthand for an abstract entity comprised of corporations, regulators, politicians, and often doctors, all with a finger in the trillion-dollar prescription pharmaceutical pie and mostly as a derogatory term.

Bioavailability: refers to the proportion of a nutritional supplement that enters the bloodstream and is able to have a biological effect in your body.

Biochemistry: the branch of science concerned with the chemical and physicochemical processes that occur within living organisms. Biochemical processes. Physiological chemistry. The chemical composition of a particular living system or biological substance.

Bioflavinoids: or flavonoids, are a large class of antioxidants. They are compounds abundant in the pulp and rinds of citrus fruits and other foods containing vitamin C. Bioflavonoids have been used in alternative medicine as an aid to enhance the action of vitamin C, to support blood circulation, as an antioxidant, and to treat allergies, viruses, or arthritis and other inflammatory conditions.

BMI: Body Mass Index. A measurement of appropriate weight, calculated by dividing weight (in kilograms) by height (in meters) squared.

Blue Zones: a concept used to identify a demographic and/or geographic area of the world where people live measurably longer lives. Blue Zones get their name from the blue pen used to draw circles on a map locating the areas.

Body fat: Adipose tissue (body fat) is a normal constituent of the human body that serves the important function of storing energy as fat for metabolic demands. Obesity is an excess of body fat frequently resulting in a significant impairment to health.

BPA: Bisphenol A is an organic synthetic compound, an estrogenic endocrine-disrupting chemical and is an unhealthy product in plastic containers, including water bottles, water pipes and lining of cans. It can increase cancer risk, thyroid dysfunction, oxidative stress, and heart disease to name a few. Avoid. If a plastic water bottle has been left in the car and has been heated up from warm weather or the sun, throw it away and do not drink, as the heated plastic may have leached into the water and is unsafe to drink.

BPH: Benign Prostatic Hyperplasia (BPH) is an enlarged prostate gland.

BPS: Bisphenol-S. In #7 plastics, typically labeled as BPA-free, but is not any better than BPA and is still an endocrine disruptor causing thyroid problems.

Cage-Free: cage-free hens are able to walk, spread their wings and lay their eggs in nests, vital natural behaviors denied to hens confined in cages. Most cage-free hens live in very large flocks that can consist of many thousands of hens who never go outside.

Calorie: The amount of heat required at a pressure of one atmosphere to raise the temperature of one kilogram of water one degree Celsius. An amount of food having an energy producing value of one calorie. Food labels refer to calories per serving.

Cancer: Cancer is a group of diseases involving abnormal cell growth with the potential to invade or spread to other parts of the body. (Metastasis). Not all tumors are cancerous; benign tumors do not spread to other parts of the body. Over 100 cancers affect humans. Most cancers form a lump called a tumor or a growth. But not all lumps are cancer. Lumps that are not cancer are called benign (be-NINE). Lumps that are cancer are called malignant (muh-LIG-nunt). There are some cancers, like leukemia (cancer of the blood), that don't form tumors. They grow in the blood cells or other cells of the body.

Candida: a fungal infection, a genus of yeast, commonly part of the normal flora of the mouth, skin, intestinal tract and vagina, but can cause a variety of diseases. Most infections are associated with predisposing factors, particularly immune suppression.

Catechins: Phytonutrients are natural, biologically active compounds found in plants. One class of phytochemicals, called flavonoids, contains over 4,000 compounds with many potential health benefits. Catechins are a type of flavonoid found in certain foods; several forms exist, but all are potent antioxidants that may help protect you from potentially damaging chemicals called free radicals.

Causation: the action of causing something. The relationship between cause and effect. Correlation does not imply causation.

CDC: center for disease control (Atlanta)

Cell: The cell is the basic structural, functional, and biological unit of all known living organisms. A cell is the smallest unit of life that can replicate independently and cells are often called the "building blocks of life." The study of cells is called cell biology.

Centenarians: a person who is 100 or more years old.

CHD: Coronary Heart Disease

Chelate: "chelate" comes from the Greek word that means "claw." That's what chelation does. The toxins are "clawed" painlessly out of your body.

Chelation is useful in applications such as providing nutritional supplements, in chelation therapy to remove toxic metals from the body. Detoxify.

Chloride: Chloride is found in many chemicals and other substances in the body. It's one of the components of salt used in cooking and in some foods. Chloride is needed to keep the proper balance of body fluids. It is an essential part of digestive stomach juices.

Chlorine: chlorine is a strong oxidizing agent. Probably the most known form of a chlorine compound is sodium chloride, otherwise known as table salt. Chlorine is found in many municipal water supplies in toxic levels.

Chlorophyll: green pigment found in algae and plants. Chlorophyll is an extremely important biochemical molecule, extremely critical in photosynthesis, which allows plants to absorb energy from light (sunshine). Drink 30 drops daily in 8oz of water to insure the transfer of light and energy from plants to your body.

Chronic: a chronic condition is a human health condition or disease that is persistent or otherwise long-lasting in its effects or a disease that comes with time or constantly recurring. The term chronic is often applied when the course of the disease lasts for more than three months, but can last a lifetime.

Circuit training: Circuit training is a form of body conditioning or resistance training using high-intensity programs. It targets strength building and muscular endurance. An exercise "circuit" is one completion of all prescribed exercises in the program. It targets strength building and muscular endurance. Traditionally, the time between exercises in circuit training is short, often with rapid movement to the next exercise station or machine.

Cohort study: are a type of medical research used to investigate the causes of disease, establishing links between risk factors and health outcomes. Cohort studies are usually forward-looking, that is, they are "prospective" studies, or planned in advance and carried out over a future period of time.

Collagen: the most abundant protein in the human body and is the substance that holds the whole body together. It is found in the bones, muscles, skin and tendons, where it forms a scaffold to provide strength and structure.

Contraindications: A contraindication is a specific situation in which a drug, procedure, or surgery should not be used because it may be harmful to the person. There are two types of contraindications: Relative contraindication means that caution should be used when two drugs or procedures are used together. (It is acceptable to do so if the benefits outweigh the risk.) Absolute contraindication means that event or substance could cause a life-threatening situation. A procedure or medicine that falls under this category should be avoided.

CoQ10: Coenzyme Q10 (CoQ10) is an antioxidant that is made in the human body. CoQ10 is needed for basic cell function. CoQ10 levels decrease with age and may be low in people with cancer, certain genetic disorders, diabetes, heart conditions, HIV/AIDS, muscular dystrophies, and Parkinson's disease. Some prescription drugs may also lower CoQ10 levels. Supplementation of COQ10 is recommended for anyone from heart attack victims, people suffering from fibromyalgia, Parkinson's disease or taking statins. If you are on statins, you must supplement with CoQ10.

Correlation: a statistical measure that indicates the extent to which two or more variables fluctuate together. A positive correlation indicates the extent to which those variables increase or decrease in parallel; a negative correlation indicates the extent to which one variable increases as the other decreases. Correlation vs. causation.

CRISPR: powerful gene-editing tool.

CT scan: an x-ray using computerized axial tomography.

CVD: Cardiovascular Disease.

CVE: Cardiovascular Event. Heart attack or stroke.

Detox: a process or period of time in which one abstains from or rids the body of toxic or unhealthy substances; detoxification.

Diabesity: diabetes and obesity together.

Diabetes: a metabolic disease in which the body's inability to produce any or enough insulin causes elevated levels of glucose in the blood.

Diet: Greek origin, a way of life or living. Food and lifestyle habits. A dietary regimen.

Dimon's 4Ds: Desire, Discipline, Determination, Dedication.

DNA: deoxyribonucleic acid, a self-replicating material present in nearly all living organisms as the main constituent of chromosomes and is the carrier of genetic information.

Double blind: In most cases, double-blind experiments are regarded to achieve a higher standard of scientific rigor than single-blind or non-blind experiments. In these double-blind experiments, neither the participants nor the researchers know which participants belong to the control group or the test group.

Drug Interactions: a drug interaction is a situation in which a substance, usually another drug, affects the activity of a drug when both are administered together. (See contraindications)

DV: daily value. The Percent Daily Value on the Nutrition Facts label is a guide to the nutrients in one serving of food. For example, if the label lists 15 percent for calcium, it means that one serving provides 15 percent of the calcium you need each day. The Percent Daily Values are based on a 2,000-calorie diet for healthy adults.

Dysbiosis: is a term for a microbial imbalance or maladaptation on or inside the body. Dysbiosis is most commonly reported as a condition in the digestive tract, particularly during small intestinal bacterial overgrowth (SIBO) or small intestinal fungal overgrowth (SIFO). Dysbiosis is when the bad guys take over. It essentially means there is an imbalance of microbial colonies in your gut.

Enteric coated: a coating that prevents absorption until a pill reaches the small intestine.

EDS: electron deficiency syndrome. Electron deficiency syndrome is a groundbreaking discovery that could be an underlying factor in all chronic disease. Industrialization and the introduction of plastics and other synthetic materials have disconnected us from the earth, which has interrupted the natural flow of electrons between the earth and you. Electron deficiency has been shown to increase inflammation in your body which is a major risk factor for disease. (See grounding.)

Electrolytes: are the body's essential ions, of which the most important are sodium, potassium, magnesium, chloride, and calcium.

EMF: Electromotive force, (denoted and measured in volt), is the voltage developed by any source of electrical energy such as a battery or dynamo. It is generally defined as the electrical potential for a source in a circuit. Includes cell phones and other wireless electronics. Possible carcinogenic radiation long-term.

Endocrine system: one of nine systems in the human body, consisting of endocrine glands that secrete hormones. There are eight glands: the pineal, pituitary, thyroid, thymus, adrenals, pancreas, ovaries (female), testes (male). (Now you know why you need an Endocrinologist specialist for optimal health.)

Endothelium: lining various organs and cavities of the body, especially the blood vessels, heart, and lymphatic vessels.

Energy: the strength and vitality required for sustained physical or mental activity.

Entropy: lack of order or predictability; gradual decline into disorder.

Enzymes: a substance produced by living organism that act as a catalyst to bring about a specific biochemical reaction. In probiotic supplements, a major help in digesting the foods we eat. Enzymes are secreted by the various parts of our digestive system and help to break down food components such as proteins, carbohydrates, and fats. There are three types of enzymes in the human body: metabolic enzymes, which run our bodies; digestive enzymes, which digest our food; and food enzymes from raw foods, which start the food digestion process. There are approximately 50,000 enzymes in the human body.

EPA: created in 1970, the EPA is an agency of the United States federal government whose mission is to protect human and environmental health.

Epidemiological (studies): Epidemiology is the study and analysis of the patterns, causes, and effects of health and disease conditions in defined populations. It is the cornerstone of public health, and shapes policy decisions and evidence-based practice by identifying risk factors for disease and targets for preventive healthcare. The branch of medical science that deals with the incidence, distribution, and possible control of diseases and other factors relating to health in the population.

Epigenetics: gene expression. Modification of gene expression rather than alteration of the genetic code itself (DNA). Ability to up-regulate or down-regulate gene expression according to disease risk through environmental or nutritional control.

Essential: absolutely necessary for survival. The body cannot synthesize on its own, or not to an adequate amount and must be provided by the diet. These nutrients are necessary for the body to function properly. The six essential nutrients include carbohydrates, protein, fat, vitamins, minerals, and water.

Estradiol: an estrogenic hormone.

Estrogen: any of a group of steroid hormones that promote the development and maintenance of female characteristics of the body.

Familial hypercholesterolemia is a genetic disorder characterized by high cholesterol levels, specifically very high levels of low-density lipoprotein LDL, in the blood and early cardiovascular disease with total cholesterol levels of 350–550 mg/dL and above. Cholesterol levels can be drastically higher in people with FH who are also obese.

F.A.S.T.: stroke acronym, used as a mnemonic to help detect and enhance responsiveness to stroke victim needs. The acronym stands for: (F) Facial drooping, (A) Arm weakness, (S) Speech difficulties and (T)Time to call 911.

FDA: Food and Drug Administration. The Food and Drug Administration is a federal agency of the United States Department of Health and Human Services, one of the United States federal executive departments.

Fermented: Fermentation is the process in which a substance breaks down into a simpler substance. Microorganisms like yeast and bacteria usually play a role in the fermentation process, creating beer, wine, bread, kimchi, yogurt and other foods. Fermentation comes from the Latin word fermentare, meaning "to leaven."

Fiber: the parts of fruits and vegetables that cannot be digested. Fiber is of vital importance to digestion; it helps the body move food through the digestive tract, reduces serum cholesterol, and contributes to disease protection. Also known as bulk or roughage. Contributes to regularity of bowel movements.

Fish Oil: Fish oil is oil derived from the tissues of oily fish. Fish oils contain the omega-3 fatty acids eicosapentaenoic acid (EPA) and docosahexaenoic acid (DHA), precursors of certain eicosanoids that are known to reduce inflammation in the body, and have other health benefits.

Fluoride: The addition of fluorides to the public water supply to reduce the incidence of tooth decay is now considered by many to be a toxin and should be filtered from tap water. Fluoride-free toothpastes are also gaining popularity.

Folic Acid: folic acid is a part of the B complex of vitamins. It is vital for red blood cells and for many other cells in the body. The form of folic acid occurring. naturally in food is called "folate," found especially in leafy green vegetables, liver, and kidney.

Frankenfoods: genetically modified foods, (GMOs), science project foods. AKA processed or manufactured foods.

Free radicals: an especially reactive atom or group of atoms that has one or more unpaired electrons; especially one that is produced in the body by natural biological processes or introduced from outside, as in tobacco smoke, toxins, or pollutants that damage cells, proteins, and DNA by altering their chemical structure. Overall, free radicals have been implicated in the pathogenesis of at least 50 diseases. Since free radicals contain an unpaired electron, they are unstable and reach out and capture electrons from other substances in order to neutralize themselves. Oxygen is a highly reactive atom that is capable of becoming part of potentially damaging molecules commonly called "free radicals." (See antioxidants.)

Free-Range: chickens that are not caged 24/7 and allowed to "range" in a small area outside of their confinement facility, but not pasture-raised.

Fructose: sugar in fruit, but not HFCS.

FTC: Federal Trade Commission. Considered by many, an attempt by the US government to regulate vitamins, minerals, and herbal supplements that the FDA cannot.

Fuel: food (nutrition) is fuel for the body.

Functional Doctor: Functional medicine is an integrative, science-based healthcare approach that treats illness and promotes wellness by focusing on the bio-chemically unique aspects of each patient, and then individually tailoring interventions to restore physiological, psychological, and structural balance. Doctors who focus on the cause, not the treatment. Alternative doctor, homeopath.

GE: genetically engineered AKA (GMO).

Genetic/Heredity: (DNA) the passing on of characteristics (genes) from one generation to the next.

GERD: Gastroesophageal Reflux Disease. Acid Reflux

Ghrelin: hunger hormone. Stimulates appetite. Secreted primarily by stomach cells and the pancreas.

GI health: in medicine, commonly used abbreviation for gastrointestinal, referring collectively to the stomach and the small and large intestine.

Glucagon: a hormone released by the pancreas that stimulates the liver to convert stored glycogen into glucose when blood glucose levels fall too low.

Glucogenesis: the conversion of glucose to glycogen for storage in the liver. A metabolic process of making glucose, a necessary body fuel, from non-carbohydrate sources such as protein (amino acids), lactate from the muscles and the glycerol component of fatty acids. Blood glucose levels must be maintained within a narrow range for optimal health.

Glutathione: Glutathione (GSH) is the most abundant intracellular thiol (sulfur-containing compound) and low molecular weight tripeptide found in living cells and is composed of the amino acids glycine, cysteine, and glutamate. Thiols such as glutathione, alpha lipoic acid, and NAC are powerful sulfur-bearing antioxidants. The antioxidant functions of Glutathione include recycling vitamins E and C and serving as a critical nucleophilic scavenger, to support antioxidation of all types of tissues. Glutathione regulates detoxification and is a naturally occurring antioxidant. As one of the primary protective molecules in the body it is found, inside and outside of all cells, in all tissues and body fluids. GSH is most highly concentrated in the liver, spleen, kidney, eye-lens, erythrocytes, and leukocytes. Higher glutathione status and/or dietary intakes have been correlated with cardiovascular, oral, and eye health, as well as increased vitality with aging. The best food sources of glutathione are fresh fruits and vegetables and newly prepared meats.

Gluten: a substance present in cereal grains, especially wheat, barley and rye, that is responsible for the elastic texture of dough. The word "gluten" comes from the Latin word for glue, and its adhesive properties hold bread and cake together. A mixture of two proteins, it causes illness in people with celiac disease and may be attributable to other autoimmune diseases, such as thyroid disease, rheumatoid arthritis, Lupus, diabetes, and multiple sclerosis. Gluten-free is recommended for optimal health.

Glycemic index: (GI) The glycemic index (GI) is a number associated with a particular type of food that indicates the food's effect on a person's blood glucose or blood sugar level.

Glycemic load: (GL) The glycemic load (GL) of food is a number that estimates how much the food will raise a person's blood glucose level after eating it. One unit of glycemic load approximates the effect of consuming one gram of glucose.

Glycogeneisis: the formation of glucose, especially by the liver, from non-carbohydrate sources, such as amino acids, (protein.)

Glyphosate: the most common weed killer in the US. It is more toxic than DDT, is a likely carcinogen and contributes to mitochondrial dysfunction. The major danger of genetically engineered foods may be related to the increased use of glyphosate, the active ingredient in Monsanto's weed killer Roundup. It can accumulate and persist in the soil for years, where it kills off beneficial microbes and stimulates virulence of pathogens. Organically-farmed fields are not doused with glyphosate. Another reason why organic foods are less prone to be contaminated with disease-causing pathogens than conventionally-grown foods. When applied to crops, glyphosate becomes systemic throughout the plant. It cannot be washed off. Once you eat this crop, the glyphosate ends up in your gut where it can decimate your beneficial bacteria. This can wreak havoc on your health as 80 percent of your immune system resides in your gut and is dependent on a healthy ratio of good to bad bacteria. Glyphosate is a strong chelator, so it immobilizes critical micronutrients, rendering them unavailable to the plant. As a result, the nutritional efficiency of genetically engineered (GE) plants is profoundly compromised. Micronutrients such as iron, manganese and zinc can be reduced by as much as 80-90 percent in GE plants. Glyphosate is in 80% of the food supply in the US. Eat organic!

GMO: genetically modified organism. A genetically modified organism (GMO) is any organism whose genetic material has been altered using genetic engineering techniques (i.e., a genetically engineered organism). GMOs are the source of medicines and genetically modified foods and are widely used in scientific research and to produce other goods.

Grain: a small, hard seed, especially the seed of a food plant such as wheat, corn, rye, oats, rice, or millet. Cereals and breads are made from grains. There is no such thing as a healthy grain.

Grain-fed: conventional, grain-fed beef animals are moved to confined feedlots after 6-12 months where they are fed grains, usually made from GMO soy or corn. This diet, along with drugs and hormones, helps them grow faster. They are also administered antibiotics to build immunity against unsanitary living conditions.

Grain-finished: most beef animals have probably eaten grass at some point in their lives, but the important thing is that they're "finished", or fattened on grain, for the 90–180 days before slaughter.

GRAS: generally regarded as safe.

Grass-fed and grass-finished: the USDA recently created a very narrow legal definition of "grass-fed," which focuses primarily on what beef animals eat. Food Alliance believes that when consumers choose grass-fed meat, they want products that come from animals raised on pasture with a forage-based diet. Grass-fed and grass-finished means a 100% grass-fed, pastured, foraged and grazed diet. (Best red-meat choice).

Green drink: green drink, sometimes referred to as juicing, is a mixture of green vegetables and often other nutrients, sometimes fruits, mixed together, usually using a juicer or a blender. Drinking a "Green" drink and the resulting juice, provides health benefits from the nutrients contained therein.

Grounding/Earthing: In electrical engineering, ground or earth is the reference point in an electrical circuit from which voltages are measured, a common return path for electric current, or a direct physical connection to the Earth.

HBOT: hyperbaric oxygen therapy

HDL: HDL cholesterol is the well-behaved or "good cholesterol." This friendly scavenger cruises the bloodstream. As it does, it removes harmful bad cholesterol (LDL) from where it doesn't belong. High HDL levels reduce the risk for heart disease. Low levels increase the risk.

Healthy fat: The body uses fat as a fuel source, and fat is the major storage form of energy in the body. Fat also has many other important functions in the body, and a higher amount is needed in the diet for good health. Good fats include fish, (wild caught sockeye salmon, anchovies and sardines, olive oil, nuts, avocados, seeds, high-quality raw dairy and grass-fed beef, pasture-raised chickens, turkey, lamb and bison. (See ketogenic)

Healthy protein: moderate. Proteins are organic compounds made up of building blocks called amino acids. There are about 20 common amino acids. Nine of them are considered essential because the body cannot make them, and therefore, they must be supplied by eating a healthy, nutritional diet.

Hemoglobin A1c: a test that measures the level of hemoglobin A1c in the blood as a means of determining the average blood sugar concentrations for the preceding two to three months.

Herbicides: herbicide(s), also commonly known as weed killers. Chemical substances that is toxic. Used to control and destroy unwanted plants and vegetation.

HFCS: high fructose corn syrup (sugar). Sugar is addictive and virtually all processed foods are loaded with HFCS. Of the 600,000 items in the US food supply, 80 percent of them contain HFCS and other added sugars. And the reason for this is because the food industry knows that when they add sugar, you eat and buy more of it, becoming fat, and sick and eventually dying.

Hidden sugar (HSC): sugar that doesn't appear on processed and manufactured food labels. Carbohydrates minus fiber = net carbs minus listed sugars = hidden sugars in grams. (Not the same as added sugar)

High Blood Pressure (Hypertension): High blood pressure is a common condition in which the long-term force of the blood against your artery walls is high enough that it may eventually cause health problems, such as heart disease or stroke.

HIIT: high intensity interval training.

Holistic: characterized by the treatment of the whole person, taking into account mental and social factors, rather than just the physical symptoms of a disease.

Homeopathy: is a medical science developed by Dr. Samuel Hahnemann (1755-1843), a German physician. It is based on the principle that any substance which can produce symptoms in a healthy person can cure similar symptoms in a sick person.

Homeostasis: Harmony, balance.

Hormones: most common: A chemical substance produced in the body that controls and regulates the activity of certain cells or organs. Many hormones are secreted by special glands, such as the thyroid gland, adrenals and pituitary.

Testosterone, estrogen, insulin, leptin, ghrelin, adrenaline, cortisol and thyroid hormones, T/3, and T/4 are all common hormones.

Hormesis: a biological phenomenon whereby a beneficial hormetic effect of improved health, stress tolerance, growth or longevity, results from exposure to resistance training type stress or an illness. Organisms like to maintain homeostasis, stability, and balance, and hormesis is ultimately about the push to maintain homeostasis in a changing environment. If the environment changes from stress due to illness or from resistance training-type stress, the body must become stronger and healthier in order to maintain homeostasis to better handle the situation the next time it occurs. Induce an adaptive response that improves your health in the long term. You get stronger, faster, healthier, and more resistant to disease than you were before. Think of hormesis as your body's hedging its bet and super-compensating just to be safe as it adapts to the imposed stresses.

HRT: Hormone Replacement Therapy. Any form of hormone therapy wherein the patient, in the course of medical treatment, receives hormones, either to supplement a lack of naturally occurring hormones, or to substitute other hormones for naturally occurring hormones. Most common, testosterone (men), estrogen (women).

hsCRP: High-sensitivity C-reactive protein (CRP) is a protein that the liver makes when there is inflammation in the body. It's also known as a marker of inflammation, and can be measured with an hsCRP (high-sensitivity C-reactive protein) blood test.

Homogenized: Homogenization is an entirely separate process that occurs after pasteurization. The purpose of homogenization is to break down fat molecules in milk so that they resist separation. Without homogenization, fat molecules in milk will rise to the top and form a layer of cream.

Hyperthyroid: overactivity of the thyroid gland, resulting in a rapid heartbeat and an increased rate of metabolism.

Hippocampus: part of a system that directs many bodily functions: the limbic system. This system is located in the brain's medial temporal lobe, near the center of the brain. The hippocampus is involved in the storage of long-term memory, which includes all past knowledge and experiences.

Hypothalamus: a region of the forebrain below the thalamus that coordinates both the autonomic nervous system and the activity of the pituitary, controlling body temperature, thirst, hunger, emotional activity, pleasure, sexual satisfaction, aggressive behavior, anger and sleep. The hypothalamus is one of the busiest parts of the brain and is mainly concerned with homeostasis.

Hypothyroid: Hypothyroidism (underactive thyroid) is a condition in which your thyroid gland doesn't produce enough of a thyroid hormone called thyroxine (T4). Thyroid hormones (T3 andT4) regulate the way in which the body uses energy metabolism and without enough thyroxine many of the body's functions slow or shut down. (Triiodothyronine-T3). There is a connection between AFib (atrial fibrillation) or Aflutter and thyroid function: Your thyroid gland is located over your voice box in your throat. It controls your metabolic rate, which means it is responsible for how fast or slow all of the processes in your body occur. If your thyroid is healthy, the processes occur at an optimal rate. Studies have shown that thyroid function has an impact on the frequency with which atrial fibrillation occurs. This is important information if you have a diagnosis of either AFib or thyroid disease. (Hypothyroidism is the most common.)

Iatrogenic: resulting from the activity of a healthcare provider or institution; said of any adverse condition in a patient resulting from treatment by a physician, nurse, or allied health professional. An iatrogenic disorder is a condition that is caused by medical personnel or procedures. Mis-prescribed pharmaceuticals. Unreadable prescription hand writing. Death by doctor. Now, the third leading cause of death in the US behind heart attack and cancer.

IGF-1: Insulin Growth Factor. Overall health and longevity marker. In several organisms such as fruit flies, worms, and rats, IGF-I is involved in the control of lifespan. When it comes to cancer, it's probably better to err on having IGF-1 lower than higher (but not too low). When it comes to autoimmunity or chronic inflammation, it's probably better to err on having IGF-1 higher than lower (but not too high). Mid-range is optimal. In the Physicians' Health Study, an IGF-1 over 185 raised the risk for prostate cancer. Higher IGF-1 (approximately 190) is associated with increased risk of cardiovascular events and deaths from cancer in elderly men (average age 75.) IGF-1 levels are about 70–80 or lower are associated with an overall increased risk of disease or death.

IF: Intermittent Fasting. A term for various diets that cycle between a period of fasting and non-fasting. Intermittent fasting can be used along with calorie restriction for weight loss.

Immune system: The immune system is the body's defense against infectious organisms and other invaders. Through a series of steps called the immune response, the immune system attacks organisms and substances that invade the body's system that causes disease. Studies show that 80% of the body's immune system is located in the digestive system. A healthy gut is paramount for maintaining optimal health. A healthy immune system is the number one defense against all disease.

Inflammation: inflammation (acute) is a protective tissue response to injury or destruction of tissues, which serves to destroy, dilute, or wall off both the injurious agent and the injured tissues. The classical signs of acute inflammation are pain, heat, redness, swelling and loss of function. Chronic or diet-induced inflammation is the cause of most all diseases, including heart attacks, cancers, strokes, diabetes, and obesity. Intracellular, inflammatory stress pathways are activated in both obesity and infection. Diabesity causes inflammation, insulin and leptin resistance, which impair glucose metabolism.

Insulin: a hormone produced in the pancreas that regulates the amount of glucose in the blood. The lack of insulin causes Type I diabetes. Too much causes insulin resistance, obesity and Type 2 diabetes. You must control insulin for optimal health.

Insulin resistance: the diminished ability of cells to respond to the action of insulin, a hormone secreted by the pancreas that regulates the level of glucose (sugar) in the body and the transporting of glucose from the bloodstream into muscle and other tissues. Insulin resistance typically develops with obesity and ushers in the onset of type 2 diabetes.

Integrative medicine: (IM) a healing-oriented medicine that takes account of the whole person, including all aspects of lifestyle. It emphasizes the therapeutic relationship between practitioner and patient, is informed by evidence, and makes use of all appropriate therapies.

Iron: The health benefits of iron mainly include carrying life-giving oxygen to human blood cells. About two-thirds of the bodily iron is found in hemoglobin. Other health benefits of iron are iron deficiency anemia, anemia of chronic disease. High-iron foods include clams, liver, sunflower seeds, nuts, beef, lamb, beans, whole grains, dark leafy greens (spinach), dark chocolate, and tofu. Do not take a multi-vitamin with iron in it. Test, don't guess.

Irradiated: food exposed to radiation for longer shelf life. Better appearance to motivate buying. Increases store profits. Bad for health. Avoid.

Irritable bowel syndrome: (IBS) is a gastrointestinal disorder, a common disorder that affects the large intestine (colon) and is characterized by the presence of a cluster of symptoms and signs in adults or children that includes cramping, abdominal pain, bloating (distention), gas, altered bowel habits, diarrhea and constipation and food intolerance. IBS is a "functional" disorder, meaning changes in the functioning of the digestive system that results in the collection of symptoms referred to as IBS. It is a problem with the movement (motility) rather than any damage to the tissues of the digestive system. IBS is a chronic condition that you will need to manage long term.

Isometric training: Isometric exercise or isometrics are a type of strength training in which the joint angle and muscle length do not change during contraction.

Ketogenic: The ketogenic diet is a high-fat, adequate-protein, low-carbohydrate diet that forces the body to burn fats rather than carbohydrates.

Laser Lithotripsy: Laser lithotripsy is a surgical procedure to remove stones from the urinary tract (i.e., kidney, ureter, bladder, or urethra).

LDL: LDL cholesterol: Low-density lipoprotein cholesterol, commonly referred to as "bad" cholesterol. Elevated LDL levels are associated with an increased risk of heart disease. Lipoproteins, which are combinations of fats (lipids) and proteins, are the form in which lipids are transported in the blood. (LDL cholesterol may not be a problem unless it's oxidized. To prevent oxidation, avoid environmental toxins, sugar, processed foods, HFCS and preservatives.)

Leaky gut syndrome: essentially, leaky gut syndrome ("intestinal hyperpermeability") is condition that happens as a consequence of intestinal tight junction malfunction. These "tight junctions" are the gateway between your intestines and what is allowed to pass into the blood stream. Possible cause of leaky gut is increased intestinal permeability or intestinal hyperpermeability. That could happen when tight junctions in the gut, which control what passes through the lining of the small intestine, don't work properly. That could let substances leak into the bloodstream.

Leptin: Leptin (from Greek, "thin"), the "satiety hormone," a protein produced by fatty tissue that regulates fat storage in the body. It's called the "obesity hormone" or "fat hormone." When scientists discovered leptin in 1994, excitement arose about its potential as a blockbuster weight loss treatment, however, to lose weight, you must have control of both leptin and insulin through what you put in your mouth.

Leukocytes: white blood cells.

Lifestyle: a healthy lifestyle leaves you fit, energetic and at reduced risk for disease, based on the choices you make about your daily habits. Good nutrition, daily exercise, stress reduction, adequate sleep and love are the foundations for optimal health. Managing stress instead of smoking or drinking alcohol, reduces inflammation on your body at the hormonal level. For longevity and a more joyous life, develop a lifestyle plan that attains your goals and live to be fit. Fit is fab. Wellness eliminates disease.

Lifestyle change: a way of living. Lifestyle changes are defined as changes that alter various lifestyle-related behaviors such as diet, physical activity, sexual behavior, smoking, alcohol consumption, substance use, and other behaviors. A more fit physique, along with enhanced self-esteem, can lead to greater self-confidence and motivation to live a healthier lifestyle.

Lipids: (fats) Lipids include fatty acids, oils, waxes, sterols, and triglycerides. They are a source of stored energy and are a component of cell membranes.

Longevity: long life. Over 85. (See centenarians and supercentenarians.)

Low-carb: low in carbohydrates.

Ls and Bs: Most probiotic supplements include Lactobacillus and Bifidobacterium, two of the most well-studied strains. Products with more bacterial strains sometimes called "mega probiotics" aren't necessarily better, but some experts say it's a good idea to switch supplement brands every month or two. Buy a minimum of 13 billion live cultures.

Macronutrients: there are only three macronutrients that the human body needs in order to function properly: carbohydrates, protein, and fats.

Micronutrients: a substance, such as a vitamin or mineral, that is essential in minute amounts for the proper growth and metabolism of a living organism. May be more important to optimal health than macronutrients.

MCT: medium chain triglycerides. (coconut oil.)

Mercury: Mercury has toxic effects on the nervous, digestive, and immune systems, and on lungs, kidneys, skin and eyes. People are mainly exposed to methylmercury, an organic compound, when they eat fish and shellfish. Eating wild-caught Alaskan sockeye salmon, anchovies, and sardines nearly eliminates methylmercury from your body. Detoxifying with chlorella and charcoal supplements will help eliminate too. Dental amalgam is a mixture of metals, consisting of liquid (elemental) mercury and a powdered alloy composed of silver, tin, and copper. Approximately 50% of dental amalgam is elemental mercury by weight. Safely remove (SMART) from a biological dentist and replace with white resin-composite filings, porcelain crowns or implants. Dental amalgam is a mixture of metals, consisting of liquid (elemental) mercury and a powdered alloy composed of silver, tin, and copper. Approximately 50% of dental amalgam is elemental mercury by weight.

Methylation: is an epigenetic mechanism used by cells to control gene expression. A number of mechanisms exist to control gene expression, but DNA methylation is a commonly used epigenetic signaling tool that can fix genes in the "off" position. Simply put, it's a biochemical process in your body that occurs during numerous other bodily processes that help you stay healthy. Methylation is a truly multi-tasking marvel that, for example, helps deter toxins, as well as helps your body repair damaged DNA and reduce inflammation. When functioning optimally methylation assures that the less desirable genes are switched off, while the preferred genes are switched on. Methylation modifies the function of DNA. Cancer and birth defects are two examples where this process has gone awry.

Methylmercury: any of various toxic compounds of mercury containing the complex

CH_3Hg. Often occur as pollutants which accumulate in living organisms (as fish) especially in higher levels of a food chain. Seafood is essentially the sole source of methylmercury. However, it's a major source of mercury, and it can be problematic if you eat a lot of seafood. The type of seafood you eat plays a big role. At the top of the food chain, shark, should be eliminated from your diet. Toward the bottom of the food chain you have sardines and anchovies, with nearly 1,000 times less mercury. Wild salmon like Coho and Sockeye can be a hundred-plus-fold lower level than high-level shark, tuna, and swordfish. Depending on the fish, there could be a thousand-fold difference between the mercury levels. Put that into perspective, that's like eating 1,000 pounds of anchovies versus 1 pound of shark. So if you eat fish on a regular basis, it's really important to look for species known to be lowest in mercury. (Inorganic mercury.)

Meta-analysis: conceptually, a meta-analysis uses a statistical approach to combine the results from multiple studies in an effort to increase power (over individual studies), improve estimates of the size of the effect and/or to resolve uncertainty when reports disagree. A subset of systematic reviews; a method for systematically combining pertinent qualitative and quantitative study data from several selected studies to develop a single conclusion that has greater statistical power.

Metabolism: The chemical processes that occur within a living organism in order to maintain life.

Metabolic syndrome: Metabolic syndrome is a clustering of several of the following medical conditions: abdominal (central) obesity, elevated blood pressure, elevated fasting plasma glucose (type 2 diabetes), high serum triglycerides, low high-density lipoprotein (HDL) levels, atherosclerosis, high cholesterol, oxidative stress and diet-induced inflammation. Metabolic syndrome is associated with the risk of developing cardiovascular disease, heart attacks, and strokes.

Methylmercury: Seafood is essentially the sole source of methylmercury. However, it's a major source of mercury, and it can be problematic if you eat a lot of seafood. The type of seafood you eat plays a big role. At the top of the food chain, shark should be eliminated from your diet. Toward the bottom of the food chain you have sardines and anchovies, with nearly 1,000 times less mercury. Wild salmon like coho and sockeye can be a hundred-plus-fold lower level than high-level shark, tuna, and swordfish. Depending on the fish, there could be a thousand-fold difference between the mercury levels. Put that into perspective, that's like eating 1,000 pounds of anchovies versus 1 pound of shark. So if you eat fish on a regular basis, it's really important to look for species known to be lowest in mercury. (Inorganic mercury.)

Microbiome: The word microbiome is defined as the collection of microbes or microorganisms that inhabit an environment (the gut and digestive system), hence gutbiome, creating a sort of "mini-ecosystem." Our human microbiome is made up of communities of symbiotic, commensal and pathogenic bacteria, along with fungi and viruses, all of which call our bodies home. Gut microbiota, AKA gut flora, is the name given today to the microbe population living in our intestine. Our gut microbiota contains tens of trillions of microorganisms, including at least 1000 different species of known bacteria with more than 3 million genes (150 times more than human genes).

Micronutrients: May be more important to optimal health than macronutrients.

Minerals: Minerals and vitamins are vital for maintaining bone health and preventing bone diseases such as osteoporosis. The hard matrix of bones is composed of minerals such as calcium, magnesium and phosphorus. Minerals the human body requires for optimal health include calcium, chloride, magnesium, phosphorus, potassium, sodium and sulfur. Different minerals have different benefits, so no mineral can be termed as more beneficial or less beneficial than another. All minerals, even trace ones, are critical for the proper functioning of the body.

Mitochondria: a spherical or elongated organelle in the cytoplasm of nearly all eukaryotic cells, containing genetic material and many enzymes important for cell metabolism, including those responsible for the conversion of food to usable energy (ATP). Healthy mitochondria are at the core of staying healthy and preventing disease.

Moderate: being within reasonable limits; not excessive or extreme. Moderate protein.

Moderation: Eating foods in moderation is a key to maintaining a healthy diet. The word moderation describes a middle ground often in either behavior or political opinions. Drink alcohol in moderation.

Morbidly obese: Morbid obesity is a medical term describing an individual who is considered morbidly obese if he or she is 100 pounds over his/her ideal body weight, has a BMI of 40 or more (man), or 35 or more (woman), and is experiencing obesity-related health conditions, such as high blood pressure, diabetes or metabolic syndrome.

MRI: Magnetic resonance imaging (MRI) is a technique that uses a magnetic field and radio waves to create detailed images of the organs and tissues within your body. Most MRI machines are large, tube-shaped magnets. When you lie inside an MRI machine, the magnetic field temporarily realigns hydrogen atoms in your body.

MSG: flavor enhancer commonly added to Chinese food, canned vegetables, soups, and processed meats. The Food and Drug Administration (FDA) has classified MSG as a food ingredient that's "generally recognized as safe" (GRAS), but its use remains controversial.

Avoid.

Mycotoxins: A mycotoxin (from Greek (mykes, mukos) "fungus" and (toxikon) "poison") is a toxic secondary metabolite produced by organisms of the fungus kingdom, commonly known as molds. The term 'mycotoxin' is usually reserved for the toxic chemical products produced by fungi that readily colonize crops.

The microfungi are capable of causing disease and death in humans and livestock. Mycotoxins occur in food and have great significance in the health of humans and animals. Since they are produced by fungi, mycotoxins are associated with diseased or moldy crops, grains and seeds.

Naturopathic: Naturopathic medicine is a distinct primary healthcare profession, emphasizing prevention, treatment, and optimal health through the use of therapeutic methods and substances that encourage individuals' inherent self-healing process.

Neurogenesis: (birth of neurons) is the process by which neurons are generated from neural stem cells and progenitor cells. It plays a central role in neural development. Neutrogenesis is most active during prenatal development and is responsible for populating the growing brain with neurons.

Neuroplasticity: the brain's ability to reorganize itself by forming new neural connections throughout life. Neuroplasticity allows the neurons (nerve cells) in the brain to compensate for injury and disease, such as after a stroke (brain attack), and to adjust their activities in response to new situations or to changes in their environment.

Neurotransmission: Latin: transmissio "passage, crossing" from transmittere "send, let through", also called synaptic transmission, is the process by which signaling molecules called neurotransmitters are released by a neuron (the presynaptic neuron), and bind to and activate the receptors of another neuron in brain communication. Electrical impulse. Brain wave. Simply, the transmission of a nerve impulse across a synapse.

Nitrates: nitrates are inorganic compounds that can be found in nature and in several foods we eat. Manufacturers add nitrates and nitrites to foods such as cured sandwich meats, bacon, salami, or sausages to give them color and to prolong their shelf life. When added to processed foods in this way, both nitrates and nitrites can form nitrosamines in the body, which can increase your risk of developing cancer. Can form during high-heat cooking of meats.

Nitrites: used to preserve and color food, especially in meat and fish products; implicated in the formation of cancer. Used interchangeably with nitrates. When we eat nitrates in plants, bacteria in our mouth convert them to nitrites. Nitrites are then absorbed and stored in our cells until they're turned into nitric oxide, a compound that's proven to relax blood vessels and increase blood flow.

(As a result of many studies, the jury is still out on whether nitrates and nitrites should be avoided at all cost. There is well-documented consensus that high consumption of processed meats can up your risk for heart disease, cancers, and death, no matter what preservatives have been added to them. Eat some bacon occasionally with your eggs and you should be fine.) (See moderation.

Nootropic/Neutraceuticals: smart drugs or supplements. Cognitive enhancers. Brain food. Substances that improve cognitive function, especially executive functions, memory, creativity and motivation. Optimal health enhancers.

Nutrition: the science or study that deals with food and nourishment in humans.

Obesity: Weight that is higher than what is considered as a healthy weight for a given height is described as overweight or obese. Body Mass Index, or BMI, is used as a screening tool for overweight or obese. Obesity has been more precisely defined by the National Institutes of Health (the NIH) as a BMI (Body Mass Index) of 30 and above. (A BMI of 30 is about 30 pounds overweight.) The BMI, a key index for relating body weight to height, is a person's weight in kilograms (kg) divided by their height in meters (m) squared. Since the BMI describes the body weight relative to height, it correlates strongly (in adults) with the total body fat content. Some very muscular people may have a high BMI without undue health risks. (I prefer body fat percentage or lean body mass to BMI, but most doctors, hospitals and insurance companies still use BMI as their barometer.)

Off-Label: Off-label use is the use of pharmaceutical drugs for an unapproved indication or in an unapproved age group, dosage, or route of administration. Both prescription drugs and over-the-counter drugs (OTCs) can be used in off-label ways, although most studies of off-label use focus on prescription drugs. Off-label use is generally legal unless it violates ethical guidelines or safety regulations. The ability to prescribe drugs for uses beyond the officially approved indications is commonly used to good effect by healthcare providers. Off-label means the medication is being used in a manner not specified in the FDA's approved packaging label or insert. Every prescription drug marketed in the US carries an individual, FDA-approved label. This label is a written report that provides detailed instructions regarding the approved uses and doses, which are based on the results of clinical studies that the drug maker submitted to the FDA.

The FDA regulates drug approval, not drug prescribing, and doctors are free to prescribe a drug for any reason they think is medically appropriate. (See iatrogenic.)

Oil pulling: a traditional Ayurveda method of oral care. It involves swishing olive oil in the mouth for 10-20 minutes as a means of preventing caries (cavities), reducing bacteria, and promoting healthy gums.

Omega-3: Omega-3 fatty acids: A class of essential fatty acids found in fish oils, especially from salmon and other cold-water fish, that acts to lower the levels of cholesterol and LDL (low-density lipoproteins) in the blood. (LDL cholesterol is considered by most as the "bad" cholesterol.) Considered anti-inflammatory.

Omega-6: Omega-6 fatty acids are a family of pro-inflammatory, polyunsaturated fatty acids. Our omega-6 to omega-3 ratio should be 1:1 to 4:1. Unfortunately, with the SAD diet Americans average 25:1 to 30:1 with a diet of McDonalds and other fast and processed foods.

Organic: Organic food is the product of a farming system that avoids the use of man-made fertilizers, pesticides, growth regulators and livestock feed additives. Irradiation and the use of genetically modified organisms (GMOs) or products produced from or by GMOs are generally prohibited by organic legislation and labels.

Organic mercury: Typically found in amalgam fillings in your mouth and environmental toxins as opposed to inorganic toxins found in fish.

OTC: Over the Counter. Non-prescription.

Oxidative stress: Oxidative stress is essentially an imbalance between the production of free radicals and the ability of the body to counteract or detoxify their harmful effects through neutralization by antioxidants. Oxidative stress causes disruptions in normal mechanisms of cellular signaling.

oxLDL: circulating oxidized low-density lipoprotein.

Oxalates: a naturally occurring molecule found in abundance in plants and humans. It is also produced as a waste product by the body. It exits the body through the urine. It's not a required nutrient for people, and too much can lead to kidney stones. In plants, oxalate helps to get rid of extra calcium by binding with the oxalate. That is why so many high-oxalate foods are from plants.

Pasteurized: To subject milk, wine, or other products to a process of partial sterilization, especially one involving heat treatment or irradiation, thus making the product have a longer shelf life for consumption

Pasture-raised: pasture-raised animals receive a significant portion of their nutrition from organically managed pasture and stored dried forages. Unlike 100% grass-fed cows, pasture-raised cows may receive supplemental organic grains, both during the grazing season and into winter months. So, always ask the butcher, "grass-fed and grass finished or grass-fed and grain finished?" Most commonly, pasture-raised is referred to chickens and their eggs. True free-range eggs, now increasingly referred to as "pasture-raised," are from hens that roam freely outdoors on a pasture where they can forage for their natural diet, which includes seeds, green plants, insects, and worms.

Pathogen: a bacterium, virus, or other microorganism that can cause disease

PCB: by chlorination of biphenyl, used as insulating materials in electrical equipment, including transformers and capacitors, and in various other industrial applications. PCBs were banned in the United States in 1979 and now are noted primarily as environmental pollutants that accumulate in animal tissue with resultant pathogenic and teratogenic effects. Teratogens may cause birth defects and disturb the development of the fetus. (PCB Free labels)

Periodontal disease: an inflammatory disease that affects the soft and hard structures that support the teeth. In its early stage, called gingivitis, the gums become swollen and red due to inflammation, which is the body's natural response to the presence of harmful bacteria.

Peripheral neuropathy: a result of damage to your peripheral nerves, often causes weakness, numbness, and pain, usually in your hands and feet. It can also affect other areas of your body. Your peripheral nervous system sends information from your brain and spinal cord (central nervous system) to the rest of your body.

Pesticides: a chemical that is used to kill animals or insects that damage plants or crops. AKA insecticides.

Pharmacokinetics: the branch of pharmacology concerned with the movement of drugs within the body.

Phlebotomist: work in hospitals, clinics, and other medical facilities drawing blood from patients in preparation for medical testing.

Phlebotomy: is the act of drawing or removing blood from the circulatory system through a cut (incision) or puncture in order to obtain a sample for analysis and diagnosis. Phlebotomy is also done as part of the patient's treatment for certain blood disorders, such as lowering hematocrit.

Phytates: (phytic acid) are antioxidant compounds found in whole grains, legumes, nuts and seeds. The chief concern about phytates is that they can bind to certain dietary minerals including iron, zinc, manganese and, to a lesser extent calcium, and slow their absorption. However, the presence of phytates in foods really isn't the worry that some individuals believe and shouldn't be an issue as long as you're practicing a well managed eating strategy. Most people consume enough minerals in common foods or supplement, to more than make up for the small amounts of these micronutrients that might be tied up by phytates. The only individuals who might need to be careful are vegetarians or those who are allergenic.

Phthalates: hormone disrupting group of chemicals used to make plastics softer, more flexible and harder to break, including plastic food wrap. They are often called plasticizers. Some phthalates are used as solvents (dissolving agents) for other materials. Fast foods increase exposure.

Phytonutrients: the term "phyto" originated from a Greek word meaning plant. Phytonutrients are certain organic components of plants and these components promote human health. Fruits, vegetables, grains, legumes, nuts and teas are rich sources of phytonutrients. Unlike the traditional nutrients (protein, fat, vitamins, minerals), phytonutrients are not "essential" for life, so some people prefer the term "phytochemical."

Pituitary gland: the pituitary is an important gland in the body and it is often referred to as the "master gland," because it controls several of the other hormone glands (e.g., adrenals, thyroid).

Plaque: a sticky deposit on teeth in which bacteria proliferate.

Plecebo: A substance containing no medication and prescribed or given to reinforce a patient's expectation to get well. An inactive substance or preparation used as a control in an experiment or test to determine the effectiveness of a medicinal drug.

Polyphenol: polyphenols are phytochemicals, meaning compounds found abundantly in natural plant food. An antioxidant, phytochemical that tends to prevent or neutralize the damaging effects of free radicals.

PQQ: a next-generation coenzyme called pyrroloquinoline quinone (or PQQ) that has been shown to induce mitochondrial biogenesis. The growth of new mitochondria in aging cells. While CoQ10 optimizes mitochondrial function, PQQ activates genes that govern mitochondrial reproduction, protection, and repair. (I use them in tandem together, which seems to synergistically improve both.)

Probiotics and Prebiotics: Probiotics are live microorganisms which, when administered in adequate amounts, confer a health benefit on the host. Prebiotics are indigestible plant fibers that already live inside the large intestine. The more food, or prebiotics that probiotics have to eat, the more efficiently these live bacteria work and the healthier your gut will be. Feed your immune system with pre and probiotics. Up to 80% of your immune system is in your gut. (Ls and Bs.)

Processed foods: Food production is the process of transforming raw ingredients into prepared food products. Food production includes industries that take raw food products and convert them into marketable food items. Big Food. Avoid.

PSA: prostate-specific antigen. A test for PSA may be used to screen for cancer of the prostate and to monitor treatment of the disease. PSA is a protein produced by the prostate gland. Although most PSA is carried out of the body in semen, a very small amount escapes into the blood stream. Test. Don't guess.

Pulse: the practice of rotating detox supplements such as chlorella and charcoal on a 4 days on, 3 days off, or 7 days on and 7 days off to enhance absorption and efficacy. There are some experts who say changing up on your brand of probiotic supplements every month or two gives you a "mega boost."

Quack: Competition.

Range: where a 100% grass-fed cows have unlimited access to forage and graze for their own fresh food and natural diet

RCT: A study design that randomly assigns participants into an experimental group or a control group. As the study is conducted, the only expected difference between the control and experimental groups in a randomized controlled trial (RCT) is the outcome variable being studied.

RDA: Required daily allowance

Renal: of or treating of the kidneys. Kidney diseases are often times referred to as chronic kidney disease.

Resistance training: resistance training is a form of exercise that improves muscular strength and endurance. During a resistance training workout, you move your limbs against resistance provided by your body weight, gravity, bands, weighted bars, or dumbbells. Circuit exercise machines are also excellent choices for resistance training. (See isometric training.)

R-Lipoic Acid: Powerful anti-oxidant. Health benefits are limitless.

RNA: (ribonucleic acid) this acid is known as being essential for creating all known forms of life.

SAD: standard American diet

Sarcopenia: age-related muscle loss

Senescence: from Latin: senescere, meaning "to grow old." The biological aging or the gradual deterioration of function

Serotonin: a neurotransmitter that is primarily found in the pineal gland, digestive tract and central nervous system. It is synthesized from the amino acid tryptophan. It plays a key role in mood and appetite and is crucial in maintaining a sense of well-being. Serotonin is sometimes called the "feel good" hormone.

Skin tags: little rice shaped, skin color or brownish, balls of smudged skin have formed somewhere on the body usually armpits or neck. A marker and strongly associated with prediabetes, insulin resistance, and Type 2 diabetes. Skin tags are inherently benign or non-cancerous.

Strength training: is a type of physical exercise specializing in the use of resistance to induce muscular contraction which builds the strength, anaerobic endurance, and size of skeletal muscles.

SOFI: skinny on the outside, fat on the inside.

Standard of Care: "First do no harm." The National Standard of Care requires a doctor to use the degree of skill and care of a reasonably competent practitioner in his or her field, under the same or similar circumstances, would have exercised. Practice guidelines assist the healthcare practitioner with patient care decisions about appropriate diagnostic, therapeutic, clinical or specific procedures for treatment. Medical negligence is always measured by the medical standard of care.

Starch: it is the most common carbohydrate in human diets and is contained in large amounts in foods such as potatoes, wheat, corn, rice, beans and many other carbohydrates. Pure starch is a white, tasteless and odorless powder that is insoluble in cold water or alcohol.

Statins: a class of lipid-lowering medications that inhibit an enzyme called HMG-CoA reductase that controls the rate of cholesterol production in the body, most notably the liver. These drugs lower cholesterol by slowing down the production of cholesterol and by increasing the liver's ability to remove the LDL-cholesterol already in the blood. Most common statins are Lipitor (atorvastatin), Crestor (rosuvastatin) and Zocor (simvastatin.)

(35 million Americans are said to be on a statin drug, with 35 million more eligible under new AMA guidelines: totaling 70 million, that's half of all adults over age 40 in the US, according to the LA Times.) Yikes! I am not a big fan of statins and don't believe the long-term benefits outweigh the long-term risks and side effects. Statins could be the biggest experiment in US history with human life at risk since the FDA Food Pyramid of the 1970's and we all know the results of that debacle! I overcame high cholesterol from my stroke and attendant metabolic syndrome without statins, even though they were prescribed for me. I got off of them early on and stayed off to this day, all attainable through proper nutrition, diet, supplementation and exercise. All naturally! These are the type of people who belong on statins, not 70 million Americans: Familial hypercholesterolemia is a genetic disorder characterized by high cholesterol levels, specifically very high levels of low-density lipoprotein LDL, in the blood and early cardiovascular disease with total cholesterol levels of 350–550 mg/dL and above. Cholesterol levels can be drastically higher in people with FH who are also obese. Research suggests statins do have anti-inflammatory properties, but there are better ways to reduce diet-induced inflammation.

Steroids: A group of molecules that includes cholesterol. The sex hormones estrogen and testosterone are built from steroids, as are many modern anti-inflammatory drugs. Synthetic hormones that are derivatives of testosterone, are used medically, especially to promote tissue growth, and are sometimes used by athletes to increase the size and strength of their muscles and improve endurance.

Strength training: is a type of physical exercise specializing in the use of resistance to induce muscular contraction which builds the strength, anaerobic endurance, and size of skeletal muscles.

Stroke: AKA brain attack. CVD. CVE. The sudden death of brain cells due to lack of oxygen, caused by blockage of blood flow or rupture of an artery to the brain. Sudden loss of speech, weakness, or paralysis of one side of the body can be symptoms. Two types: ischemic and hemorrhagic. (See TIA)

Structured water: Live water. Structured water is water in nature. If you take a gallon or ten gallons of water and pour it into a mountain stream at the top of the mountain and then collect it at the bottom, the water is structured. Structured water is free of memory. It has a balanced pH.

Subcutaneous fat: is fatty tissue lying directly under the skin.

Sucrose: table sugar, carbohydrate. Chief component of cane or beet sugar.

Sugar: The term sugar is the generic term for any disaccharides (e.g., sucrose) and monosaccharides (e.g., fructose, glucose). One hundred and fifty-six pounds: that's how much added sugar Americans consume each year on a per capita basis, according to the US Department of Agriculture (USDA). More addictive than cocaine. Avoid at all costs. (See hidden sugar calculator-HSC)

Supercentenarians: A supercentenarian (sometimes hyphenated as super-centenarian) is someone who has lived to or passed his or her 110th birthday. This age is achieved by about one in 1,000 centenarians. The number of supercentenarians is forecast to rise rapidly over the next 25 years.

Supplementation: intended for ingestion that contains a "dietary ingredient" intended to add further nutritional value to (supplement) the diet. A "dietary ingredient," supplements: include vitamins, minerals, fiber, fatty acids, or amino acids, an herb or other botanical, among other substances. US authorities define dietary supplements as foods, while elsewhere they may be classified as drugs or other products. There are more than 50,000 dietary supplements available. Contains a "dietary ingredient" intended to add further nutritional value to (supplement) the diet. Not controlled by the FDA, but, FTC has some jurisdiction.

Tap water: (municipal water) from all over the world (including the US). is contaminated with heavy metals and toxins that can cause cancer and other serious illnesses. Every informed person knows you should NEVER drink the tap water. Nearly all bottled water is just filtered tap water!

Telomeres: Inside the nucleus of a cell, our genes are arranged along twisted, double-stranded molecules of DNA called chromosomes. At the ends of the chromosomes are stretches of DNA called telomeres, which protect our genetic data, make it possible for cells to divide and hold some secrets to how we age and get cancer. As telomere length shortens, our life span shortens.

Testosterone: a steroid hormone that stimulates development of male secondary sexual characteristics, produced mainly in the testes, but also in the ovaries and adrenal cortex. (TRT) testosterone replacement therapy is a class of hormone replacement therapy in which androgens, often testosterone, are replaced. TRT is often prescribed to counter the effects of male aging.

Thyroid: gland that makes and stores hormones that help regulate the heart rate, blood pressure, body temperature, and the rate at which food is converted into energy. Thyroid hormones are essential for the function of every cell in the body. The body's master switch.

TIA: Transient Ischemic Attack. While TIA is often labeled a "mini-stroke," it is more accurately characterized as a warning stroke that should be taken very seriously. TIA is still caused by a clot, the only difference between a TIA and major stroke is the blockage is transient (temporary.) TIA symptoms occur rapidly and last a relatively short time, less than 5 minutes. When a TIA is over, usually, causes no permanent damage or injury to the brain.

TOFI: thin on outside, fat on the inside.

Toxin: A toxin is a poisonous substance produced within living cells or one produced by bacteria. Biological toxins are toxic substances produced by microorganisms, animals, and plants that have the capability of causing harmful effects when inhaled, ingested, injected or absorbed. Toxins are not just pesticides or hazardous waste. A toxin is anything that damages the body. Toxins can be from food, wheat, nuts, legumes, etc., the air, water, mold, clothing, or even your cell phone.

tPA: (tissue plasminogen activator) stroke clot buster. The only FDA approved treatment for ischemic strokes is tissue plasminogen activator. tPA works by dissolving the clot and improving blood flow to the part of the brain being deprived of blood flow.

Trans fat: An unhealthy substance, also known as trans fatty acid, made through the chemical process of hydrogenation of oils. Hydrogenation solidifies liquid oils and increases the shelf life and the flavor stability of oils and foods that contain them. The main constituents of natural fats and oils and high concentrations in the blood indicate an elevated risk of stroke. Avoid. (Example: McDonalds French fries.)

Triglycerides: a type of fat (lipid) found in your blood. When you eat, your body converts any calories it doesn't need to use right away into triglycerides. The triglycerides are stored in your fat cells. Later, hormones release triglycerides for energy. High triglycerides are unhealthy.

TRT: testosterone replacement therapy.

TSH: thyroid stimulating hormone is a pituitary hormone that stimulates the thyroid gland to produce thyroxine (T4), and then triiodothyronine (T3) which stimulates the metabolism of almost every tissue in the body.

Type 2 diabetes: diabetes mellitus type 2 is a long term metabolic disorder that is characterized by high blood sugar, insulin resistance and relative lack of insulin. Common symptoms include increased thirst, frequent urination, and unexplained weight loss. Type 2 diabetes is 100 percent reversible through diet, nutrition, supplementation, exercise and lifestyle change.

Ultrasound: diagnostic ultrasound, also called sonography or diagnostic medical sonography, is an imaging method that uses high-frequency sound waves to produce images of structures within your body. No radiation.

USDA: United States Department of Agriculture

Ureteroscopy: an upper urinary tract endoscopy performed most commonly with an endoscope passed through the urethra, bladder, and then directly into the upper urinary tract. Kidney stone removal procedure.

VHR: variable heart rate syndrome

Visceral fat: Visceral fat is body fat that is stored within the abdominal cavity and is therefore stored around a number of important internal organs such as the liver, pancreas, and intestines.

Vitamins: any of a group of substances that are found naturally in many foods, are necessary in small quantities for good health and normal development and functioning, and are designated by a capital letter and sometimes a number: (Vitamin B6, vitamin B12, vitamin C, vitamin E.) Deficiencies of vitamins produce specific disorders.

VLDL: very low density lipoprotein, the damaging form of cholesterol. VLDL contains the highest amount of triglycerides, about 50%. VLDL is considered a type of bad cholesterol, because it helps cholesterol build up on the walls of arteries. Lipoproteins are made up of cholesterol, triglycerides and proteins. They move cholesterol, triglycerides, and other lipids (fats) around the body.

Well formulated eating strategy: A well-managed eating strategy is one that helps to maintain or improve overall health. A healthy diet provides the body with essential nutrition, fluids, adequate essential amino acids from protein, essential fatty acids, vitamins, minerals, and adequate calories.

Wellness: the quality or state of being healthy in body and mind, especially as a result of your deliberate effort. An approach to healthcare that emphasizes preventing illness and prolonging life, as opposed to emphasizing disease treatment.

Wild-caught: wild-caught fish come from seas, rivers, and other natural bodies of water; farm-raised fish are raised in tanks, irrigation ditches, and ponds and fed an omega-6 rich diet, pesticides, herbicides, hormones and antibiotics.

WLPB: Weight loss plateau buster. Intermittent fasting (IF), plus calorie restriction.

X-Ray: X-rays are electromagnetic radiation that differentially penetrates structures within the body and creates images of these structures on photographic film or a fluorescent screen. These images are called diagnostic X-rays. Diagnostic X rays are useful in detecting abnormalities within the body. They are a painless, non-invasive way to help diagnose problems such as broken bones, tumors, dental decay, and the presence of foreign bodies. When participating in dental X-rays, ask for a thyroid shield to protect your "master switch." Most all dentists provide. If not, you need a new dentist.

Yoga: Hatha yoga texts emerged around the 11th century with origins in tantra. Yoga gurus from India later introduced yoga to the west, following the success of Swami Vivekananda in the late 19th and early 20th century. In the 1980s, yoga became popular as a system of physical exercise across the Western world. An ancient art based on a harmonizing system of development for the body, mind, and spirit. The continued practice of yoga will lead you to a sense of peace and well-being, mentally, physically and spiritually balanced and also a feeling of being at one with the environment.

Bibliography/References/Suggested Reading

365 Ways to Boost Your Brain Power, Adams Media, 2009

A Consumer Guide to Interpreting Your Blood Work, CreateSpace, Dr. Daniel T. Wagner, 2016

A Low Carbohydrate, Ketogenic Diet Manual, Eric C. Westman, M.D., MHS, 2013

After a Stroke, Cleo Hutton, Demos Medical Publishing, 2005

After the Stroke, Mark McEwen, Daniel Paisner, Gotham Books, 2008

American Physical Therapy Association, Book of Body Maintenance and Repair, Marilyn Moffat, PT, PhD, FAPTA, Steve Vickery, Henry Holy and Company,1999

Anatomy of an Illness, Norman Cousins, Bantam Books, 1981

Antifragile, Nassim Nicholas Taleb, Random House, 2014

Appetite for Profit, Michelle Simon, NMation Books, 2006

Are You Insulin Resistant? Gary M. Larsen, Sound & Simple Lifestyle Publishing, 2014

Beat The Heart Attack Gene, Bradley Bale, M.D., Amy Doneen, ARNP, Lisa Collier Cool, Wiley, 2014

Body by Science, Doug McGuff, M.D., John Little, McGraw-Hill Education, 2009

Boost Your Brainpower, Frank Minirth, M.D., Revell, 2007

Brain Candy, Theodore I. Lidsky, PhD, Jay S. Schneider, PhD, Simon & Schuster, 2001

Brain, Heal Thyself, Madonna Siles, Lawrence J. Beuret, M.D., Hampton Road Publishing Company, 2006

Cancer as a Metabolic Disease, Wiley, 2012, Thomas N. Seyfried, PhDChange Your Brain Change Your Life, Daniel G. Amen, M.D., Harmony, 2015

Changing For Good, James O. Prochaska, PhD, John C. Norcross, PhD, Carlo C. Diclemente, PhD, Quill, 1994

Cholesterol Clarity, Jimmy Moore, Eric C. Westman, M.D., Victory Belt Publishing, 2013

Conquering Stroke, Valerie Greene, John Wiley & Sons, 2008

David and Goliath, Malcolm Gladwell, Little, Brown and Company, 2013

Dead Doctors Don't Lie, Dr. Joel Wallach, Dr. Ma Lan, Wellness Publication, Inc., 2015

Death by Food Pyramid, Denise Minger, Primal Blueprint Publishing, 2013

Death by Medicine, Gary Null, PhD, Martin Feldman, M.D., Debra Rasio, M.D., Carolyn dean, M.D., N.D., Praktikos Books, 2011

Diet Wise, Dr. Keith Scott-Mumbry Mb, ChB, MD, PhD, FCRP, Mother Whale, Inc., 2005

Different Strokes, Steven Boorstein, Skyhorse Publishing, 2011

Disease Proof, David L. Katz, M.D., MPH, Stacey Colino, Plume, 2014

Doctoring Data, Dr. Malcolm Kendrick, Columbus Publishing, 2014

Earthing: The most important health discovery ever! By Clinton Ober, Stephen T. Sinatra, M.D., Martin Zucker, Basic Health Publications, Inc. 2014

Eat More, Weigh Less, Dr. Dean Ornish, HarperPaperbacks, 1999

Eat Right for Your type, Dr. Peter J. D'Adamo, Catherine Whitney, Berkley, 1996

Eat to live, Joel Fuhrman, M.D., Little, Brown & Company, 2011

Eating for Optimal Health, Edward Swartzberg, M.D., F.A.C.P., University of California, Berkley School of Public Health, 2015

Eating Well For Optimum Health, Andrew Weil, M.D., William Morrow Paperbacks, 2001

Fast Exercise, Dr. Michael Mosley, Pet Bee, Atria, 2012

Fat Chance, Robert H. Lustig, M.D., M.S.L., Plume, 2013

Fix It!, Chauncey Crandall, M.D., Newsmax Health, 2012

Food Forensics, Mike Adams, BenBella Books, 2016

Food Politics: How the Food Industry Influences Nutrition and Health, Dr. Marion Nestle, University of California Press, 2013

Fooled by Randomnes, Nassim Nicholas Taleb, Random House, 2004

Grain Brain, David Perlmutter, M.D., Kristin Loberg, Little, Brown & Company, 2013

Hormone Harmony, Alicia Stanton, M.D. & Vera Tweed, Healthy Life Library, 2009

How Not To Die, Michael Greger, M.D., Gene Stone, Flatiron Books, 2015

Inflammation Nation, Floyd H. Chilton, PhD, Laura Tucker, Simon & Schuster, 2006

Juicing, Fasting and Detoxing For Life, Cherie Calbom, MS, John Calbom, MA, Grand Central Life & Style, 2014

Kate's Journey: Triumph Over Adversity, Kate Adamson, Nosmada Press, 2004

Keto Clarity, Jimmy Moore, Eric C. Westman, M.D., Victory Belt Publishing, 2014

Live Life aggressively, Mike Mahler, A Mahler's Aggressive Strength, 2011

Living Lo-Carb, Jonny Bowden, Phd, CNS, Sterling, 2013

Mastering Leptin, Byron J. Richards, CCN. Mary Guignon Richards, Wellness Resources Books, 2009

Medicine & Culture, Lynn Payer, Henry Holt & company, 1996

Mind Boosters, Ray Sahelian, M.D., St, Martin's Griffin, 2000

Mind Over Medicine, Lissa Rankin, M.D., Hay House, Inc. 2014

My Stroke of Insight, Jill Bolte Taylor, PhD, Penquin Group, 2006

My Stroke of Luck, Kirk Douglas, HarperCollins, 2002

Natural Cures "They" Don't Want You To Know About, Kevin Trudeau, Alliance Publishing Group, 2004.

Nutrition Almanac, John D. Kirschman, McGraw-Hill, 2007

Nutritional Supplements Professional edition, Lyle MacWilliam, MSc, FP, Northern Dimension Publishing, 2007

Outliers, Malcomb Gladwell, Penquin Books, 2011

Oxidative Stress, Matthew Jordan, 2012

Paleo for Beginners, Rockridge Press, 2013

Paralyzed but not Powerless, Kate Adamson, Nosmada Press, 2007

Peeling the Onion, Reversing the Ravages of Stroke, Robin Robinson, SORA Publishing, 2005

Prescription for Nutritional healing, Phyllis A. Balch, CNC, Stacy Bell, DSC, Avery, 2010

Protein Power, Michael R. Eades, M.D., Mary Dan Eades, M.D., Bantam Books, 1998

Rewire Your Brain Rewire Your Life, Bob Guns, PhD, WingSpan Publishing, 2008

Rise Above, Ralph W. Braun, The Braun Corporation, 2010

Smart Drugs & Nutrients, Ward Dean, M.D., John Morgenthaler, Health freedom Publications, 1991

Smart Fat, Steven Masley, M.D., FAHA, FACN, FAAFP, CNS, Jonny Bowden, Ph.D., CNS, HarperOne, 2016

Soda Politics: Taking on Big Soda (and Winning), Dr. Marion Nestle, Oxford University Press, 2015

Stronger After Stroke, Peter G. Levine, Demos Health, 2013

Sugar Impact Diet, JJ Virgin, Hachette Book Group, 2014

Super Immunity, Joel Fuhrman, M.D., HarperCollins, 2011

Testosterone: A Man's Guide, Nelson Vergel, BsChE, MBA, Milestones Publishing, 2011

The 120-Year Diet, Roy L. Walford, M.D., Simon and Schuster, 2000

The 150 Healthiest Foods on Earth, Jonny Bowden, PhD, C.N.S., Fair Winds Press, 2007

The Advanced Guide to Longevity Medicine, Mitchell J. Ghen, D.O., PhD, IMPAKT Communications, Inc., 2001

The Anti-Aging Plan, Roy L. Walford, M.D., Lisa Walford, Marlowe & Company, 2005

The Anti-Inflammation Zone, Dr. Barry Sears, Harper Collins, 2005

The Anti-inflammation Zone, Dr. Barry Sears, William Morrow Paperbacks, 2005

The Antioxidant Miracle, Lester packer, PhD, Carol Coleman, Wiley, 199

The Art and Science of Low Carbohydrate Living, Jeff S. Volek, PhD, RD, Stephen D. Phinney, M.D., PhD, Beyond Obesity, LLC, 2011

The Big Fat Surprise, Nina Teicholz, Simon & Schuster Paperbacks, 2014

The Black Swan, Nassim Nicholas Taleb, Random house, 2010

The Cholesterol Conspiracy, Ladd McNamarra, M.D., OrthoMolecular Medicine, Inc., 2006

The Complete Thyroid Book, Kenneth Ain, M.D., M. Sara Rosenthal, PhD, McGraw-Hill Education, 2010

The Fast diet, Dr. Michael Mosley, Mimi Spencer, Atria, 2014

The Fat Switch, Richard J. Johnson, M.D., Mercola.com, 2012

The Food Babe Way, Vani Hari, Little, Brown & Company, 2016

The Gabriel Method, Jon Gabriel, Atria Books, 2008

The Game of Life, Florence Scovel Shinn, DeVorss & Company, 1925

The good Gut, Justin Sonnenburg, PhD, Erica Sonnenburg, PhD, Penguin Press, 2015

The Great Cholesterol Myth, Jonny Bowden, PhD, C.N.S., Stephen Sinatra, M.D., F.A.C.C., Fair Winds Press, 2015

The Guide to a Dairy-Free Diet, David Brownstein, M.D., Sheryl Shenfelt, C.N., Medical alternative Press, 2011

The Guide to a Gluten-Free Diet, David Brownstein, M.D., Sheryl Shenfelt, C.N., Medical Alternative Press, 2011

The guide to Healthy Eating, David Brownstein, M.D., Sheryl Shenfelt, C.N., Medical Alternative Press, 2010

The Life Plan, Jeffry S. Life, M.D., PhD, Atria, 2011

The Mediterranean Zone, Barry Sears, PhD, Zink Ink, 2014

The Metabolic Effect Diet, Jade Teta, ND, CSCS, Keoni Teta, ND, Lac, CSCS, HarperCollins, 2010

The Metabolic Typing Diet, William Wolcott, Trish Fahey, Harmony, 2002

The Micronutrient Miracle, Jayson Calton, PhD, Mira Calton, CN, Rodale Books, 2015

The Mind & The Brain, Jeffrey M. Scwartz, M.D., Sharon Begley, HarperCollins, 2002

The Most effective Ways to Live Longer, Jonny Bowden, PhD, C.N.S., Fair Winds Press, 2010

The Obesity Epidemic, Zoe Harcombe, BA, MA, Columbus Publishing, 2010

The Oxygen Revolution, Paul G. Harch, M.D., Virginia McCullough, Hatherleigh Press, 2010

The Perfect Gene Diet, Pamela McDonald, N.P., Hay House, 2010

The Rave Diet & Lifestyle, Mike Anderson, RaveDiet.com, 2009

The Rosedale Diet, Dr. Ron Rosedale and Carol Colman, Harper Collins, 2004

The Self Health Revolution, J. Michael Zenn, Atria Books, 2012

The Sharp Brains Guide to Brain Fitness, Alvaro Fernandez, Elkhonon Goldberg, PhD, Pascale Michelon, PhD, SharpBrains, Inc., 2013

The Simple Heart Cure, Chauncey Crandall, M.D., Humanix Books, 2013

The Skinny Gut Diet, Brenda Watson, Leonard smith, M.D., Harmony, 2016

The Soy Deception, David Brownstein, M.D., Sheryl Shenefelt, C.N., Medical Alternatives Press, 2011

The Sugar Fix, Richard J. Johnson, M.D., Timothy Gower, Elizabeth Gollub, PhD, RD, Rodale, 2008

The Supplement pyramid, Michael a. Smith, M.D., Sara Lovelady, Basic Health Publications, Inc., 2014

The Testosterone Syndrome, Eugene Shipper, M.D., William Fryer, M. Evans & Company, Inc., 1998

The Truth About Statins, Barbara H. Roberts, M.D., Rocket books, 2012

The Ultimate Metabolism Diet, Scott Rigden, M.D., Hunter House, 2008

The Ultimate pH solution, Michelle Schoffro Cook, DMN, DAc, CNC, HarperCollins, 2008

The World's Greatest Treasury of Health Secrets, Bottom Line Publications, 2009

Toxic Fat, Barry Sears, Ph.D., Thomas Nelson, 2008

Tripping Over The Truth, Travis Christofferson, CreateSpace, 2014

True Strength, Kevin Sorbo, Da Capo Press, 2011

Turn Up the Heat, Dr. Philip Goglia, PhD, BookSurge Publishing, 2009

Virgin Coconut Oil, Brian & Marianita Shilhavy, Sophia Media, 2004

Vitamin K2, Dennis Goodman, M.D., AuthorHouse, 2015

Vitamin, Minerals and Supplements, Helen Pensanti, M.D., Barbara A. Hoffman, Siloam Press, 2002

Wheat Belly, William Davis, M.D., Rodale Books, 2014

Why We Get Fat, Gary Taubes, Anchor, 2011

Notes/Comments/Questions

(Blank Pages)

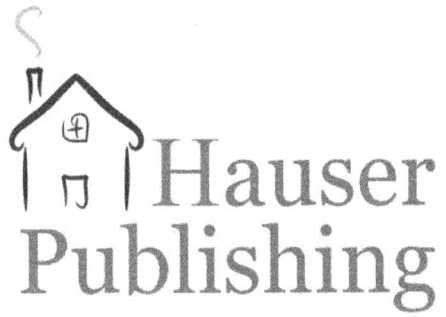

Hauser
Publishing

www.ingramcontent.com/pod-product-compliance
Lightning Source LLC
Chambersburg PA
CBHW080810280326
41926CB00091B/4141